Lung Connective Tissue: Location, Metabolism, and Response to Injury

Editor:

John A. Pickrell, D.V.M., Ph.D.
Scientist
Department of Pathobiology
Lovelace Inhalation Toxicology Research Institute
Albuquerque, New Mexico

CRC Press, Inc.
Boca Raton, Florida

Library of Congress Cataloging in Publication Data

Main entry under title:

Lung connective tissue--location, metabolism, and
response to injury.

Bibliography: p.
Includes index.
1. Lungs--Diseases. 2. Connective tissues--
Diseases. 3. Connective tissues. I. Pickrell,
John A. [DNLM: 1. Connective tissue--Metabolism.
2. Connective tissue--Physiopathology. 3. Lung--
Anatomy and histology. 4. Lung--Metabolism. 5. Lung
diseases--Physiopathology. WF600.3 L961]
RC756.L835 616.2'4 79-17910
ISBN 0-8493-5749-7

This book represents information obtained from authentic and highly regarded sources. Reprinted material is quoted with permission, and sources are indicated. A wide variety of references are listed. Every reasonable effort has been made to give reliable data and information, but the author and the publisher cannot assume responsibility for the validity of all materials or for the consequences of their use.

Direct all inquiries to CRC Press, Inc., 2000 N.W. 24th Street, Boca Raton, Florida, 33431.

International Standard Book Number 0-8493-5749-7

Library of Congress Card Number 79-17910
Printed in the United States

PREFACE

Our understanding of pulmonary interaction with the environment has progressed dramatically over the past years. The importance of pulmonary connective tissue in this interaction has become increasingly evident. Many of the tools and even the facts necessary to understand the role of pulmonary connective tissue in health and disease exist or are being gathered. The need to think about these diverse facts, collate them, and form them into cohesive patterns describing pulmonary interactions for the benefit of the pulmonary patient are becoming increasingly apparent. It is the purpose of this book to consider each fact carefully in each facet of lung connective tissue, structure, metabolism, and response to injury. Following this consideration of what is known the authors will speculate to varying degrees as to how this set of facts relates to the particular aspect of pulmonary biology or pathology. This book presupposes some basic knowledge of biology, medicine, biochemistry, and immunology which have been discussed at length in many fine books or monographs on the subjects. However, the relevance to each aspect of the lung is discussed in some detail.

The authors hope that this volume serves the purpose of collating facts and ideas concerning pulmonary connective tissue and its interaction with other lung elements in health and disease. It would certainly be presumptuous to claim that all or even a large part of the answers are contained herein. We do hope that these facts and ideas may provide the basis upon which further progress can be made in this new but rapidly developing field. Finally, we hope that such progress will be reflected in improved health of patients, not only in therapeutic manipulation, but in prevention of lung disease.

John A. Pickrell
Albuquerque, New Mexico

THE EDITOR

John A. Pickrell, D.V.M., Ph.D., is a Scientist in the Department of Pathobiology at The Inhalation Toxicology Research Institute in Albuquerque, New Mexico. He formerly held an NIH post-professional fellowship at the University of Illinois, Urbana, Illinois. He graduated in 1965 with a D.V.M. degree from The University of Illinois, and obtained his Ph.D. degree in Veterinary Medicine Science with a sole minor in biochemistry from the same institution in 1968.

Dr. Pickrell is a member of The American Physiological Society and The Federation of American Societies for Experimental Biology. Membership in other professional societies include: Phi Zeta, Phi Kappa Phi, American Veterinary Medical Association, American Society of Veterinary Clinical Pathologists, American Society of Veterinary Physiologists and Pharmacologists, American Association of Clinical Chemists, American Thoracic Society, American Association for Advancement of Science, Society for Experimental Biology and Medicine, and Toastmasters International. Dr. Pickrell has given more than 30 scientific presentations or invited lectures and published more than 30 research papers. His major research interests include pulmonary connective tissue pathobiology and clinical pathology.

ACKNOWLEDGMENTS

In early 1975, our director, Dr. R. O. McClellan, the associate director, Dr. Robert K. Jones, and my project coordinator, Dr. David O. Slauson, made me "an offer I couldn't refuse" and convinced me to begin work on an in-depth review article concerning lung connective tissue in health and disease. None of us had any idea of the nature of such an undertaking, nor of its value to me. I am grateful for being convinced to stick with the project long enough to realize its scientific value to me.

I must thank the response of our library staff during this time span, Ms. Joan Stoddart, Lynn Merritt, Susan Small, and Frank Kellerman, who so enthusiastically and magnificently responded to my request of everything on connective tissue that I soon had collected several hundred references. Mr. Frank Kellerman verified references used in the text. This extensive task was greatly appreciated. I could see that this effort was beginning to resemble a monograph, book, or very long review article.

Thanks go to the critical comments and intellectual stimulation of my colleagues who reviewed parts of the manuscript: Drs. Charles Mitchell and Bob Carpenter (structure), Drs. Rogene Henderson and Ray Pfleger (metabolism), and Dr. Hartwig Muhle, Joe Mauderly, and Ron Wolff (diseases and parts of the rest). A special note of thanks to Dr. F. F. Hahn for his work on the pathology aspects of the disease chapters is given. Thanks are also due to the nameless reviewers solicited by CRC Press who gave me several ideas. The typing by Ms. Elsie Spencer was invaluable; her reading of the "sanskrit" of the principal author was noteworthy and done under trying circumstances. Thanks go also to Ms. Carol Garcia, Tanna Callaway, and Victoria Gonzales, who typed portions of the manuscript. We appreciate the efforts of Ms. Judy Miller in coordinating production and assembly of the final manuscript. The graphics and illustration of Mr. E. E. Goff are gratefully acknowledged.

The principal author especially wishes to acknowledge the superb technical assistance of those people performing work in his laboratory which was cited in this book: Mr. J. J. Belasich, Ms. Patricia Lynn Bryant, Ms. Dorothy Harris, Mr. Gary Jones, Dr. Catherine Lustgarten, Mr. David McCamey, Mr. Ralph Rodriquez, Ms. Kathy Sass, Ms. Janette Shafer, Ms. Carol T. Schnizlein, Ms. Karen Servilla, Ms. Frances Straus, Ms. Debora Villa, Mr. David Wesselman, and Ms. Susan Wilson. Without you there would have been little to report. Thanks for the intellectual stimulation provided over the years. Thanks especially for the enthusiastic encouragement of Ms. Frances Straus and Kathy Sass in this and associated projects.

A special note of thanks goes to my family, Bonnie, Debbie, and Greg, for their understanding, encouragement, and interest. My belated apologies to them for many lost evenings, some days, and an occasional weekend. Thanks, Bonnie and Deb, for your help in collating and checking references. Thanks to all of the people who helped me in this project. Without your help there would not have been a book.

Finally, the editorial assistance provided by CRC Press is recognized and sincerely appreciated. Research was supported in part by the U.S. Department of Energy Contract Number EY-76-C-04-1013 in facilities accredited by the American Association for Accreditation of Laboratory Animal Care.

DEDICATION

To Bonnie, Debbie and Greg and to Frances and Kathy

CONTRIBUTORS

Robert Burrell, Ph.D.
Professor of Microbiology
West Virginia University
Morgantown, West Virginia

Joseph O. Hill, Ph.D.
Microbiologist
Lovelace Inhalation Toxicology
Research Institute
Albuquerque, New Mexico

Joe L. Mauderly, D.V.M.
Physiologist
Lovelace Inhalation Toxicology
Research Institute
Albuquerque, New Mexico

John A. Pickrell, D.V.M., Ph.D.
Scientist
Department of Pathobiology
Lovelace Inhalation Toxicology
Research Institute
Albuquerque, New Mexico

Ron Wolff, Ph.D.
Associate Scientist
Lovelace Inhalation Toxicology
Research Institute
Albuquerque, New Mexico

TABLE OF CONTENTS

Chapter 1

INTRODUCTION

J. A. Pickrell

Connective tissue supports most of the body's cells. In recognition of this, the literature concerning connective tissue has increased markedly. Connective tissue is discussed exclusively at the Gordon Conference concerning Structural Macromolecules. Several books,[1-3,9,12-14] a review series,[6] and a journal[8] are a small indication of the increase. Lung connective tissue is also being intensely studied. It has been the subject of a recent book[4] and held an important position in discussions at the Gordon Conference concerning Non-respiratory Lung Function and the 1975 Aspen Lung Conference.[10] Pulmonary connective tissue supports other lung tissues and is important to both respiratory and nonrespiratory lung function. Several papers[5, 7, 11, 15] have reviewed pulmonary connective tissue in health and disease. The location of each connective tissue constituent, collagen, elastin, and proteoglycans, provides understanding of its role in lung molecular biology. The metabolism of each constituent in normal lung provides a basis for predicting which component will be altered by injury.

The lung responds to injury in a limited number of ways; the response of each constituent to specific injury patterns determines the biochemistry, physiology, and anatomy of the response which constitutes a specific disease entity. Since such diseases or injuries are often specialized end-stage expressions of lung injury, the response of injured lung to therapy may imply important pathogenetic information about the process being studied, in addition to defining improved methods of treatment. The understanding of pathogenesis is especially important because not only the three connective tissue constituents, collagen, elastin, and proteoglycans, but also the response of these constituents to injury is heterogeneous. Likewise, the interaction of responses leading to late-occurring degeneration or neoplasia is of great interest. The relation of local pulmonary fibrosis to the heterogeneity of collagen remains intriguing. The purpose of this book is to review evidence defining the location, the metabolism, and the response to injury of each constituent of pulmonary connective tissue. Attention will also be given to therapeutic manipulation of specific injury responses and to major voids toward which research should be directed to define more adequately the areas covered in this review.

Chapters 2, 3, and 4 relate what is known concerning the structure of pulmonary collagen, elastin, mucoproteins, and proteoglycans. Some speculation is offered regarding function of these constituents. Likewise, the way these four constituents interact to form their portion of the extracellular matrix is discussed. Consideration is given as to how each constituent helps to preserve the pulmonary structural integrity.

Chapters 5, 6, 7, and 8 record what is known concerning the metabolism (biosynthesis and degradation) of collagen, elastin, proteoglycans, and mucoproteins. The greatest effort is expended on collagen metabolism, where most is known. The significance of the variety of post-translational modifications is considered. In the cases of elastin and proteoglycans and mucoproteins known facts are combined with speculative parallels drawn to or differing from collagen metabolism. At each point, the relation of the process to the control of that connective tissue constituent was considered.

Chapters 9, 10, and 11 consider lung cells, kinetics and immunology. These chapters constitute a beginning of the bridge between morphology and physiology and biochemistry. Chapter 9 indicates briefly the complex nature of pulmonary cellular composition, but limits discussion mostly to those cells producing connective tissue, especially fibroblasts, on which most in vitro data exist. Interactions of cells with substratum and other cells were considered. Soluble factors which influence cell proliferation were evaluated. Special attention was given to phosphatidyl inositol, and a section was devoted to the interaction of cells with fibronectin and other connective tissue constituents of the extracellular matrix. In Chapter 10 an attempt is made to describe interaction of mesenchymal cells with matrix as a control of relative numbers of different lung cells present. Speculation concerning possible transcriptional and translational control of collagen production is discussed. The role of recently discovered collagen bound collagenase is considered. A speculative model is described and some evidence against it evaluated. In Chapter 11, Hill and Burrell briefly review mechanisms of pulmonary connective tissue injury. They discuss connective tissue injury by cytotoxic antibody, immune complex injury, nonspecific activation of complement, and cell-mediated immune injury. Attempts are made to speculate on potential interactions of the immune system and connective tissue, based on what is known concerning the two systems and concerning such interaction.

In Chapter 12, Pickrell attempts to describe a general view of pulmonary response to injury from a variety of sources. The primary thesis is that the lung responds to injury in only a limited number of ways. Four examples of chronic lung injury, fibrosis, emphysema, bronchitis, and neoplasia, may represent a single type but different intensity of injury.

In Chapters 13—16, the authors attempt to discuss each of these disease entities in turn. In Chapter 13, Pickrell and Mauderly deal with fibrosis, describing anatomic changes and causes, limited discussion of physiology changes, description of altered collagen metabolism, changes in proteoglycan metabolism, and attempts at therapeutic manipulation. An attempt is made at cellular-molecular description based on Chapters 10 and 12. In Chapter 14, Pickrell and Mauderly discuss anatomic, physiologic, and biochemical changes of connective tissue in emphysema. They also describe briefly attempts at therapeutic manipulation. Again an attempt is made at describing cellular-molecular interactions in light of Chapters 10 and 12. In Chapter 15, Wolff, Mauderly, and Pickrell describe bronchitis and asthma, i.e., the lung's response to upper airway injury. Special attention is given to physiology of clearance, essential to an understanding of changes in bronchitis. In Chapter 16, Pickrell attempts to discuss specific aspects of neoplasia, i.e., anatomy, physiology, and biochemistry. It must be understood that this chapter constitutes only an initial attempt at such understanding which may be regarded as speculative and controversial. The authors hope this first step will provide the groundwork and stimulate further speculation and answers to experimental questions. Thus we will begin to understand pulmonary neoplasia at somewhere near the level of the other diseases.

Chapter 17 attempts to summarize the foregoing chapters. This chapter states the important aspects of what is known, opinions speculating what may be deduced, and finally the major areas where progress is needed.

REFERENCES

1. **Balazs, E. A.,** *Chemistry and Molecular Biology of the Intercellular Matrix,* Vol. 1—3, Academic Press, New York, 1970.

2. **Burleigh, P. M. C. and Poole, A. R., Eds.,** Dynamics of connective tissue macromolecules, *American Elsevier,* New York, 1975.
3. **Chvapil, M.,** *Physiology of Connective Tissue,* Butterworths, London, 1967.
4. **Crystal, R. G.,** The biochemical basis of pulmonary function, in *Lung Biology in Health and Disease,* Vol. 2, Marcel Dekker, New York, 1976.
5. **Crystal, R. G.,** Lung collagen: definition, diversity and development, *Fed. Proc.,* 33, 2248, 1974.
6. **Hall, D. A. and Jackson, D. S.,** *International Review of Connective Tissue Research,* Vol. 1—7, Academic Press, New York, 1963—1976.
7. **Hance, A. J. and Crystal, R. G.,** The connective tissue of lung, *Am. Rev. Respir. Dis.,* 112, 657, 1975.
8. **Mandl, I. Ed.,** *Connective Tissue Research,* Vol. 1—6, Gordon and Breach Science Publishers, New York, 1973—1979.
9. **Pérez-Tamayo, R. and Rojkind, M.,** Molecular pathology of connective tissues, in *The Biochemistry of Disease,* Vol. 3, Marcel Dekker, New York, 1973.
10. **Petty, T. L. and Filley, G. F., Eds.,** Interstitial lung diseases, *Chest,* 69(2), 251, 1976.
11. **Pickrell, J. A., Harris, D. V., Mauderly, J. L., and Hahn, F. F.,** Altered collagen metabolism in radiation-induced interstitial pulmonary fibrosis, *Chest,* 69, 311, 1976.
12. **Ramachandran, G. N. and Reddi, A. H.,** *Biochemistry of Collagen,* Plenum Press, New York, 1976.
13. **Ramachandran, G. N. and Gould, B. S.,** *Treatise on Collagen,* Vol. 1, 2a, 2b, Academic Press, New York, 1967 and 1968.
14. **Slavkin, H. C. and Greulich, R. C., Eds.,** *Extracellular Matrix Influences on Gene Expression,* Academic Press, New York, 1975.
15. **Turino, G. M., Rodriquez, J. R., Greenbaum, L. M., and Mandl, I.,** Mechanisms of pulmonary injury, *Am. J. Med.,* 57, 493, 1974.

Chapter 2

COLLAGEN STRUCTURE

J. A. Pickrell

TABLE OF CONTENTS

I. LOCATION

Collagen provides support to tissues throughout the lung, is composed of different molecular types, and may influence the pattern of lung growth. In large and most smaller airways it is located in the interstitium, in cartilagenous plates, and as a component of basement membrane. Irregular cartilagenous plates extend to near the terminal bronchioles; therefore, cartilage collagen probably extends to that point. Vessels also contain interstitial and basement membrane collagen, as does each alveolar unit.[11] Since collagen must perform a variety of functions to support the lung as it grows and after it reaches maturity, it is not surprising to find that pulmonary collagen is heterogeneous (composed of different molecular types), and that different lung cells can make collagen.[13, 24, 42] Moreover, the preliminary finding that the species of origin of mesoderm determines pattern of lung growth[87, 103] indicates collagen's importance. Alescio's[2] finding that azetidine-2-carboxylic acid interferes with collagen synthesis and lung epithelial budding indicates how important collagen is to lung growth. Although lung collagen is incompletely characterized, evidence to date indicates many similarities to collagen from other tissues.

II. GENERAL STRUCTURE

Tropocollagen, which forms the backbone or subunit of polymeric native collagen (Figure 1), is comprised of three α-chains, each weighing 95,000 to 100,000 daltons,[83] and has a unique repeating triplet sequence which causes it to form a 3000-by-14 Å rod-like structure. Basement membrane collagen, which will be discussed subsequently, differs. Of the approximately 1050 amino acids in an α-chain, over 1000 amino acids are present in the repeating triplet sequence of (gly-X-Y) where X is often proline but may be another amino acid and where X is not equivalent to Y. Proline is either not hydroxylated in this (#2) position or it is hydroxylated as 3-hydroxyproline rather than 4-hydroxyproline. In the Y (#3) position proline is frequently present and hydroxylated in the 4 position.[31, 34, 37] Proline in either position 2 or 3 (whether hydroxylated or not) limits rotation of the polypeptide chains.[79a, 104] Three-hydroxyproline is not thought to be present in the Y position. This long repeating sequence of amino acids forms a rod-like structure, an α-chain. Three α-chains bind in a right-handed helical arrangement to form a tropocollagen molecule.[83]

Tropocollagen is triple helical; thermal helix stability is influenced by a number of parameters; the helix may contain areas of differing thermal stability. Stability of the helix is dependent upon the amount and location of proline and its degree of hydroxylation, upon polar and hydrophobic amino acid locations, and upon glycosylation and other undefined factors.[32] The helix is additionally stabilized by intramolecular cross-links formed between complementary regions of the three chains which are not in the repeating triplet sequence, but rather at the N and C terminal ends of tropocollagen and are called telopeptides.[83, 104] Hydroxyproline/proline within a given collagen type also influences stability of the triple helix.[30,91,112] As the ratio increases, the melting temperature (T_m) rises. This ratio varies with collagen type: [α_1 (IV)], 1.5; [α_1 (I)], 0.7—0.8. Careful analysis of the α_1(I)CB2 (the second cyanogen bromide peptide of the α_1 chain of type I collagen) fragment reveals a T_m of 36 or 62°C depending upon different degrees of hydroxylation of proline.[112] The implication that the collagen helix contains regions of differing heat stability is in agreement with Burdzhanadze[16] who suggests that despirilization of collagen is not an "all or none" event and is likewise in agreement with the primary structure of type I collagen.[32] Although hydroxyproline apparently stabilizes the collagen triple helix, the mechanism is unclear. However,

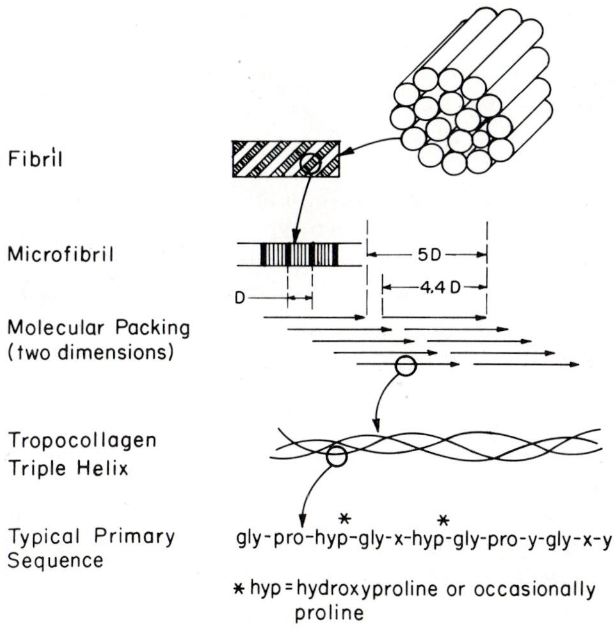

FIGURE 1. Collagen structural elements are shown. These include primary sequence, triple helical tropocollagen, molecular packing, microfibril, fibril, and fiber. These elements are part of the supramolecular collagen structural hierarchy.

studies in the nonaqueous solvents tend to rule out the water bonding proposed by Ramachandarin and Ramakrishnan,[86] and other studies tend to eliminate hydrogen bonding.[85] Both groups agree with Bhatnagar[9] who ascribes the stability to non-bonded interactive stacking of imino acids. Future work will add definition to this intriguing area.

Lung collagen not in helical form is attacked and degraded by nonspecific proteases to low molecular weight hydroxyproline peptides that are rapidly cleared through the kidney. Thus collagen not in the triple helix can provide no support because it is metabolized before it can be cross-linked, possibly before it becomes extracellular.[10] Hydroxylysine is present in collagen and C1Q (a part of the first component of collagen) exclusively and relates to both intramolecular cross-linking and to glycosylation, but its significance is undefined. Likewise, defects in intra- and intermolecular collagen cross-linking lead to a friable type of tissue which functions poorly at best,[59] probably being inordinately susceptible to collagenase in vivo.

Collagen fibrils form by a series of intricate patterns including limitation of lateral growth; the means of supporting tissue is undefined. Collagen triple helical trimers form side to side and head to tail associations in a quarter-stagger array to form collagen fibrils and, in some tissues, fibers.[31, 32, 83] Trelstad et al.[106] has suggested that fibrillogenisis occurs by accretion of incremental aggregates or subassemblies. In fact, when one considers the structure of the extracellular matrix,[11a] a combination of these mechanisms seems feasible. Experimental differentiation between them would seem to require further work. The differential equations for fibril association predict "cigar shaped" tactoid formation, and such an effect has been observed,[8] especially when the c-terminal telopeptide is removed. However, Bard and Chapman[8] observed limitation of lateral growth and resultant fibril and fiber formation, indicating formation of new fibrils to be less probable as fibril growth proceeded. Thus, as lateral growth is limited, fibrils presumably lengthen into those present in biological systems. An intriguing question has always concerned the rigidity conferred by collagen to the surrounding tissue. The molecular nature of the rigidity of the triple stranded "ropelike" collagen helix or fibril is as yet incompletely explained, not totally unlike that of the old Indian Rope Trick. Presumably future investigations will further enlighten this mystery.

Although tropocollagen molecules have many similarities, recently they have been noted to be heterogeneous. These collagen types have different amino acid compositions and presumably different primary sequences and may come from different structural genes.[34, 74] Nomenclature for these collagens includes type I collagen $[(\alpha_1(I)]_2 [\alpha_2(I)]_1$, type II collagen $[(\alpha_1(II)]_3$, type III collagen $[\alpha_1(III)]_3$, and type IV collagen $[\alpha_1(IV)]_3$. Other types of collagen[1, 44] or variants of collagen types have been noted.[20]

A. Type I Collagen

Type I collagen $[(\alpha_1(I)]_2(\alpha_2)$ (two α_1 and one α_2 chains) is distributed throughout the body and the lung, being a most common type in bone, tendon, skin and other tissues.[12, 42, 63, 74, 105] It presumably constitutes a large portion of the interstitial collagen of lung, located in airways, alveoli, and blood vessels.

Type I collagen is well defined chemically. Structural features may relate to a slow biological turnover and possibly reflect its specialization. Type I collagen may have a slow biological turnover. It may, in light of its more complex structure and slow turnover, be regarded as the most specialized form of collagen, although the relation of structure, turnover, and specialization may be specious. Its primary amino acid sequence has been elucidated by Fietzek and Kuhn.[31] Type I collagen has ≃33% glycine. It also has a 4-hydroxyproline/proline ratio of 0.7—0.8 for the 22% imino acids. It has no cystine, one residue of 3-hydroxyproline, and a $T_m \simeq 38°C$.[74] This T_m indicates that the triple helix is stable at body temperature. The glycine content and collagen sequence data indicate a near maximum number of triplet repeating units.[31] The regularity of the triplet repeat and relative absence of intrachain non-triplet segments or "buckles" are consistent with the slow metabolic turnover of type I collagen and collagen of bone or tendon.

The many different pulmonary cells which make type I collagen constitute most of the lung cells. This collagen provides most of the lung tissue support and accumulates in some lung diseases. The idea that cells adjacent to certain collagens synthesize and secrete them has long been popular. Cell types capable of making type I collagen continue to be of interest. The interstitial cell, the fibroblast, the contractile cell, and the pericyte of lung have similar morphology and are referred to as mesenchymal cells.[42, 49, 54] These cells constitute a large proportion of total lung cells,[33] and are capable of synthesizing type I collagen.[36, 43] Likewise, a cat lung cell of epithelial origin has been used to synthesize type I collagen.[41] Other nonpulmonary, nonmesenchymal cells, some of which are of epithelial origin,[38, 55, 92] can also synthesize collagen. Since interstitial collagen provides major bronchial and vascular support and a slow turnover, it is important to understand the qualitative and quantitative aspects of its production, breakdown, and accumulation in health and disease. The fate of excess accumulations of type I collagen in idiopathic pulmonary fibrosis[94] and their effect on pulmonary function are undefined.

B. Type II Collagen

Type II collagen has three identical chains $[(\alpha_1(II)]_3$. It is found nearly uniquely in cartilage,[24, 74] although it has been reported in the vitreous humor[100] and synthesized by the retina of the eye.[98] It does not form prominent fibrils,[99] possibly because of its tendency to form a unique in vitro staggered banding pattern which may be associated with the major collagen helix.[15] The reason for the high hydroxylysine content[65, 67, 72, 74] relative to that of type I collagen is unclear. However, that hydroxylysine residues are glycosylated[15, 28] has suggested the intriguing possibility that interaction of the nonhelical glycosylated regions with a helical collagen portion may constitute a functionally important difference from other collagen types. Miller[69] suggests that hydroxyallysine precursors may condense with helical hydroxylysine-forming stable keto-amine cross-links, making type II collagen less soluble than type I. Type II collagen has a tendency to form very fine fibrils.[99] Possibly the bulky carbohydrate groups restrict deposition of additional molecules once a certain diameter is achieved.[69] Perhaps this is why high concentrations of sodium chloride[65] or ammonium sulfate[106] are necessary to precipitate it in vitro once it has been solubilized by pepsin.

Type II collagen is synthesized by chondrocytes[75] in about the same time as type I collagen.[110, 111] Bronchial slices in the lung also synthesize type II collagen,[13, 14, 24] indicating that tracheal and bronchial cartilage may synthesize type II collagen in lung. However, quantity of lysosomal enzymes may alter the type of collagen produced.[25] Since bronchiole irregular cartilage plates extend to near the terminal bronchioles,[11] cartilage collagen may be present at multiple pulmonary levels. Future measurements will define its location. Measurements of relative proportions of the type II collagen present in a mixture of collagen types have used differential salt precipitation[62] and CNBr marker peptides.[28, 70] They have been used on relatively large amounts of collagen in cartilage.

C. Type III Collagen

Pulmonary type III collagen has (1) the same thermal stability, but (2) more hydroxyproline and glycine, (3) finer fibrils, and (4) in vitro precipitation at lower salt concentrations than does type I collagen. This type III collagen is found in skin, blood vessels, and lung, usually in conjunction with type I collagen.[3, 4, 17, 19, 21, 24, 27, 35, 46, 48a, 59, 60, 63, 94, 113] Type III collagen is composed of three identical α-chains $[(\alpha_1(III)]_3$, with a uniquely high hydroxyproline/proline ratio (>1), high glycine, some cystine, and lacks 3-hydroxyproline.[3, 17, 19, 46, 63] Although type III collagen has a high hydroxylation of peptidyl proline which would stabilize the collagen triple helix, it has a high content of glycine[19, 46, 59, 63] which might destabilize it. Thus, the type III collagen helix has the same T_m as type I collagen.[17] The possibility that the excess glycine might interrupt and "slightly buckle" the helix is currently undefined. If true, this would predispose collagen toward lattice precipitate formation at lower concentrations of NaCl as reported by Chung and Miller[21] or $(NH_4)_2SO_4$ as observed by Trelstad et al.[106] than type I collagen. Type III collagen forms much finer fibrils than type I collagen.[64] Increased susceptibility of type III collagen to trypsin proteolysis was noted by Miller et al.[71] Type III collagen has been referred to as "fetal" collagen, since it is present in higher concentrations in younger animals.[27] Whether it has a more rapid turnover than type 1 remains to be determined.

Disulfide bonds in pulmonary type III collagen are unreactive and may form interhelical cross-links important to helical stability. Although the importance of disulfide bonds is undefined, Schneir and Miller[93] have demonstrated the presence of no sulfhydryl group reactivity in type III collagen. This raised the question of function of the SH groups in type III collagen. McLees et al.[63] demonstrated intramolecular disulfide cross-links in the helical portion of the molecule. The sulfhydryl groups may relate to the insolubility of type III collagen relative to type I collagen noted by Chung et al.[21] Likewise, the formation of intrachain disulfide bonds near the areas of high glycine content should be considered and may relate to the as yet undefined molecular function of type III collagen. Modest irregularities in the triple helix caused by high glycine content and stabilized by hydroxyproline or disulfide bonds might induce type III collagen to remain triple helical in the denatured but unreduced state.[19] Chung et al.[21] indicated that disulfide bonds were important in maintaining the type III, γ-collagen (triple helical collagen), although the in vivo significance of such bonds was unclear. Type III collagen has also been measured by marker CNBr peptides.[70] LaPiere et al.[56] have shown that association of type III with type I collagen monomers slows the in vitro fibril formation and gives it more of the properties of type III gel formation. Fibers are of intermediate size relating to the portion of type III added. This may have important implications in response of tissue to injury.[56]

Type III collagen may lie beneath and support epithelium and endothelium, which places it in a location to be active in coagulation. It is located with and produced by the same mesenchymal cells as type I collagen. Type III collagen has been found only in tissues containing type I collagen and which also support epithelium and endothelium.[42] Bailey et al.[4] noted the presence of high amounts of type III collagen in hypertrophic scars; Huang[46] reports that most of the alveolar collagen fibers are type III collagen. Although localization of type III collagen in lung has not yet been accomplished, its location beneath the vascular endothelium as indicated by the immunohistochemical techniques[35] place it in a crucial position for damage to lungs induced by inhaled toxicants.[81, 97] Likewise, the report by Hugues et al.[47] that type III collagen may be the main collagen in aggregating platelets suggests a reason for this location. Gay et al.[36] have recently suggested that type III procollagen may undergo no or incomplete cleavage prior to formation of the microfibril. Although the relation of this to in vivo function is undefined, the report of Fessler et al.[29] that procollagen will form thin fibrils in vitro suggests a method by which in vivo function may occur. Lung mesenchymal cells are capable of synthesizing type III collagen as well as type I collagen. Likewise, certain cultured lung cells of epithelial origin may synthesize type I and III collagen,[42, 43] as may fibroblasts.[36]

D. Type IV Collagen

Type IV collagen found in various basement membranes throughout the body has several differences from types I, II, and III collagen. Early work[50] indicates that the triple helix contains three α_1 chains (>110,000 daltons each) with distinct chemical features called $[\alpha_1(IV)]$. Chung et al.[20] isolated three collagens probably of basement membrane origin. One of these was 55,000 daltons and primarily of endothelial origin. The remaining two were somewhat larger than α chains (>110,000) and came from epithelial or smooth muscle basement membrane. Kresina et al.[52] from the same laboratory isolated several basement membrane collagen chains suggesting a family of different but related polypeptides. Miller[69a] reports the isolation of at least two genetically distinct types of basement membrane collagen. Seyer[93a] has isolated at least five basement membrane collagens from lung, some having the same molecular weights as those of Chung et al.[20] Seyer[93a] indicates that the amino acid composition of each is distinct, with relatively low alanine values and high amounts of hydroxylysine. The amino acid contents and structural features of these collagens are similar to those described in the remainder of this section. Greenberg[38a] reports the in vitro synthesis of type IV collagen in lung. Specific chemical features of such collagen isolated from lens capsule, lomerulus, and parietal yolk sac include high hydroxylation of proline and lysine relative to type I collagen.[23, 50, 78] The high hydroxylysine content is present presumably to allow subsequent glycosylation, which is also higher than that in type I collagen.[108] However, in vitro fibril formation is undefined, leaving open the question of what function this carbohydrate serves. The reason for the high hydroxyproline content probably differs from type III collagen, since glycine contents are usually equal to or slightly less than type I collagen, while being substantially higher in type III. Moreover, type IV collagen T_m remains undefined, probably because type IV collagen is not routinely isolated in the amounts required for the measurement.

3-Hydroxyproline, which is present in higher amounts in type IV collagen than in type I collagen[24, 50] or type II collagen[72] and is usually located in the most stable triplet, has no defined function. Although it is spread relatively uniformly throughout the CNBr peptides of Bovine lens capsule (1 to 2 residues, CNBr peptides 6 to 12; 6000 to 20,000 daltons), some of the smaller ones (500 to 6000 daltons; CNBr peptides 1 to 5) lack 3-hydroxyproline. Moreover, it usually occurs in the sequence gly-3hyp-4hyp[39] which even without the 3-hyp represents the triplet which stabilizes the triple helix most effectively.[31] Since no functional role has been defined for 3-hydroxyproline, the significance of its presence or lack of it is unclear. Collagenous protein isolated from lung parenchyma by techniques which solubilized other basement membranes seemed to lack 3-hydroxyproline,[51] although the amino acid composition suggested some contamination with noncollagenous protein.[42] Bradley et al.[14] observed the presence of 3-hydroxyproline in isolated lung collagen, but have not yet identified its source.

The presence of large amounts of cysteine[50] in type IV collagen is largely unexplained. For instance, whether the cystine groups are reactive is undetermined. If they are not, as in type III collagen, the question of the formation of intrachain disulfide bonds and, in a more general way, of cystine function must be further explored. The recent finding[76] that the procollagen type IV triple helix of parietal yolk sac is incorporated directly into fibrillar collagen without extracellular cleavage by procollagen peptidease raises the question of how type IV fibrils are formed, compared to type I collagen. The possibility that this different polymerization if present may relate to the specific biological function of type IV collagen must be considered, especially in light of Fessler et al.'s[29] observation that procollagen forms fibrils in vitro.

Type IV collagen produced by the cells it anchors may play an important role in developing pulmonary fibrosis. Type IV collagen comprises a significant portion of the basement membrane which anchors epithelial and endothelial cells.[50] These cells apparently synthesize basement membrane collagen[45, 114] in proportions analogous to the more specialized chick lens cells and parietal yolk sac cells.[50, 76, 78] This makes it tempting to speculate that lung epithelial and endothelial cells would likewise synthesize type IV collagen. Whether the collagenous vascular anchoring filaments[57] represent type IV collagen or form connection with the more common type I collagen, the arrangement plays a central role in pulmonary lymph, and hemodynamics and edema formation[40, 80] and thus a central role in lung disease. Liebow[61] indicates that the anatomy of observed pulmonary fibrosis depends upon whether the basement membrane is interrupted. The role of the interruption in or layering of basement membrane[109] is undetermined, although its pathogenesis suggests that it represents an injury response. Basement membranes from different tissues may differ in molecular weight and perhaps in function, as indicated by intriguing but preliminary data.[20] Further information concerning isolation, characterization, and measurement of type IV collagen will elucidate these interesting facets.

E. Summary

One can see that we have at least four types of collagen requiring four different DNA sequences, which are probably coded on different genes. Different cell types favor the synthesis of one or two collagen types, although some systems if stressed can make nearly all types of collagen.[1] Unique physical characteristics probably lead to different aggregations and fibril formation in the case of type II or III collagen compared to type I collagen. Likewise, other unique features of type III collagen compared to type I collagen may affect turnover. Finally, the proposed lack of proteolysis prior to fibril formation in type III and IV collagen must have some effect on supramolecular collagen organization, although this effect is as yet undelineated. Whether this relates to the increased susceptibility of type III collagen to proteolysis (see Chapters 5 and 6 for discussion) remains to be seen. Different aggregations and turnover times of the respective collagens presumably lead to their being optimal to support different physiological functions. It is anticipated that these functions are uniquely suited to the evolution or function of the organ or tissue in which these collagen types are located. Future research will more completely define the complex relationships of interaction between collagen and associated parenchymal tissue. Since the lung has a wide variety of tissue types, one might anticipate the presence of many different interactions. The presence of all four collagen types in lung[42] is consistent with this variety. The normal human lung contains collagen of types I, II, and III identical to that found elsewhere in the body.

III. C1Q

A fraction of complement's first component (C1Q) has a triple helical portion, less imino acid content, and more hydroxylysine and carbohydrate moieties. The A chain of C1Q has a collagen-like portion consisting of 26 gly-X-Y triplets or 78 amino acid residues which is susceptible to collagenase.[88] The presence of proline in the X position four times and hydroxyproline in the Y position five times lends some stability to a triple helix if one is formed.[31] The imino acid content (13%) is much lower than most vertebrate collagen (22%); thus, any helix formation might be less stable in the absence of additional stabilizing factors.[88] The high degree of hydroxylation of lysine relative to collagen types by itself presumably lends little stability to the complement helix. However, it is consistent with a degree of glycosylation similar to type IV collagen; glycosylated hydroxylysine stabilizes the collagen helix. Likewise, the carbohydrate moieties of C1Q are similar to those of glomerular basement membrane. Whether this implies a function of the collagenous portion of C1Q which might be construed to be similar to basement membrane collagen is not defined. For example, epithelial cells rest upon and are supported by basement membrane. C1Q recognizes immune complexes and thereby initiates the complement reaction.[79] Perhaps this is due to an apical triple helical portion of slightly less stability combining three monomers and leaving both the longer noncollagenous c terminal ends and the shorter noncollagenous N terminal ends of the chain free to form the specific complement interaction.[88] Although the proportions are different, C1Q is not totally unlike procollagen in overall structure. Investigation of this or similar hypotheses represents potential future achievements. Work reported by Müller-Eberhard[79] indicated the presence of similar amino acids and sugars, although compositions of his C1Q and of the B, C, and D chains of C1Q reported by Reid[88] both differed from the more extensively studied A chain. Complement represents an important component of the immunologic reaction in various organs including the lung. Eeckhout et al.[26] report that C1Q and native collagen react similarly to IgG. Minor structural differences are suggested by an insensitivity of C1Q to mouse bone collagenase but a sensitivity to bacterial collagenase.

IV. CROSS-LINKING

Although collagen triple helices and subsequently fibrils can form without cross-links, such fibrils provide little structural stability and break down more rapidly than fibers with cross-links. These cross-links form from selected lysines and hydroxylysines with the aid of lysyl oxidase. Piez[82] reviewed the formation of collagen cross-links and noted the importance of the formation of the aldehyde, allysine, and subsequently lysinonorleucine. The subsequent isolation of lysyl oxidase which forms allysine[84, 95, 96] preceded its characterization.[84, 94, 96] Likewise, blockage by beta amino proprionitrile (BAPN), a lysyl oxidase inhibitor,[95, 96] increases collagen breakdown, probably because the collagen is inherently less cross-linked and, thus, less stable. Veis and Anesey[107] noted an enhancement of molecular bonding between α_1-chains with increasing maturation of collagen. Kuboki et al.[53] noted the presence of the collagen cross-link δ,δ dihydroxylysinonorleucine. Likewise, several different collagen cross-links were detected in basement membrane collagen.[101]

The presence of other collagen cross-links, notably hydroxylysinonorleucine and fraction C,[5, 6, 89, 102] was noted; subsequently they were partially characterized.[48, 90] The predominant collagen cross-link changes with age.[6] Cannon and Davison[18] reviewed aging and cross-linking in mammalian collagen. They note that reducible cross-links decrease with time, correlating with cessation of growth. They conclude that reducible cross-links are converted to a stable non-reducible state and that persistence of low level reducible crosslinks may be indicative of low level collagen turnover in the tissue. Changes in ratios of reducible cross-links are of doubtful functional significance and may simply reflect variation in post-translational lysine modification.[18] Perhaps in injured tissue (lung), levels of reducible cross-links would increase, reflecting an increased turnover of collagen. These might be detected by ion exchange chromatography, by reduction with sodium borotritide, or a combination of these procedures. Bailey and Robbins[89] suspect that histidinohydroxymerodesmosine (compound C) results from the *Michael* addition of histidine across the α,β unsaturated double bond of the previously formed aldimine. Further, both hydroxy- and dihydroxylysinonorleucine are formed by a condensation involving an Amaddori rearrangement. Age-related changes in reduced collagen compounds show dihydroxylysinonorleucine to be an important fetal cross-link.[89] By 1 year, hydroxylysinonorleucine predominates. This is shortly followed by histidinohydroxymerodesmosine and finally by hexitol lysines, which are probably not involved in collagen cross-linking.[89] Nearly complete formation of the cross-links is supported by the minor nature of lysinonorleucine, aldol histidine, hydroxymerodesmosine, and hexitol lysine, presumed intermediates in the cross-link formation. The disappearance of all noted cross-links with increasing age of the animals[89] is in potential disagreement with the seeming increase of collagen stability during advancing collagen maturity.[167] Perhaps this can be explained.[18] A modified Strecker reaction has been used by Pereyra (cited in Tanzer[102]) to establish independently the chemical structure of carbonyl-derived compounds and point the way to additional unidentified substances. However, these two conflicting findings have been observed preliminarily before and may be at least partially explained by a more stable cross-link formation.[95, 96] Further work will shed increasing light on this complex area.

REFERENCES

1. **Adli, F. A., Burgeson, R. E., Kaitila, I. I., and Hollister, D. W.,** Identification of two new collagen alpha chains in human fetal membranes, paper presented at the meeting of West Coast Connective Tissue Workers, Heber, Utah, March 5 to 7, 1976.
2. **Alescio, T.,** Effect of a proline analogue, azetidine-2-carboxylic acid, on the morphogenesis *in vitro* of mouse embryonic lung, *J. Embryol. Exp. Morphol.,* 29, 439, 1973.

3. **Anesey, J., Scott, P. G., Veis, A., and Chyatte, D.,** The isolation of a soluble type III collagen precursor from rat skin, *Biochem. Biophys. Res. Commun.*, 62, 946, 1975.
4. **Bailey, A. J., Bazin, S., Sims, T. J., LeLous, M., Nicoletis, C., and Delaunay, A.,** Characterization of the collagen of human hypertrophic and normal scars, *Biochim. Biophys. Acta*, 405, 412, 1975.
5. **Bailey, A. J. and Lapiere, C. M.,** Effect of an additional peptide extension of the N-terminus of collagen from dermatosparactic calves on the cross-linking of the collagen fibers, *Eur. J. Biochem.*, 34, 91, 1973.
6. **Bailey, A. J. and Robins, S. P.,** Development and maturation of the crosslinks in the collagen fibers of skin, *Front. Matrix Biol.*, 1, 130, 1973.
7. **Bailey, A. J., Sims, T. J., Le Lous, M., and Bazin, S.,** Collagen polymorphism in experimental granulation tissue, *Biochem. Biophys. Res. Commun.*, 66, 1160, 1975.
8. **Bard, J. B. L. and Chapman, J. A.,** Diameters in collagen fibrils grown *in vitro, Nature (London), New Biol.*, 246, 83, 1973.
9. **Bhatnagar, R. S.,** Role of non-bonded interactions in the stability of the collagen triple helix, paper presented at the meeting of West Coast Connective Tissue Workers, Gleneden Beach, Ore., March 25 to 27, 1977.
10. **Bienkowski, R. S., Cowan, M. J., McDonald, J. A., and Crystal, R. G.,** Degradation of newly synthesized collagen, *J. Biol. Chem.*, 253 (12), 4356, 1978.
11. **Bloom, W. and Fawcett, D. W.,** Respiratory system, in *A Textbook of Histology*, W. B. Saunders, Philadelphia, Pa., 1975, 743.
11a. **Bornstein, P., Duksin, D., Balian, G., Davidson, J. M., and Crouch, E.,** Organization of extracellular protein on the connective tissue surface: relevance to cell-matrix interaction *in vitro* and *in vivo*, *Ann. N.Y. Acad. Sci.*, 312, 93, 1978.
12. **Bornstein, P. and Piez, K. A.,** The nature of the intramolecular cross-links in collagen. The separation and characterization of peptides from the cross-link region of rat skin collagen, *Biochemistry*, 5, 3460, 1966.
13. **Bradley, K., McConnell-Breul, S., and Crystal, R. G.,** Lung collagen heterogeneity, *Proc. Natl. Acad. Sci. U.S.A.*, 71, 2828, 1974.
14. **Bradley, K. H., McConnell, S. D., and Crystal, R. G.,** Lung collagen composition and synthesis: characterization and changes with age, *J. Biol. Chem.*, 249, 2674, 1974.
15. **Bruns, R. R., Trelstad, R. L., and Gross, J.,** Cartilage collagen: a staggered substructure in reconstituted fibrils, *Science*, 181, 269, 1973.
16. **Burdzhanadze, T. V.,** Certain features of the process of despiralization of collagen, *Biofizika*, 19, 356, 1974.
17. **Byers, P. H., McKenney, K. H., Lichtenstein, J. R., and Martin, G. R.,** Preparation of type III procollagen and collagen from rat skin, *Biochemistry*, 13, 5243, 1974.
18. **Cannon, D. J. and Davison, P. F.,** Aging, and crosslinking in mammalian collagen, *Exp. Aging Res.*, 3(2), 87, 1977.
19. **Chung, E., Keele, E. M., and Miller, E. J.,** Isolation and characterization of the cyanogen bromide peptides from the alpha-1 (III) chain of human collagen, *Biochemistry*, 13, 3459, 1974.
20. **Chung, E., Rhodes, R. K., and Miller, E. J.,** Isolation of three collagenous components of probable basement membrane origin from several tissues, *Biochem. Biophys. Res. Commun.*, 71(4), 1167, 1976.
21. **Chung, E. and Miller, E. J.,** Collagen polymorphism: characterization of molecules with the chain composition $[\alpha 1(III)]_3$ in human tissues, *Science*, 183, 1200, 1974.
22. **Chung, E., Rhodes, R. K., and Miller, E. J.,** Characterization of basement membrane collagens, *Fed. Proc. Abstr.*, 35, 1520, 1976.
23. **Clark, C. C., Minor, R. R., Koszalka, T. R., Brent, R. L., and Kefalides, N. A.,** The embryonic rat parietal yolk sac; changes in the morphology and composition of its basement membrane during development, *Dev. Biol.*, 46, 243, 1975.
24. **Crystal, R. G.,** Lung collagen: definition, diversity and development, *Fed. Proc.*, 33, 2248, 1974.
25. **Deshmukh, K., Just, M., and Nimni, M. E.,** A defect in the intramolecular and intermolecular cross-linking of collagen caused by penicillamine. III. Accumulation of acid soluble collagen with a high hydroxylysine content in bone, *Clin. Orthop. Relat. Res.*, 91, 186, 1973.
26. **Eeckhout, Y., Riccomi, H., Cambiaso, C., Vaes, G., and Masson, P.,** Studies on properties common to collagen and C1Q, *Arch. Int. Physiol. Biochim.*, 84 (Abstr.), 611, 1976.
27. **Epstein, E. H.,** $[\alpha_1(III)]_3$ Human skin collagen. Release by pepsin digestion and preponderance in fetal life, *J. Biol. Chem.*, 249, 3225, 1974.
28. **Eyre, D. R. and Muir, H.,** Type III collagen: a major constituent of rheumatoid and normal human synovial membrane, *Connect. Tissue Res.*, 4, 11, 1975.

29. **Fessler, J. H., Doege, K. J., Siegel, R. C., and Fessler, L. I.,** Procollagen associations into supramolecular structures, *Fed. Proc. Abstr.,* 36, 680, 1977.
30. **Fessler, L. I. and Fessler, J. H.,** Protein assembly of procollagen and effects of hydroxylation, *J. Biol. Chem.,* 249, 7637, 1974.
31. **Fietzek, P. P. and Kuhn, K.,** Information contained in the amino acid sequence of the α 1(I)-chain of collagen and its consequences upon the formation of the triple helix, of fibrils and crosslinks, *Mol. Cell. Biochem.,* 8, 141, 1975.
32. **Fietzek, P. P. and Kuhn, K.,** The primary structure of collagen, *Int. Rev. Connect. Tissue Res.,* 7, 1, 1976.
33. **Fulmer, J. D. and Crystal, R. G.,** The biochemical basis of pulmonary function, in *The Biochemical Basis of Pulmonary Function,* Crystal, R. G., Ed. Marcel Dekker, New York, 1976, 419.
34. **Gallop, P. M., Blumenfeld, O. O., and Seifter, S.,** Structure and metabolism of connective tissue proteins, *Annu. Rev. Bioch.,* 41, 617, 1972.
35. **Gay, S., Balleisen, L., Remberger, K., Fietzek, P. P., Adelmann, B. C., and Kuhn, K.,** Immunohistochemical evidence for the presence of collagen type III in human arterial walls, arterial thrombi, and in leucocytes, incubated with collagen in vitro, *Klin. Wochenschr.,* 53, 899, 1975.
36. **Gay, S., Martin, G. R., Müller, P. K., Timpl, R., and Kühn, K.,** Simultaneous synthesis of types I and III collagen by fibroblasts in culture, *Proc. Natl. Acad. Sci. U.S.A.,* 73, 4037, 1976.
37. **Grant, M. E. and Prockop, D. J.,** The biosynthesis of collagen (I, II and III), *N. Engl. J. Med.,* 286, 194, 242, 291, 1972.
38. **Green, H. and Goldberg, B.,** Synthesis of collagen by mammalian cell lines of fibroblastic and non-fibroblastic origin, *Proc. Natl. Acad. Sci. U.S.A.,* 53, 1360, 1965.
38a. **Greenberg, D.,** Synthesis of type IV collagens by rat lungs in vitro, presented at The Western Connective Tissue Society Meeting, Seattle, Wash., February 9 to 11, 1979.
39. **Gryder, R. M., Lamon, M., and Adams, E.,** Sequence position of 3-hydroxyproline in basement membrane collagen, *J. Biol. Chem.,* 250, 2470, 1975.
40. **Guyton, A. C., Taylor, A. E., and Brace, R. A.,** A synthesis of interstitial fluid regulation and lymph formation, *Fed. Proc.,* 35(8), 1881, 1976.
41. **Hance, A. J., Bradley, K., and Crystal, R. G.,** Lung collagen heterogeneity. Synthesis of type I and type III collagen by rabbit and human lung cells in culture, *J. Clin. Invest.,* 57, 102, 1976.
42. **Hance, A. J. and Crystal, R. G.,** The connective tissue of lung, *Am. Rev. Respir. Dis.,* 112, 657, 1975.
43. **Hance, A. J. and Crystal, R. G.,** Collagen, in *The Biochemical Basis of Pulmonary Function,* Crystal, R. G., Ed., Marcel Dekker, New York, 1976, 215.
44. **Harvey, W., Cheung, H. S., Benya, P., and Nimni, M. E.,** Rabbit articular chondrocytes in culture synthesize a variety of collagen species, *Fed. Proc. Abstr.,* 35, 714, 1976.
45. **Howard, B. V., Macarak, E. J., and Gunson, D.,** Characterization of the collagen synthesized by endothelial cells in culture, *Fed. Proc. Abstr.,* 35, 1519, 1976.
46. **Huang, T. W.,** Chemical and histochemical studies of human alveolar collagen fibers, *Am. J. Pathol.,* 86, 81, 1977.
47. **Hugues, J., Herion, F., Nusgens, B., and Lapiere, C. M.,** Type III collagen and probably not type I collagen aggregates platelets, *Thromb. Res.,* 9, 223, 1976.
48. **Hunt, E. and Morris, H. R.,** Collagen cross-links. A mass-spectrometric and 1H- and ^{13}C-nuclear-magnetic-resonance study, *Biochem. J.,* 135, 833, 1973.
48a. **Hurst, D. J., Kilburn, K. H., Baker, W. M.,**Normal newborn and adult human lung collagen — analysis of types, *Connect. Tissue Res.,* 5, 117, 1977.
49. **Kapanci, Y., Assimacopoulos, A., Irle, C., Zwahlen, A., and Gabbiani, G.,** "Contractile interstitial cells" in pulmonary alveolar septa: a possible regulator of ventilation/perfusion ratio? Ultrastructural, immunofluorescence, and *in vitro* studies, *J. Cell Biol.,* 60, 375, 1974.
50. **Kefalides, N. A.,** Structure and biosynthesis of basement membranes, *Int. Rev. Connect. Tissue Res.,* 6, 63, 1973.
51. **Kefalides, N. A. and Denduchis, B.,** Structural components of epithelial and endothelial basement membranes, *Biochemistry,* 11, 4613, 1969.
52. **Kresina, T. F., Rhodes, R. K., and Miller, E. J.,** A further evaluation of the collagenous components derived from basement membrane-rich tissues, *Fed. Proc. Abstr.,* 37(6), 1528, 1978.
53. **Kuboki, Y., Tanzer, M. L., and Mechanic, G. L.,** Isolation of polypeptides containing the intermolecular cross-link $\delta\delta'$-dihydroxylysinonorleucine from dentin collagen, *Arch. Biochem. Biophys.,* 158, 106, 1973.
54. **Kuhn, C.,** The cells of the lung and their organelles, in *The Biochemical Basis of Pulmonary Function,* Crystal, R. G., Ed., Marcel Dekker, New York, 1976, 3.

55. **Langness, U. and Udenfriend, S.,** Collagen biosynthesis in nonfibroblastic cell lines, *Proc. Natl. Acad. Sci. U.S.A.,* 71, 50, 1974.
56. **Lapiere, C. M., Nusgens, B., and Pierard, G. E.,** Interaction between collagen Type I and Type III in conditioning bundles organization, *Connect. Tissue Res.,* 5, 21, 1977.
57. **Leak, L. V.,** The structure of lymphatic capillaries in lymph formation, *Fed. Proc.,* 35, 1863, 1976.
58. **Lenaers, A., Ansay, M., Nusgens, B. V., and Lapiere, C. M.,** Collagen made of extended α-chains, procollagen, in genetically-defective dermatosporactic calves, *Eur. J. Bioch.,* 23, 533, 1971.
59. **Lenaers, A. and Lapiere, C. M.,** Type III procollagen and collagen in skin, *Biochim. Biophys. Acta,* 400, 121, 1975.
60. **Lichtenstein, J. R., Byers, P. H., Smith, B. D., and Martin, G. R.,** Identification of the collagenous proteins synthesized by cultured cells from human skin, *Biochemistry,* 14, 1589, 1975.
61. **Liebow, A. A.,** Definition and classification of interstitial pneumonias in human pathology, in Alveolar Interstitum of the Lung, Int. Symp., Paris, 1974, *Prog. Respir. Res.,* 8, 1, S. Karger, Basel, 1975.
62. **Mayne, R., Vail, M. S., and Miller, E. J.,** The effect of embryo extract on the types of collagen synthesized by cultured chick chondrocytes, *Dev. Biol.,* 54, 230, 1976.
63. **McLees, B. D., Schleiter, G., and Pinnell, S. R.,** Isolation of type III collagen from human adult parenchymal lung, *Biochemistry,* 16, 185, 1977.
64. **Miller, A.,** Molecular packing in collagen fibrils, in *Biochemistry of Collagen,* Ramachandran, G. N., and Reddi, A. H., Eds., Plenum Press, New York, 1976, 85.
65. **Miller, E. J.,** Isolation and characterization of a collagen from chick cartilage containing three identical α chains, *Biochemistry,* 10, 1652, 1971.
66. **Miller, E. J.,** Isolation and characterization of the cyanogen bromide peptides from the α 1(II) chain of chick cartilage collagen, *Biochemistry,* 10, 3030, 1971.
67. **Miller, E. J.,** Structural studies on cartilage collagen employing limited cleavage and solubilization with pepsin, *Biochemistry,* 11, 4903, 1972.
68. **Miller, E. J.,** A review of biochemical studies on the genetically distinct collagens of the skeletal system, *Clin. Orthop.,* 92, 260, 1973.
69. **Miller, E. J.,** Biochemical characteristics and biological significance of the genetically-distinct collagens, *Mol. Cell. Biochem.,* 13(3), 165, 1976.

69a. **Miller, E. J., Kresina, T. F., Gay, S., and Rhodes, R. K.,** Recent developments in the chemistry of basement membrane collagens, presented at The Western Connective Tissue Society Meeting, Seattle, Wash., February 9 to 11, 1979.

70. **Miller, E. J., Epstein, E. H., Jr., and Piez, K. A.,** Identification of three genetically distinct collagens by cyanogen bromide cleavage of insoluble human skin and cartilage collagen, *Biochem. Biophys. Res. Commun.,* 42, 1024, 1971.
71. **Miller, E. J., Finch, J. E., Jr., Chung, E., and Butler, W. T.,** Specific cleavage of the native type III collagen molecule with trypsin, *Arch. Biochem. Biophys.,* 173, 631, 1976.
72. **Miller, E. J. and Lunde, L. G.,** Isolation and characterization of the cyanogen bromide peptides from the α 1(II) chain of bovine and human cartilage collagen, *Biochemistry,* 12, 3153, 1973.
73. **Miller, E. J. and Mathews, M. B.** Characterization of notochord collagen as a cartilage-type collagen, *Biochem. Biophys. Res. Commun.,* 60, 424, 1974.
74. **Miller, E. J. and Matukas, V. J.,** Biosynthesis of collagen — the biochemist's view, *Fed. Proc.,* 33, 1197, 1974.
75. **Miller, E. J., Woodall, D. L. and Vail, M. S.,** Biosynthesis of cartilage collagen: use of pulse labeling to order the cyanogen bromide peptides in the α1 (II) chain, *J. Biol. Chem.,* 248, 1666, 1973.
76. **Minor, R. R., Clark, C. C., Strause, E. L., Koszalka, T. R., Brent, R. L., and Kefalides, N. A.,** Basement membrane procollagen is not converted to collagen in organ cultures of parietal yolk sac endoderm, *J. Biol. Chem.,* 251, 1789, 1976.
77. **Minor, R. R., Hoch, P. S., Koszalka, T. R., Brent, R. L., and Kefalides, N. A.,** Organ cultures of the embryonic rat parietal yolk sac. I. Morphologic and autoradiographic studies of the deposition of the collagen and the noncollagen glycoprotein components of basement membrane, *Dev. Biol.,* 48, 344, 1976.
78. **Minor, R. R., Strause, E. L., Koszalka, T. R., Brent, R. L., and Kefalides, N. A.,** Organ cultures of the embryonic rat parietal yolk sac. II. Synthesis, accumulation, and turnover of collagen and noncollagen basement membrane glycoproteins, *Dev. Biol.,* 48, 365, 1976.
79. **Müller-Eberhard, H. J.,** Complement, *Annu. Rev. Biochem.,* 44, 697, 1975.

79a. **Peréz-Tamayo, R.,** Pathology of collagen degradation — a review, *Am. J. Pathol.,* 92, 509, 1978.

80. **Permutt, S. and Caldini, P.,** Tissue pressures and fluid dynamics of the lungs, *Fed. Proc.,* 35, 1876, 1976.

81. **Pickrell, J. A., Harris, D. V., Mauderly, J. L., and Hahn, F. F.**, Altered collagen metabolism in radiation-induced interstitial pulmonary fibrosis, *Chest*, 69, 311, 1976.
82. **Piez, K. A.**, Cross-linking of collagen and elastin, *Annu. Rev. Biochem.*, 37, 547, 1968.
83. **Piez, K. A. and Miller, A.**, The structure of collagen fibrils, *J. Supramol. Struct.*, 2, 121, 1974.
84. **Pinnel, S. R. and Martin, G. R.**, The crosslinking of collagen and elastin: enzymatic conversion of lysine in peptide linkage to α-aminoadipic-δ-semialdehyde (allysine) by an extract of bone, *Proc. Natl. Acad. Sci. U.S.A.*, 61, 708, 1968.
85. **Prockop, D. J., Berg, R. A., Kivirikko, K. I., and Uitto, J.**, Intracellular steps in the biosynthesis of collagen, in *Biochemistry of Collagen*, Ramachandran, G. N. and Reddi, A. H., Eds., Plenum Press, New York, 1976, 163.
86. **Ramachandran, G. N. and Ramakrishnan, C.**, Molecular structure, in *Biochemistry of Collagen*, Ramachandran, G. N. and Reddi, A. H., Eds., Plenum Press, New York, 1976, 45.
87. **Reddi, A. H.**, Collagen and cell differentiation, in *Biochemistry of Collagen*, Ramachandran, G. N. and Reddi, A. H., Eds., Plenum Press, New York, 1976, 449.
88. **Reid, K. B.**, A collagen-like amino acid sequence in a polypeptide chain of human C1Q (a subcomponent of the first component of complement), *Biochem. J.*, 141, 189, 1974.
89. **Robins, S. P. and Bailey, A. J.**, The chemistry of collagen cross-links: the characterization of fraction C, a possible artifact produced during the reduction of collagen fibres with borohydride, *Biochem. J.*, 135, 657, 1973.
90. **Robins, S. P. and Bailey, A. J.**, The chemistry of the collagen cross-links: the mechanism of stabilization of the reducible intermediate cross-links, *Biochem. J.*, 149, 381, 1975.
91. **Rosenbloom, J., Harsch, M., and Jimenez, S.**, Hydroxyproline content determines the denaturation temperature of chick tendon collagen, *Arch. Biochem. Biophys.*, 158, 478, 1973.
92. **Ross, R. and Glomset, J. A.**, Atherosclerosis and the arterial smooth muscle cell, *Science*, 180, 1332, 1973.
93. **Schneir, M. and Miller, E.**, The absence of sulfhydryl group reactivity in type III collagen , paper presented at the meeting of West Coast Connective Tissue Society, Heber, Utah, March 5 to 7, 1976.
93a. **Seyer, J. M.**, Basement membrane associated collagens of human lung, *Fed. Proc. Abstr.*, 37(6), 1527, 1978.
94. **Seyer, J. M., Hutcheson, E. T., and Kang, A. H.**, Collagen polymorphism in idiopathic chronic pulmonary fibrosis, *J. Clin. Invest.*, 57, 1498, 1976.
95. **Siegel, R. C.**, Collagen cross-linking, synthesis of collagen cross-links *in vitro* with highly purified lysyl oxidase, *J. Biol. Chem.*, 251, 5786, 1976.
96. **Siegel, R. C. and Fu, J. C. C.**, Collagen cross-linking; purification and substrate specificity of lysyl oxidase, *J. Biol. Chem.*, 251, 5779, 1976.
97. **Slauson, D. O., Hahn, F. F., Benjamin, S. A., Chiffelle, T. L., and Jones, R. K.**, Inflammatory sequences in acute pulmonary radiation injury, *Am. J. Pathol.*, 82, 549, 1976.
98. **Smith, G. N., Linsenmayer, T. F., and Newsome, D. A.**, Synthesis of type II collagen *in vitro* by embryonic chick neural retina tissue, *Proc. Natl. Acad. Sci. U.S.A.*, 73, 4420, 1976.
99. **Strawich, E. and Nimni, M. E.**, Properties of a collagen molecule containing three identical components extracted from bovine articular cartilage, *Biochemistry*, 10, 3905, 1971.
100. **Swann, D. A., Constable, I. J., and Harper, E.**, as cited in *Invest. Opthalmol.*, 11, 735, 1972; **Eyre, D. R., and Muir, H.**, *Biochem. J.*, 151, 595, 1975.
101. **Tanzer, M. L. and Kefalides, N. A.**, Collagen crosslinks: occurrence in basement membrane collagens, *Biochem. Biophys. Res. Commun.*, 51, 775, 1973.
102. **Tanzer, M. L.**, Crosslinking, in *Biochemistry of Collagen*, Ramachandran, G. N., and Reddi, A. H., Eds., Plenum Press, New York, 1976, 137.
103. **Thurlbeck, W. M.**, Postnatal growth and development of the lung, *Am. Rev. Respir. Dis.*, 111, 803, 1975.
104. **Traub, W. and Piez, K. A.**, The chemistry and structure of collagen, *Adv. Protein Chem.*, 25, 243, 1971.
105. **Trelstad, R. L., Kang, A. H., Toole, B. P., and Gross, J.**, Collagen heterogeneity: high resolution separation of native $[\alpha 1(I)]_2\alpha_2$ and $[\alpha 1(II)]_3$ and their component α chains, *J. Biol. Chem.*, 247, 6469, 1972.
106. **Trelstad, R. L., Hayashi, K., and Gross, J.**, Collagen fibrillogenesis: intermediate aggregates and suprafibrillar order, *Proc. Natl. Acad. Sci. U.S.A.*, 73, 4027, 1976.
107. **Veis, A. and Anesey, J.**, Modes of intermolecular crosslinking in mature insoluble collagen, *J. Biol. Chem.*, 240, 3899, 1965.
108. **Veis, A. and Brownell, A. G.**, Collagen biosynthesis, *Crit. Rev. Biochem.*, 2, 417, 1975.
109. **Vracko, R.**, Basal lamina scaffold-anatomy and significance for maintenance of orderly tissue structure, *Am. J. Pathol.*, 77, 314, 1974.

110. **Vuust, J. and Piez, K. A.,** A kinetic study of collagen biosynthesis, *J. Biol. Chem.*, 247, 856, 1972.

111. **Vuust, J. and Piez, K. A.,** Biosynthesis of the α chains of collagen studied by pulse-labeling in culture, *J. Biol. Chem.*, 245, 6201, 1970.

112. **Ward, A. R. and Mason, P.,** Influence of proline hydroxylation upon the thermal stability of collagen fragment α 1CB2, *J. Mol. Biol.*, 79, 431, 1973.

113. **Weiss, J. B., Shuttleworth, C. A., Brown, R., Sedowfia, K., Baildam, A., and Hunter, J. A.,** Occurrence of type III collagen in inflamed synovial membranes: a comparison between non rheumatoid, rheumatoid and normal synovial collagens, *Biochem. Biophys. Res. Commun.*, 65, 907, 1975.

114. **Wilken, D. R., Hanson, W. H., Dyar, R. E., Klemencic, J. M., Butz, M. E., and Turk, T. L.,** Basement membrane synthesis by cultured canine kidney tubule cells, *Fed. Proc. Abstr.*, 35, 1519, 1976.

Chapter 3

ELASTIN LOCATION AND STRUCTURE

J. A. Pickrell

TABLE OF CONTENTS

I. LOCATION

Elastic tissue (elastin) provides resiliency to lung tissue by its composition and its unique anatomic location. Elastin has an amorphous component which provides elasticity and a microfibrillar component which may serve as scaffolding to align and cross-link amorphous elastin (Figure 1).[6, 13, 37] The alveolar system is designed so that changes in volume are not accompanied by changes in surface area.[55] Sobin et al.[45] observed minimal accumulation of elastic fibers in the intersection of alveolar walls. Thurlbeck[49] reviewed postnatal lung growth and indicated that elastic tissue played a central role in alveolar development. The consolidation of elastic tissue into an almost "fishnet" type of elastic structure preceded the subdivision of alveoli into spiral walls.[55] Bundles of elastin fibers fan out from alveolar ducts and alveolar margins in sweeping patterns, passing across a number of alveoli, although a fine network similar to collagen is not apparent.[45] These findings not only support, but elegantly describe, the location of interstitial alveolar elastin, relating it to early subdivision of alveoli. The vascular sheet of blood which passes by alveoli to be aereated may be contained in capillary "sinuses".[9, 10, 35, 39, 46] These sinuses are likened to an underground parking garage containing support posts in a hexagonal array which have a collagen exterior, a microfibrillar elastin middle, and an amorphous elastin core representing an elastic fiber (Figure 1). This elastin provides elasticity for the pulmonary vascular system and assists in maintaining the low pulmonary arterial pressure compared to systemic pressures. Additionally, it maximizes the efficiency of blood-gas exposure and resultant exchange.

Elastin is associated with smooth muscle cells, a dense network of accompanying small blood vessels in bronchial walls, prevents excess bronchodilation,[11, 33] and is critical to pulmonary distensibility and collapsibility. The central fiber which spirals the alveolar duct is thought to consist of elastin and collagen.[55] Digestion of lungs with elastase seems to reduce the compliance or elastic recoil, but not to affect the maximal inflation volume.[19, 22, 51] In vitro reactions with tracheal segments agree and are consistent with a reduction of Young's modulus of elastin disproportionately larger than the protein loss.[51a]

II. STRUCTURE

Amorphous elastin, although poorly characterized, seems to be a random network which is partially constrained. Amorphous elastin is a poorly characterized protein, chiefly because of its insolubility in substances which do not break peptide bonds and its lack of a clear X-ray diffraction pattern.[15] Although complex and poorly defined, the X-ray diffraction pattern of elastin suggested that hydrated elastin is essentially an amorphous random network, (Figure 1).[17] Gray et al.[15] have proposed an oiled coil model, and Urry and Long[54] provided support for a fibrillar model; (Figure supports the desmosine cross-link. NMR techniques indicated that the rotational correlation time of water-swollen elastin was slower than collagen denatured in 2 *M* KCNS, suggesting elastin to be partially constrained. Torchia and Piez[50] noted a sharpening of side chain methyl carbon resonance when water-swollen elastin was "denatured" with 2 *M* KCNS, indicating that KCNS may be acting to remove constraints on these hydrophobic side chains.

Disruption of hydrophobic forces alters several properties of elastin. Alcohols increased the rate of alkaline hydrolysis of elastin, probably by disrupting hydrophobic forces.[23] Although the results of Kagan et al.[20] indicated sodium dodecyl sulfate (SDS) to have a similar increase of elastase-induced elastolysis, this was complicated by the apparently increased elastin affinity for elastase induced by the SDS. Whether this is

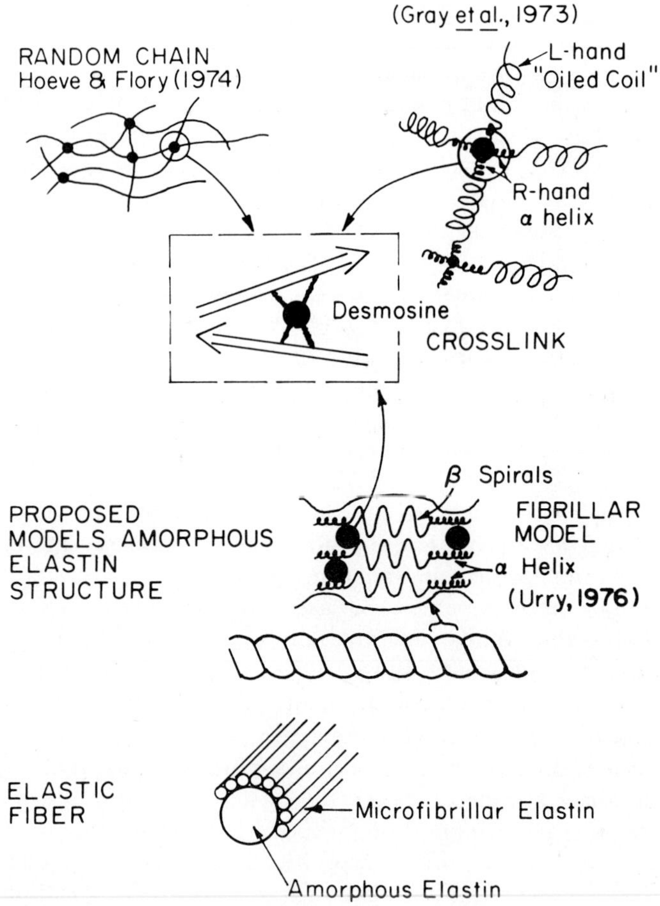

FIGURE 1. Diagrams of proposed models of amorphous elastin structure include the random chain of Hoeve and Flory,[17] the "oiled coil" of Gray et al.,[15] and the fibrillar model of Urry.[53] Definition of elastin structure remains to be resolved. The elastic fiber is composed of amorphous and microfibrillar elastin.

due to disruption of hydrophobic forces and thus germane to this mechanism is unclear. Gosline[13] reported that stretching elastin to which alpha napthylsulfonate (ANS) is bound greatly reduces the ANS fluorescence, indicating that the dye is responding to an increase in polarity as the elastin is stretched, possibly from exposure to aqueous solvent. However, whether the reduced ANS fluorescence is due to an altered geometry of the elastin fibers was not determined.

Elastin may represent a random network (Figure 1) swollen by an extremely poor solvent. The volume change of resilin tendon with increasing temperature is negligible. Water-swollen elastin increases in volume with concomitant temperature increases, but elastin swollen in 30% glycol or other alcohols does not.[13] The second virial coefficient of light scattering of α-elastin swollen in water is negative. Elastin is thus constrained by adverse polymer solvent interactions and possibly hydrophobic forces and, when stretched, some constraints are removed. Schein et al.[41] demonstrated that tropoelastin was a random coil. Although these results do not necessarily mean random coil formation is maintained after the chains are incorporated into the elastic fiber, the present findings must be taken into account in any proposed mechanism of fiber formation.

Urry points out in discussing this article that small regions of β-spiral would not be detected.[41] Elastin provides resistance to lung tissue because oscillation occurs at low frequencies. Although elastin has excellent resilience properties at low frequencies, at higher frequencies, such as that produced by hummingbird or insect wings, resilience falls profoundly. Thus, elastin is not found in such situations. Franzblau[8] reported that it was not found in the avian lung in appreciable quantities since the muscular diaphragm is responsible for the avian substitute for elastic recoil. However, Rucker et al.[38a] characterized elastin synthesis using chick lungs. Mammalian lungs have a slower frequency of respiration (≤ 1/sec) and only one diaphragm and contain modest amounts of elastin, which is ideally suited for and provides pulmonary elastic recoil.

Amorphous elastin is a large, resilient, relatively insoluble polymer whose primary structure is being elucidated using a soluble elastin component (no cross-links because of inhibition of the cross-linking enzyme, lysyl oxidase, which requires copper cofactor) from copper deficient swine.[5, 44] Tryptic peptides were used for sequencing elastin fragments since elastin lacks methionine; thus, CNBr fragmentation would not occur. These analyses provided data to define 730 of 850 amino acid residues in an elastin mononer. Although elastin has a glycine content similar to that of collagen, the sequential arrangement of glycine is quite different.[5] Elastin glycine residues are not subject to the constraint present in collagen, specifically a repeating triplet gly-X-Y. Instead, Foster et al.[5] report repetitions of a tetrapeptide, gly-gly-val-pro, a pentapeptide, pro-gly-val-gly-val, and a hexapeptide, pro-gly-val-gly-val-ala. In elastin, proline rarely precedes glycine, but often follows it. Foster et al.[5] report hydroxyproline to be a constituent of elastin, not just a contaminant. Uitto et al.[52] report the level of prolyl hydroxylase will influence considerably the hydroxylation of proline in in vitro elastin synthesis without affecting the rate of elastin synthesis. Thus, hydroxyproline is not necessary to maintain elastin structure.

Elastin has cross-links which are thought to confer some of the properties of elastin which differ from most other proteins, specifically elasticity (Figure 1). These cross-links are reported[28, 48] to be quite similar to tetrasubstituted pyridinum compounds. The two isomers (1,3,4,5 and 1,2,5,6 substituted compounds) were named desmosine and isodesmosine, respectively. Considerable α helical content was reported by Gray et al.[15] and some evidence exists for the β-turn or helix being central in elastin function.[15, 54]

Different proposals for specific linking of peptide chains to these cross-links have been given. The cross-links are the condensation product of four lysine residues.[25, 26] This process may be inhibited by inducing a copper deficiency or by administering BAPN[25] which blocks the cross-linking enzyme lysyl oxidase.[32, 43] The peptide sequences lys-ala-ala-lys and lys-ala-ala-ala-lys were noted frequently in the cross-link regions. Foster et al.[4] and Gray et al.[15] propose that two uninterrupted chains are connected by one cross-link and that the region near the cross-link is α helix and the remainder an oiled β coil. Alternative hypotheses reviewed by Sandberg[40] include three other similar models. The random chain with cross-links[17] is not inconsistent with the data of Foster et al.,[4] although the α helix near the cross-links will allow the lysine residues to be separated by two or three alanines without distortion.[40] Thus the presence of the α helix seems consistent with Foster's data. Hoeve and Flory[17] indicate the oiled coil to have similar problems to Partridge's[27] corpuscular theory. Specifically, tightly packed globular polypeptide chains or extensive fixed structures in these models could not have the short relaxation time observed.[50] Whether macromolecular fibrils form as proposed by Urry[53] and supported by electron microscopic work[3, 14] remains undefined. All models involve extensive hydrophobic regions. However, if such regions alone are expected to provide the elasticity, Young's modulus for elastin would be much higher;[40] thus, other mechanisms must be involved (Figure 1).

III. SUMMARY

Elastin is composed of two compounds, (1) amorphous elastin, which is linked and perhaps "cloaked", and (2) microfibrillar elastin, an elastic fiber (Figure 1). Amorphous elastin has elastic properties at low resonance frequencies which are conferred on it by its unique cross-linking pattern involving the tetrafunctional desmosines and by its molecular constraints, some of which are removed by stretching. Microfibrillar elastin probably facilitates the formation of these unique cross-links, their patterns, and the resulting constraints of amorphous elastin. Much controversy surrounds the exact nature of the elastin molecule. Likewise, its mode of formation is, at present, nearly completely obscured. Since elastin provides the resiliency or "spring" to many organs, this property is of considerable interest. The question concerning molecular homogeneity of elastin has intrigued investigators for considerable time, although it remains undefined. One school of thought says that most elastin functions are quite similar, differing only in intensity. Nature could logically conserve information by dictating molecular homogeneity in the case of elastin. Alternatively, different tissues may require different elastins. Since no one has ever accused Mother Nature of evolving systems which we would consider logical (especially with incomplete understanding), resolution of this intriguing question must await collection of further data.

Numerous investigators[7, 11, 12, 31, 40] have reviewed the pathway by which the cross-links form, and these will be detailed in the elastin metabolism section. Cox et al.[3] believe that hydrophobic bonding alone can accomplish this registration function. However, Sherr et al.[42] noted the resemblance of the microfibrillar component of elastin to the collagen registration peptides. If analogous, this finding suggests that microfibrillar elastin may serve as a scaffold from which amorphous elastin can be properly cross-linked. Perhaps the cross-linking enzyme is brought into aposition with tropoelastin by microfibrils. The similarity of microfibrillar elastin to structural glycoproteins of elastin, while intriguing, sheds no further light upon the role of microfibrillar elastin.[34]

IV. LUNG

Lung elastin is similar to aortic elastin in the rabbit and likewise similar in the central and peripheral area of dog and hamster.[8] Parenchymal lung tissue (and subsequently elastin) was separated from bronchial tissue by brief passage of a disintegrated mince through a fine mesh screen.[18] Hot alkali extractions seem to damage the elastin cross-links so that abnormally low values of desmosine and isodesmosine are apparently obtained.[12] Gallop and Paz[12] values for elastin which were not extracted in hot alkali are higher than most reported, as reviewed by Sandberg.[40] Likewise the roughly equal ratio of desmosine/isodesmosine reviewed by Sandberg[40] is not observed in Gallop and Paz's[12] work on lung elastin, with desmosine being higher than isodesmosine. Lung elastin may have a unique structural configuration requirement fulfilled by cross-linking in this unusual manner. This may differ from that reviewed by Sandberg[40] for ligamentum nuchae (2-dimensional stress) or aorta (3-dimensional stress). These differing requirements still both produced approximately equimolar amounts of the two desmosine isomers.[40] Further work will increasingly elucidate this fascinating area.

The question of which cells synthesize elastin is still open. Two mesenchymal cells seem to participate in elastin synthesis,[36, 38] the smooth muscle cell and the fibroblast. However, few definitive studies indicating cell type have been performed. Other cell types may participate as well.[16] Cells free of the extracellular matrix of embryonic aorta are capable of synthesizing collagen and elastin.[52] Elastin has been quantitated by desmosine measurement in tissue hydrolysates from normal and injured lungs.[24, 29, 30, 47] Total elastin, regardless of its degree of maturation, has been measured[16a] by the amount of val-pro (found in uniquely high concentrations in elastin),[5,40] although this method still has to be proven.[16] The intriguing question of whether the "contractile interstitial cell" of Kapanci et al.,[21] which resembles both the smooth muscle cell and the fibroblast, is an important producer of pulmonary elastin awaits cloning of this cell from lung. Subsequent to such cloning, the immunologic detection of intracellular soluble elastin should provide the technology to define this problem.[2]

REFERENCES

1. **Bloom, W. and Fawcett, D. W.,** Respiratory system, in *A Textbook of Histology,* W. B. Saunders, Philadelphia, 1975, 743.
2. **Christner, P., Dixon, M., Cywinski, A., and Rosenbloom, J.,** Radioimmunological identification of tropoelastin, *Biochem. J.,* 157, 525, 1976.
3. **Cox, B. A., Starcher, B. C., and Urry, D. W.,** Coacervation of alpha-elastin results in fiber formation, *Biochim. Biophys. Acta,* 317, 209, 1973.
4. **Foster, J. A., Rubin, L., Kagan, H. M., and Franzblau, C.,** Isolation and characterization of cross-linked peptides from elastin, *J. Biol. Chem.,* 249, 6191, 1974.
5. **Foster, J. A., Bruenger, E., Gray, W. R., and Sandberg, L. B.,** Isolation and amino acid sequences of tropoelastin peptides, *J. Biol. Chem.,* 248, 2876, 1973.
6. **Foster, J. A., Mecham, R. P., and Franzblau, C.,** A high molecular weight species of soluble elastin, *Biochem. Biophys. Res. Commun.,* 72, 1399, 1976.
7. **Francis, G., John, R. and Thomas, J.,** Biosynthetic pathway of desmosines in elastin, *Biochem. J.,* 136, 45, 1973.
8. **Franzblau, C.,** Lung Elastin, report for Natl. Heart Lung Institute, distr. by Natl. Technical Information Serv., U.S. Department of Commerce, Springfield, Va., PB248387, 1975.
9. **Fung, Y. C. and Sobin, S. S.,** Theory of sheet flow in lung alveoli, *J. Appl. Physiol.,* 26, 472, 1969.
10. **Fung, Y. C., Zweifach, B. F., and Intaglietta, M.,** Elastic environment of the capillary bed, *Circ. Res.,* 19, 441, 1966.
11. **Gallop, P. M., Blumenfeld, O. O., and Seifter, S.,** Structure and metabolism of connective tissue proteins, *Annu. Rev. Biochem.,* 41, 617, 1972.
12. **Gallop, P. M. and Paz, M. A.,** Post-translational protein modifications, with special attention to collagen and elastin, *Physiol. Rev.,* 55, 418, 1975.
13. **Gosline, J. M.,** The physical properties of elastic tissue, *Int. Rev. Connect. Tissue Res.,* 7, 211, 1976.
14. **Gotte, L., Giro, M.G., Volpin, D., and Horne, R. W.,** *J. Ultrastruct. Res.,* 46, 23, 1974; as cited in **Sandberg, L. B.,** Elastin structure in health and disease, *Int. Rev. Connect. Tissue Res.,* 7, 208, 1976.
15. **Gray, W. R., Sandberg, L. B., and Foster, J. A.,** Molecular model for elastin structure and function, *Nature (London),* 246, 461, 1973.
16. **Hance, A. J. and Crystal, R. G.,** The connective tissue of lung, *Am. Rev. Respir. Dis.,* 112, 657, 1975.

16a. **Hauschka, P. V. and Gallop, P. M.,** Elastin biosynthesis in mouse lung, *Fed. Proc. Abstr.,* 33, 1536, 1974.

17. **Hoeve, C. A. and Flory, P. J.,** The elastic properties of elastin, *Biopolymers,* 13, 677, 1974.
18. **Hospelhorn, V. D.,** Separation and Characterization of Lung Elastin, report for Natl. Heart Lung Institute, distr. by Natl. Technical Information Serv., U.S. Department of Commerce, Springfield, Va., PB248390, 1975.
19. **Johanson, W. G. and Pierce, A. K.,** Effects of elastase, collagenase and papain on structure and function of rat lungs *in vitro, J. Clin. Invest.,* 51, 288, 1972.
20. **Kagan, H. M., Crombie, G. D., Jordan, R. E., Lewis, W., and Franzblau, C.,** Proteolysis of elastin-ligand complexes. Stimulation of elastase digestion of insoluble elastin by sodium dodecyl sulfate, *Biochemistry,* 11, 3412, 1972.
21. **Kapanci, Y., Assimacopoulos, A., Irle, C., Zwahlen, A., and Gabbiani, G.,** "Contractile interstitial cells" in pulmonary alveolar septa: a possible regulator of ventilation/perfusion ratio? Ultrastructural, immunofluorescence, and in vitro studies, *J. Cell Biol.,* 60, 375, 1974.

22. **Karlinsky, J. B., Snider, G. L., Franzblau, C., Stone, P. J., and Hoppin, F. G.,** *In vitro* effects of elastase and collagenase on mechanical properties of hamster lungs, *Am. Rev. Respir. Dis.*, 113, 769, 1976.
23. **Kornfeld-Poullain, N. and Robert, L.,** Effet de différents solvants organiques sur la dégradation alcaline de l'elastine, *Bull. Soc. Chim. Biol.*, 50, 759, 1968.
24. **Kuhn, C. and Starcher, B.,** The significance of connective tissue repair in elastase-induced emphysema, *Am. Rev. Respir. Dis.*, 113 (Abstr.), 209, 1976.
25. **Miller, E. J., Martin, G. R., Mecca, C. E., and Piez, K. A.,** The biosynthesis of elastin cross-links: the effect of copper deficiency and a lathyrogen, *J. Biol. Chem.*, 240, 3623, 1965.
26. **Narayanan, A. S. and Page, R. C.,** Demonstration of a precursor-product relationship between soluble and cross-linked elastin, and the biosynthesis of the desmosines *in vitro, J. Biol. Chem.*, 251, 1125, 1976.
27. **Partridge, S. M.,** Biosynthesis and nature of elastin structures, *Fed. Proc.*, 25, 1023, 1966.
28. **Partridge, S. M., Elsden, D. F., and Thomas, J.,** Constitution of the cross-linkages in elastin, *Nature (London)*, 197, 1297, 1963.
29. **Pickrell, J. A., Harris, D. V., Pfleger, R. C., Benjamin, S. A., Belasich, J. J., Jones, R. K., and McClellan, R. O.,** Biological alterations resulting from chronic lung irradiation. II. Connective tissue alterations following inhalation of ^{144}Ce fused clay aerosol in Beagle dogs, *Radiat. Res.*, 63, 299, 1975.
30. **Pickrell, J. A. and Shafer, J.,** Lung connective tissue measurements. I. Amino acid analysis procedures for determination of canine lung connective tissue, *Arch. Intern. Med.*, 127, 891, 1971.
31. **Piez, K. A.,** Cross-linking of collagen and elastin, *Annu. Rev. Biochem.*, 37, 547, 1968.
32. **Pinnel, S. R. and Martin, G. R.,** The crosslinking of collagen and elastin: enzymatic conversion of lysine in peptide linkage to α-aminoadipic-δ-semi-aldehyde (allysine) by an extract of bone, *Proc. Natl. Acad. Sci. U.S.A.*, 61, 708, 1968.
33. **Radford, E. P.,** Static mechanical properties of mammalian lungs, in *Handbook of Physiology*, Respiration, Sec. 3, Vol. 1, Fenn, W. O., and Rahn, H., Eds., American Physiological Society, Washington, D.C., 1964, 429.
34. **Robert, B., Szigeti, M., Derouette, J. C., and Robert, L.,** Studies on the nature of the "microfibrillar" component of elastic fibers, *Eur. J. Biochem.*, 21, 507, 1971.
35. **Rosenquist, T. H., Bernick, S., Sobin, S. S., and Fung, Y. C.,** The structure of the pulmonary interalveolar microvascular sheet, *Microvasc. Res.*, 5, 199, 1973.
36. **Ross, R.,** The smooth muscle cell. II. Growth of smooth muscle in culture and formation of elastic fibers, *J. Cell Biol.*, 50, 172, 1971.
37. **Ross, R. and Bornstein, P.,** The elastic fiber. I. The separation and partial characterization of its macromolecular components, *J. Cell Biol.*, 40, 366, 1969.
38. **Ross, R. and Klebanoff, S. J.,** The smooth muscle cell. I. *In vivo* synthesis of connective tissue proteins, *J. Cell Biol.*, 50, 159, 1971.

38a. **Rucker, R. B., Heng, C. S., Murray, J., and Buckingham, K.,** Putative forms of soluble elastin and their relationship to the synthesis of fibrous elastin, paper presented at the meeting of West Coast Connective Tissue Society, Gleneden Beach, Ore., February 25 to 27, 1977.

39. **Ryan, S. F., Ciannella, A., and Dumais, C.,** The structure of the interalveolar septum of the mammalian lung, *Anat. Rec.*, 165, 467, 1969.
40. **Sandberg, L. B.,** Elastin structure in health and disease, *Int. Rev. Connect. Tissue Res.*, 7, 159, 1976.
41. **Schein, J., Carpousis, A., and Rosenbloom, J.,** Evidence that tropoelastin exists as a random coil, in *Elastin and Elastic Tissue*, Sandberg, L. B., Gray, W. R., and Franzblau, C., Eds., Plenum Press, New York, 1977, 727.
42. **Sherr, C. J., Taubman, M. B., and Goldberg, B.,** Isolation of a disulfide-stabilized, three-chain polypeptide fragment unique to the precursor of human collagen, *J. Biol. Chem.*, 248, 7033, 1973.
43. **Siegel, R. C.,** Collagen cross-linking, synthesis of collagen cross-links *in vitro* with highly purified lysyl oxidase, *J. Biol. Chem.*, 251, 5786, 1976.
44. **Smith, D. W., Weissmann, N., and Carnes, W. H.,** Cardiovascular studies on copper deficient swine. XII. Partial purification of a soluble protein resembling elastin, *Biochem. Biophys. Res. Commun.*, 31, 309, 1968.
45. **Sobin, S. S., Bernick, S., Tremer, H. M., Rosenquist, T. H., Lindal, R., and Fung, Y. C.,** The fibroprotein network of the pulmonary interalveolar wall, *Chest*, 65 (Suppl.), 4S, 1974.
46. **Sobin, S. S., Fung, Y. C., Tremer, H. M., and Rosenquist, T. H.,** Elasticity of the pulmonary alveolar microvascular sheet in the cat, *Circ. Res.*, 30, 440, 1972.
47. **Starcher, B. C. and Galione, M. J.,** A large scale procedure for purification of desmosine and isodesmosine, *Prep. Biochem.*, 5, 455, 1975.

48. **Thomas, J., Elsden, D. F., and Partridge, S. M.,** Partial structure of two major degradation products from the cross-linkages in elastin, *Nature (London),* 200, 651, 1963.
49. **Thurlbeck, W. M.,** Postnatal growth and development of the lung, *Am. Rev. Respir. Dis.,* 111, 803, 1975.
50. **Torchia, D. A. and Piez, K. A.,** Mobility of elastin chains as determined by 13 C nuclear magnetic resonance, *J. Mol. Biol.,* 76, 419, 1973.
51. **Turino, G. M. and Lourenco, R. V.,** The connective tissue basis of pulmonary mechanics, in *Pulmonary Emphysema and Proteolysis,* Academic Press, New York, 1972, 509.

51a. **Turino, G. M., Rodriguez, J. R., Greenbaum, L. M., and Mandl, I.,** Mechanisms of pulmonary injury, *Am. J. Med.,* 57, 493, 1974.

52. **Uitto, J., Hoffman, H. P., and Prockop, D. J.,** Synthesis of elastin and procollagen by cells from embryonic aorta: differences in the role of hydroxyproline and the effects of proline analogs on the secretion of the two proteins, *Arch. Biochem. Biophys.,* 173, 187, 1976.
53. **Urry, D. W.,** *Adv. Exp. Med. Biol.,* 43, 211, 1974; as cited in **Sandberg, L. B.,** Elastin structure in health and disease, *Int. Rev. Connect. Tissue Res.,* 7, 210, 1976.
54. **Urry, D. W. and Long, M. M.,** Conformations of the repeat peptides of elastin in solution: an application of proton and carbon-13 magnetic resonance to the determination of polypeptide secondary structure, *Crit. Rev. Biochem.,* 3, 1, 1976.
55. **Whimster, W. F.,** The microanatomy of the alveolar duct system, *Thorax,* 25, 141, 1970.

Chapter 4

PROTEOGLYCANS AND MUCOPROTEINS

J. A. Pickrell

TABLE OF CONTENTS

I. LOCATION

Proteoglycans are located throughout the pulmonary tree, in the alveolar parenchyma, and in the bronchial airways and vessels. Specific proteoglycans interact with collagen and possibly elastin; their role is not clear. Specifically, Romanova and Boikov[29] have described a proteoglycan glycocalyx covering the entire alveolar airspace epithelium. Moreover, they have shown that it may participate in active transfer across type I alveolar epithelial cells. No endothelial hypocalyx was noted. Proteoglycans are the combination of proteins and glycosaminoglycans (GAG) (formerly called acid mucopolysaccharides).[11] They are interspersed between collagen and elastin in bronchial and vessel walls. The interaction with collagen and elastin is currently unelucidated, although speculation concerning a structural role continues. For instance, dermatan sulfate interacts more strongly with collagen than does chondroitin sulfate.[19] The close association of amounts of GAG and collagen has been frequently noted.[10] Although collagen and GAG seem to be controlled differently, an extracellular association occurs. Reports concerning the effect of proteoglycans on fibroblast synthesis of collagen raises a question concerning a potential synthetic role.[25] Lippman and Matthews[22] indicate that this role is far from understood. The potential combination with the hydroxylysyl carbohydrate attachments of cartilage and basement membrane collagen and their potentially slower biosynthesis again suggest a possible role for proteoglycans. To date, no specific role for lung proteoglycans has been elucidated, although characterization has been initiated.[11]

Mucoproteins or glycoproteins are secretory products of the goblet cells and submucosal glands and accompany cilia down the bronchial tree, sometimes to the end of the terminal bronchioles.[1] They provide the mucus blanket necessary to sweep particles upward to be cleared on the mucociliary escalator. This mucus blanket is composed of an upper "gel" layer and a lower "sol" layer which facilitates clearance.[38] The glycoprotein moiety is responsible for its rheologic behavior.[23] Davis et al.[7] discuss the potential influence of active transport on water movement and the subsequent alteration of mucus rheology. Thus, mucus is located on the surfaces of branching and conducting airways but not to any great concentration in normal alveoli. Although a clearance role has been assigned to mucoproteins, only preliminary characterization has begun.[3,9,16]

II. STRUCTURE

Proteoglycans have unique structural features. They are composed of proteins and specific glycosaminoglycans (GAG) (Figure 1). Serine is usually the amino acid for the 30—100 attachment points for the GAG, although in keratan SO_4 attachment may also be through threonine.[8,28] Except for the keratan-chondroitin sulfate-protein complex of cartilage,[30] one uniform GAG is attached to the protein. Thus, proteoglycans are named for their GAG: hyaluronic acid, chondroitin 4 and 6 sulfate, dermatan sulfate, heparin, heparan sulfate, and keratan sulfate.[8] Hance and Crystal[11] have reviewed the structural features of GAG. They find all GAG except keratan sulfate to be present in lung. The predominnce of heparin + heparan sulfate in adults' pulmonary GAG synthesis is in agreement with White et al.[35] who reported heparin to be the main GAG in lung. Also Wusteman[36] reported heparin and heparan sulfate in bovine parenchyma and pleura to predominate in a mixture which contains all GAG except keratan sulfate.

Some evidence of pulmonary GAG heterogeneity has been observed.[11] Heparan sulfate from beef-lung tissue is indicated by proton magnetic resonance (p.m.r.) spectra

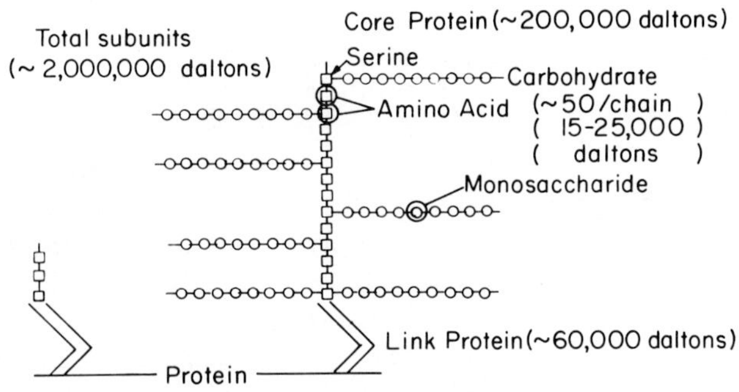

FIGURE 1. Proteoglycan structure is comprised of a protein, a link protein of ∿60,000 daltons, a core protein of ∿200,000 daltons, and carbohydrate side chains containing sufficient monosaccharide residues (∿50/chains) to have 15—25,000 daltons/side chain and ∿2,000,000 daltons/proteoglycan subunit.

to be heterogeneous. Likewise, heparan sulfate from other tissues has been shown to have different acetamido/sulfamino ratios as well as D-glucuronic/L-iduronic acid ratios.[5, 34] Moreover, beef-lung heparin reported to have only low amounts of *N*-acetylglucosamine has been observed to have some fractions with as high as 9%.[5]

Proteoglycans are "space fillers" (resistant to compression) which impede or channel liquid flow through tissue. They bind to collagen in the extracellular matrix and compete in this binding with other molecules.[6,12,18,24] The physiologic function of proteoglycans is elegantly reviewed by Comper and Laurent.[6] Hyaluronic acid is a random coil with a large volume and can be affected by other substances, such as urea. There is no general agreement as to whether these proteoglycans are covalently bound to other proteins in the extracellular matrix. Heparin is present on the surface of cells and competes with fibronectin for binding to collagen.[6, 18] Proteoglycans are gel-like. This property allows them to entangle and form polymeric networks — that is, maintain or organize structure. The solution domains or hydrodynamic volumes of proteoglycans are 100 to 1000 times as large as protein when a small amount of protein is present. They are viscoelastic at low strain and elastic at high strain frequency. Other proteoglycans can aggregate on hyaluronate. In light of the shift in rapid cell proliferation to predominantly hyaluronate,[17] one wonders if the tissue is not (1) using the most efficient "space filler" resistant to compression and (2) preparing for binding to other proteoglycans and ultimately to collagen in the extracellular matrix. The use of hyaluronate vs. dermatan SO_4 to indicate mesenchymal cell proliferation or collagen synthesis in injured lung is probably doomed to failure. This is because of the complicated nature of the proteoglycan complex and the diverse nature of the pulmonary response. Proteoglycans very strongly affect osmotic pressure. Because of the nature of their location, the effect is on local osmotic pressure. Comper and Laurent[6] state that the relatively high concentration of hyaluronate in very young brain may function to retain large amounts of water so that neuronal migration may take place and develop.

This may be applied hypothetically to the lung, since young lungs have much more hyaluronate.[11, 12] Perhaps this hyaluronate retains large amounts of water so that maximum differentiation and growth may take place. Later a more rigid extracellular matrix is provided both by the dermatan-hyaluronate binding and fibronectin.[2] In this environment, more collagen is produced which binds to the proteoglycan. Heparin ordinarily on the surface of mesenchymal cells competes (as a polyanion) for binding of collagen (probably procollagen in the in vivo situation) with fibronectin.[18] It is possible that both extracellular cleavage of procollagen and cross-linking into fibrils take place when bound to either fibronectin or proteoglycan. This is theorized because of the relationships described and the observation by Siegel[32] that the cross-linking enzyme for collagen and elastin (lysyl oxidase) prefers particulate to soluble substrate. This will be discussed in more detail in Chapter 5. One can readily see that the presence or concentration of specific proteoglycans could have a profound effect on pulmonary structure and function. Methods quite important to the elucidation of pulmonary structural glycoproteins are being developed. Simple methods for study of GAG quantities are reviewed and a thin layer chromatographic method is discussed along with cetylpyridinum chloride precipitation.[26] Identification and quantitation of connective tissue hexosamines have been performed by amino acid analysis[27] and by a combination of gas liquid chromatographic and colorimetric procedures[4, 14, 15] The uronic acid composition[34] and their linkages[20] have been studied. Hovingh and Linker[13] report a disaccharide repeating unit in heparin sulfate. The development of an automated procedure for the determination of glucuronic acid free of most interferences is a major advance.[31] Likewise, electrophoretic separation of GAGs,[17, 21] should prove useful in the study of proteoglycan structure and metabolism. Whether circular dichroism[33] will become a quantitative analytical tool, or a qualitative one awaits further refinement of the procedure. It will provide valuable data on proteoglycan-protein interactions.

Although chemically similar to proteoglycans, mucin glycoproteins have shorter carbohydrate side chains, lack uronic acids, are resistant to hyaluronidase, and are somewhat more neutral than proteoglycans.[11, 37] Jones et al.[16] used a histologic procedure to quantitate the amount of pig bronchial epithelium staining for neutral or acid glycoproteins. In addition, Boat et al.[3] studied the mucous glycoprotein secretions from nasal polyp epithelium maintained in organ culture. Separation into three fractions by DEAE cellulose chromatography revealed similar amino acid compositions, but different contents of sialic acid and fucose as well as $^{35}SO_4$ incorporation relative to ^3H-glucosamine. The significance of this data is unclear. However, work continues to suggest promise for monitoring disease processes involving mucous glycoproteins.

REFERENCES

1. **Bloom, W. and Fawcett, D. W.,** Respiratory system, in *Textbook of Histology,* W. B. Saunders, Philadelphia, 1975, 743.
2. **Bornstein, P., Duksin, D., Balian, G., Davidson, J. M., and Crouch, E.,** Organization of extracellular protein on the connective tissue cell surface: relevance to cell-matrix interactions *in vitro* and *in vivo, Ann. N.Y. Acad. Sci.,* 312, 93, 1978.
3. **Boat, T. F., Kleinerman, J. I., Carlson, D. M., Maloney, W. H., and Matthews, L. W.,** Human respiratory tract secretions. I. Mucous glycoproteins secreted by cultured nasal polyp epithelium from subjects with allergic rhinitis and with cystic fibrosis, *Am. Rev. Respir. Dis.,* 110, 428, 1974.
4. **Braund, K. G., Ghosh, P., Taylor, T. K. F., and Larsen, L. H.,** The identification and quantitation of connective tissue hexosamines using a combination of gas liquid chromatographic and colorimetric procedures, *Anal. Biochem.,* 64, 10, 1975.
5. **Cifonelli, J. A. and King, J.,** Structural studies on heparins with unusually high *N*-acetylglucosamine contents, *Biochim. Biophys. Acta,* 320, 331, 1973.
6. **Comper, W. D. and Laurent, T. C.,** Physiological function of connective tissue polysaccharides, *Physiol. Rev.,* 58(1), 255, 1978.
7. **Davis, B., Marin, M. G., Olver, R. E., and Nadel, J. A.,** Active ion transport across canine tracheal epithelium: a possible control system for mucociliary transport, *Chest,* 67 (Suppl.), 57s, 1975.
8. **Dorfman, A. and Matalon, R.,** The mucopolysaccharidoses, in *The Metabolic Basis of Inherited Disease,* 3rd ed., Stanbury, J. B., Wyngaarden, J. B., and Fredricks, D. S., Eds., McGraw-Hill, New York, 1972, 1218.

9. **Francis, G. and Thomas, J.,** Isolation and characterization of acidic structural glycoproteins in pulmonary tissues, *Biochem. J.,* 145, 299, 1975.
10. **Hall, B. K.,** Correlations between the concentrations of acid mucopolysaccharide and collagen in the tibia of the embryonic chick, *Can. J. Zool.,* 51, 771, 1973.
11. **Hance, A. J. and Crystal, R. G.,** The connective tissue of lung, *Am. Rev. Respir. Dis.,* 112, 657, 1975.
12. **Horwitz, A. L., Elson, N. A., and Crystal, R. G.,** Proteoglycans and elastic fibers, in *The Biochemical Basis of Pulmonary Function,* Crystal, R. G., Ed., Marcel Dekker, New York, 1976, 273.
13. **Hovingh, P. and Linker, A.,** The disaccharide repeating-units of heparan sulfate, *Carbohydr. Res.,* 37, 181, 1974.
14. **Inoue, S.,** The determination of iduronic acid and glucuronic acid in heparins by a new technique: re-evaluation of the variable hexuronic acid composition of mammalian heparins, *Biochim. Biophys. Acta,* 329, 264, 1973.
15. **Inoue, S. and Miyawaki, M.,** Quantitative analysis of iduronic acid and glucuronic acid in sulfated galactosaminoglycuronans by gas chromatography, *Anal. Biochem.,* 65, 164, 1975.
16. **Jones, R., Baskerville, A., and Reid, L.,** Histochemical identification of glycoproteins in pig bronchial epithelium: a) normal and b) hypertrophied from enzootic pneumonia, *J. Pathol.,* 116, 1, 1975.
17. **Kawamoto, T. and Nagai, Y.,** Developmental changes in glycosaminoglycans, collagen and collagenase activity in embryonic chick skin, *Biochim. Biophys. Acta,* 437, 190, 1976.
18. **Kleinman, H. K., McGoodwin, E. B., Martin, G. R., and Klebe, R. J.,** Binding of cell attachment protein to collagen: effects of chemical modifications, *Ann. N.Y. Acad. Sci.,* 312, 436, 1978.
19. **Laurent, T. C.,** Interaction between proteins and glycosaminoglycans, *Fed. Proc.,* 36, 24, 1977.
20. **Linker, A.,** The uronidic linkages of heparitin sulfate, *Connect. Tissue Res.,* 3, 33, 1975.
21. **Linker, A. and Hovingh, P.,** The uses of degradative enzymes as tools for identification and structural analysis of glycosaminoglycans, *Fed. Proc.,* 36, 43, 1977.
22. **Lippman, M. M. and Mathews, M. B.,** Heparins: varying effects on cell proliferation *in vitro* and lack of correlation with anticoagulant activity, *Fed. Proc.,* 36, 55, 1977.
23. **Litt, M.,** Rheological aspects of mucociliary flow, *Ann. N.Y. Acad. Sci.,* 221, 212, 1974.
24. **Motomiya, M., Arai, H., Sato, H., Yokosawa, A., Nagai, H., and Konno, K.,** Increase of dermatan sulfate in a case of pulmonary fibrosis, *Tohoku J. Exp. Med.,* 115, 361, 1975.
25. **Norrby, K.,** Effect of heparin, histamine and serotonin on the density-dependent inhibition of replication in two fibroblastic cell lines, *Virchows Arch. B,* 15, 75, 1973.
26. **Pennock, C. A.,** A review and selection of simple laboratory methods used for the study of glycosaminoglycan excretion and the diagnosis of the mucopolysaccharidoses, *J. Clin. Pathol.,* 29, 111, 1976.
27. **Pickrell, J. A. and Shafer, J.,** Lung connective tissue measurements. I. Amino acid analysis procedures for determination of canine lung connective tissue, *Arch. Intern. Med.,* 127, 891, 1971.
28. **Rodén, L., Baker, J. R., Cifonelli, J. A., and Mathews, M. B.,** Isolation and characterization of connective tissue polysaccharides, in *Methods in Enzymology,* Vol. 28, Colowick, S. P., and Kaplan, N. O., Eds., Academic Press, New York, 1972, 73.
29. **Romanova, L. K. and Boikov, A. K.,** Detection of the mucopolysaccharide component of the supraplasmalemmal covering of cells lining the alveoli of the rat lung, *Bull. Exp. Biol. Med.,* 77, 198, 1974.
30. **Rosenberg, L., Margolis, R., Wolfenstein-Todel, C., Pal, S., and Strider, W.,** Organization of extracellular matrix in bovine articular cartilage, in *Extracellular Matrix Influences on Gene Expression,* Slavkin, H. C., and Greulich, R. C., Eds., Academic Press, New York, 1975, 415.
31. **Rosenthal, H. G., Bentley, J. P., and Albin, E. E.,** A sensitive automated procedure for the determination of glucuronic acid, *Connect. Tissue Res.,* 4, 155, 1976.
32. **Siegel, R. C.,** Biosynthesis of collagen cross-links: increased activity of purified lysyl oxidase with reconstituted collagen fibrils, *Proc. Natl. Acad. Sci. U.S.A.,* 71, 4826, 1974.
33. **Stone, A. L.,** Optical conformation of heparin and heparin complexes with cationic dyes, amines and protein models, *Fed. Proc.,* 36, 101, 1977.
34. **Taylor, R. L., Shively, J. E., Conrad, H. E., and Cifonelli, J. A.,** Uronic acid composition of heparins and heparan sulfates, *Biochemistry,* 12, 3633, 1973.
35. **White, A., Handler, P., and Smith, E. L.,** *Principles of Biochemistry,* 5th ed., McGraw-Hill, New York, 1973, 412.
36. **Wusteman, F. S.,** Glycosaminoglycans of bovine lung parenchyma and pleura, *Experientia,* 28(8), 887, 1972.
37. **Yeager, H.,** Tracheobronchial secretions, *Am. J. Med.,* 50, 493, 1971.
38. **Yoneda, K.,** Mucous blanket of rat bronchus. An ultrastructural study, *Am. Rev. Respir. Dis.,* 114, 837, 1976.

Chapter 5

COLLAGEN BIOSYNTHESIS

J. A. Pickrell

TABLE OF CONTENTS

I. THE BIOSYNTHETIC SYSTEM

Biosynthesis of collagen may be regarded as encompassing all events between transcription and the formation of collagen fiber (Figures 1 and 2). These events include (1) transcription of the appropriate collagen genome; (2) translation of the collagen messenger ribonucleic acid (m-RNA) and several unique post translational events; (3) hydroxylation of proline and lysine residues; (4) glycosylation of hydroxylysine residues; (5) registration of pro-alpha chains; (6) disulfide bond and triple helix formation; (7) packaging and secretory vessicle formation in the Golgi apparatus; (8) transcellular movement and secretion of collagen and cleavage of the amino terminal procollagen extension; (9) fibril formation and cleavage of C terminal procollagen extension; and (10) intramolecular and intermolecular cross-linking. An excellent review[64] of this area is highly recommended for the reader. Information relating to control of this complex biosynthetic system is sparse and often indirect.

A. Transcription of Collagen Genome

Although little is known about transcription of collagen DNA, Miller and Matukas[124] and Prockop et al.[160] reviewed the collagen types elucidated at that time and speculated concerning the possibility of separate genomes for each collagen type. Fessler and Fessler[64] reviewed considerable evidence suggestive that different genes carried information for different collagens. The most convincing evidence cited in that review was the finding by Raj et al.[162] that genes for human type I and III collagens were on different chromosomes. They segregated independently in human-mouse somatic cell hybrids. Both Prockop et al.[160] and Miller and Matukas[124] indicated the lack of delineation of total potential for collagen synthesis in a tissue, but commented upon the diverse types of tissues having apparently similar collagens, comprised almost entirely of alpha-1 chains. These four types of collagen have been reviewed[41, 80, 124] and discussed in this paper. Likewise recently reported data indicate another type of collagen[2] and indicate that several potential collagen types may be produced by chondrocyte culture. Crystal[41] has pointed to the similarity of lung collagen and other vertebrate collagens. His laboratory[22, 23, 41] has demonstrated polymorphism in lung collagen. This line of evidence suggests that synthesis of collagen types is under genome control. The data are consistent with the suggestion of Miller and Matukas[124] and the preliminary evidence of Raj et al.[162] that the genome for type I collagen may be distinct from that of type III and other collagens.

The controls of collagen transcription are as yet poorly understood, but may be related to amount and type of membrane bound procollagen. Probes of c-DNA to collagen message may help in analyzing problems of the occurrence and transcriptional control of a family of collagen genes.[64] Type III collagen relative to type I changes from fetal to adult in skin and in vessels. This data must be considered with those reviewed by Gefter[69a] who suggested that DNA transcription might be modulated by the cell membrane. Whether this can be the same mechanism as that reviewed by Revel and Groner,[165] where a cell membrane interaction increased cell porosity and led to preferential translation of m-RNA optimum to the new salt concentration, remains to be elucidated. Kao et al.[93] noted that procollagen added to tendon fibroblast cultures increases the portion of membrane bound ribosomes and the production of procollagen. This finding is consistent with both Gefter's hypothesis and with Kao's speculation concerning the possible role of membrane-bound procollagen in modulating collagen biosynthesis within the cell. Thus, specific collagen biosynthesis may be modulated at the cellular or genome level. The biological significance of the recent report of Miller et al.[122] indicating pepsin digested type III collagen helices to be sen-

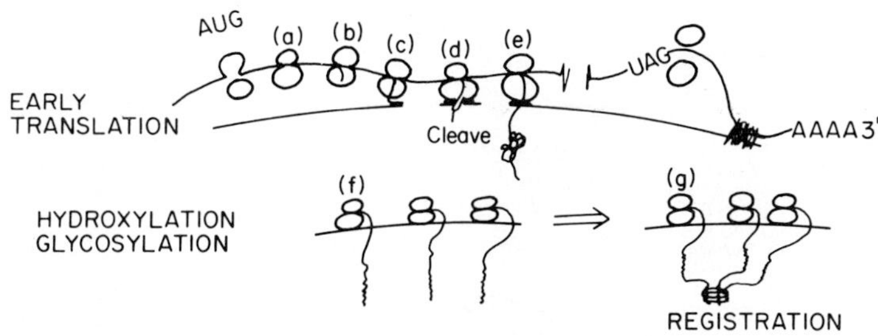

FIGURE 1. Early intracellular events of collagen synthesis include attachment of m-RNA-bound polysmal complexes to the endoplasmic reticulum. The newly synthesized chain is vectorially secreted into the cisternae of the rough endoplasmic reticulum while undergoing hydroxylation of proline and lysine, glycosylation of hydroxylysine, and registration in rapid but as yet incompletely defined succession.

sitive to trypsin was not discussed. Klein and Chandrarajan[98] report them to have similar in vivo turnover, raising doubt as to influence in cross-linked collagen. However, type III procollagen may be the molecule which is more sensitive in vivo. Since procollagen quantity influences rate of procollagen production, type I procollagen, which may be less sensitive, may cause increased production of type I collagen. Heparin is largely on the surface of cells,[40a] and it (as a polyanion) competes with fibronectin for the binding of collagen or procollagen.[99] Speculatively, this could provide the mechanism whereby procollagen attaches to the cell and thereby modulates collagen synthesis. Since it presumably requires intact procollagen, this could be the mechanism for the relative increase of type I collagen noted by Seyer et al.,[176] that is, the cleavage of type III procollagen by proteolysis noted by Miller et al.[121] This might be viewed as a competition phenomenon between fibronectin and heparin with the proportions playing a role in the transcription rate of each collagen type. This theory is supported qualitatively with the observation[80, 86] that increased pulmonary heparin is present near birth, the precise time collagen synthesis is highest relative to other proteins. It is later at ≃6 months that dermatan sulfate is increased.[86] Such conjecture must be substantiated by further experimentation, but this area is beginning to yield useful data concerning transcriptional mechanisms and modulations of collagen biosynthesis.

B. Translation of the Collagen Messenger Ribonucleic Acid (m-RNA)

Proteins destined for cellular export are thought to be translated on ribosomes bound to the rough endoplasmic reticulum[195] by attachment of the nascent chain to a specific site on the membrane. A small peptide whose length approximates membrane width (12 to 15 amino acids) is cleaved[32] and the nascent chain transported vectorially through the membrane and released.[15, 102, 172] WI38 cells, diploid fibroblasts, are known to secrete large amounts of collagen. They also secrete large amounts of noncollagenous proteins.[152a] Diegelman et al.[48] and Pritchard et al.[158] have presented evidence suggesting this mechanism to be logical for collagen biosynthesis, since 70 to 90% of the fibroblast or osteoblast activity toward collagen synthesis is localized on membrane-bound rather than free polysomes.

Message translation and protein synthesis begin before ribosomal attachment to a specific site of RER (Figure 2)[102, 172]. Their sequence make chain alignment possible very early in the synthesis of collagen. Two things are important to this initiation in other protein systems. First is the 5-terminal methylation of m-RNA,[177] which facilitates efficient binding of mixed m-RNA to the ribosome. Lande et al.[102] report evidence suggesting that the m-RNA is attached to the ER near its 3′ end. Second is the

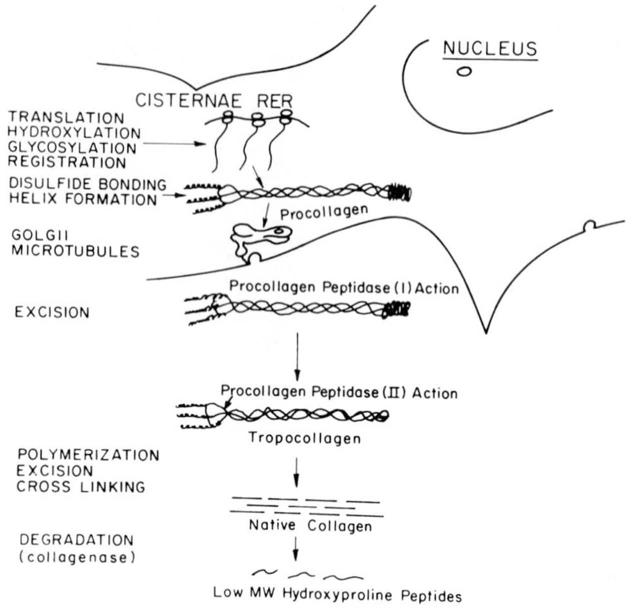

FIGURE 2. Collagen biosynthesis (type I) includes translation, hydroxylation, glycosylation, and registration as described in Figure 1. Disulfide bonding and helix formation are thought to follow. Triple helical collagen is secreted, involving golgii and microtubules, undergoes limited excision, is cross-linked into fibrils and fibers, and may undergo degradation.

prevention of inhibition of the initiation complex by some substance such as hemin.[111] The amino terminal sequence may contain a peptide with information sufficient for advantageous attachment or just attachment to the RER. At least preproinsulin contains a peptide of 23 amino acids which is cleaved prior to secretion into the cisternae of the RER.[32] Possibly this cleavage is what commits the protein to be secreted, although further work will more completely define this concept. Other proteins such as myeloma light chain precursor, pretrypsinogen, prealbumin, and preproparathormone may also be in this category.[32, 160] An early function of the amino terminal extension of each pro-alpha chain may be to attach in a location appropriate to the interaction of two companion pro-alpha chains. Alternatively, this extension may merely facilitate membrane attachment. In either event, chain registration alignment of the three collagen chains may be accomplished or facilitated very soon after the nascent chains penetrate the ER.

Collagen chain messenger RNAs are probably translated as three separate monocistronic RNAs. Analysis of the data of Vuust and Piez[195a, 195b] and more recently of Fessler et al.[63] indicates that the m-RNA of alpha-1 and alpha-2 are probably translated simultaneously, although translation via a series of permuted polycistronic messages is not excluded. These chains are most likely assembled by sequential addition of individual amino acids and not as shorter chains to be assembled later.[124] Lazarides and Lukens[105] report identification of polysomes synthesizing alpha-1 and alpha-2 chains by means of an in vitro system for completion and release of nascent polypeptides. Their experiments indicated collagen polysomes to be larger than a 23 S ribosome but smaller than a 50 to 60 S ribosome aggregate. This size was in good agreement with that calculated for a monocistronic m-RNA molecule coding for a single alpha chain, but too small to be consistent with coding for a di- or polycistronic message. Boedtker et al.[18] estimate the non-ribosomal rapidly labelled RNA to migrate in the 28 to 30 S region and thus have a molecular weight of at least 1,600,000. A prominently labelled peak of such radioactivity migrated with an apparent molecular weight of 1,800,000. Other systems[13] have yielded similar results. This compound had the ability to program the synthesis of collagenase-sensitive protein in reticulocyte lysates.

Partially purified collagen polysomes may help characterize translation of m-RNA to collagen. Message size awaits isolation of complete procollagen or m-RNA. Pawlowski et al.[147] succeeded in partially purifying collagen polysomes by specifically sedimenting them after treatment with anti-collagen antibodies followed by goat anti-rabbit antibodies. Moreover, the amount of ^{125}I anticollagen antibodies bound to a mixture of polysomes correlated to the amount of collagen being synthesized in a particular tissue. Assuming specificity of the collagen antibodies, the application of this system to measure quantity of collagen m-RNA translation is obvious. It would also lend specificity for synthesized collagen in the Sabatini et al.[172] system as well as providing advantages over the determination of membrane-bound vs. free polysomes performed by Kao et al.[93] Pritchard et al.[158] reported in vitro synthesis of collagen polypeptides on rat skin polysomes using reticulocyte definitive initiation factors. Similarly, cell free collagen synthesis has been performed in lung,[39, 40, 81] although definitive estimates of polysome size have not yet been made. The characterization of either pro-alpha-one or its respective m-RNA is an interesting question. This question must be answered prior to the determination of whether the pro-alpha-1 m-RNA will translate a protein larger than the current translated sequence of pro-alpha-one. Slow progress in this area may be due to the extremely long message, the high content of guanosine and cytosine of the RNA, and the possibility that the m-RNA may fold upon itself. These factors contribute to artifactual degradation, and to a difficulty in separation from an m-RNA of a similar size. Further definition of this area will enable one to study different perturbations of the collagen synthesizing machinery.

Procollagen lies between two extension peptides and is translated amino to carboxyterminal at ≃200 residues per minute for the helical portion. Vuust and Piez[195a, 195b] indicate the rate of translation of type I collagen in bone to approximate 200 amino acid residues (approximately 600 nucleic acid residues) per minute, requiring 6.0 min to synthesize a chain of what was probably P_N- collagen, procollagen in which the c terminal nonhelical extension is not present (Figure 3). They indicate that insufficient time existed for synthesis of the COOH piece. However, Fessler et al.,[63] using bone type I collagen, suggest that the assumption of a faster translating rate (similar to that of globin) for the non-helical portion of procollagen related to its lower imino acid content. This renders their data on bone type I collagen compatible with Vuust and Piez[195a, 195b] and with Miller et al.[125] for cartilage (type II collagen). Fessler et al.[63] data indicate procollagen to be translated from amino to carboxy terminal as a collagen chain lying between two extension peptides. The translating rate of pulmonary collagen m-RNAs has not as yet been elucidated. However, since the main product of pulmonary polysome translation is type I collagen,[81] one can expect the translating rates to approximate those determined previously for type I and II collagen from bone and cartilage.

Control of collagen synthetic rate may reside at the translational level. Adams et al.[1] have shown that in transformed fibroblasts, m-RNAs for collagen and fibronectin are reduced dramatically. This presumably reflects the lack of extracellular matrix being produced in neoplasia and reflects the ability of the cell to interact with its matrix in a way most suited to its own ends. Carpousis et al.[30] have shown a preferential usage of one t-RNA isoaccepting species cognate to GGU and GGC in collagen synthesis with polysomes. There is an absence of such selectivity in noncollagen protein synthe-

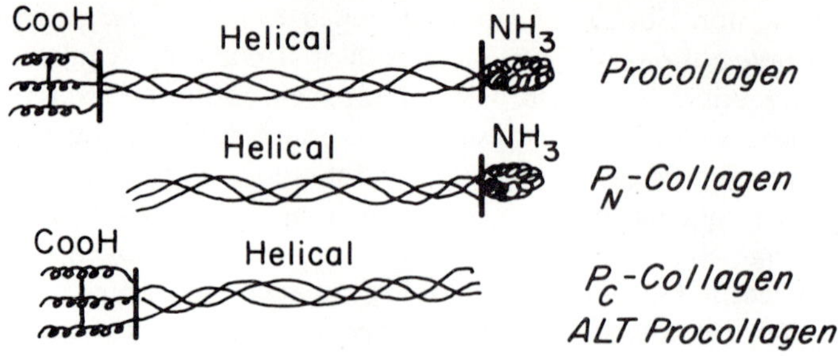

FIGURE 3. Procollagen contains an amino and a carboxy terminal extension which probably comprise between them at least 50,000 daltons. P_N collagen undergoes cleavage of the C terminal extension and has only an amino terminal extension (∿15,000 daltons), while P_C collagen (ALT procollagen) has undergone N terminal cleavage and has only the C terminal extension (∿35,000 daltons) in addition to tropocollagen (∿100,000 daltons). In type I procollagen in vivo cleavage of extensions occur by two separate peptideases[44, 64, 192a] which do not attack the tropocollagen molecule.

sis. Fessler and Fessler[64] review evidence which indicates no clear-cut control of collagen synthesis can be affected by availability of t-RNAs prevalent in collagen. Christner and Rosenbloom[35] suggest that simple usage of more glycine does not produce an increase in glycyl t-RNA. Silk gland synthesis of fibroin produced an increase in t-RNA similar to that of collagen, except that the codon response for the t-RNA species differed.[30] This coincides with the work of Zilberstein (cited in Carpousis et al.[30]) who showed that a minor isoaccepting species of t-PNA could determine the translation rate (reviewed by Lodish[110]). Potential control points at initiation factor, phosphorylation, m-PNA maturation, and the sensitivity of the translating ribosomal complex to ionic strength should be considered.[165] However, these have not been specifically related to collagen synthesis. The role assigned to the finding that cyclic AMP can modulate collagen synthesis in vitro in normal fibroblasts[8] has yet to be defined. However, Revel and Groner[165] indicate that cyclic AMP inhibits the inhibition of protein synthesis by phosphorylation of eIf_2. This could be production of non-collagen protein at the expense of collagen. R. Crystal[40b] indicates the cyclic AMP response to be tied to a β-adrenergic response of lung cells in an as yet undefined manner. More work in this area should yield valuable information. Finally, the role of procollagen in modulating the level of collagen synthesis need not act at a transcriptional level. However, if it controls collagen types, it is difficult to see how this specificity could be built into translational control. Further work in this area should prove very enlightening. The possibility that collagen has both transcriptional and translational controls should be considered.

C. Hydroxylation

1. Proline

Certain prolyl residues in nascent peptides are enzymatically hydroxylated until the triple helix forms. Prolyl residues preceeding glycine in the sequence of nascent pro-alpha chains are the natural substrate for hydroxylation by an enzyme (prolyl hydroxylase) located on the non-translating side of the membrane-bound protein translation aggregate.[29,20,47,71,73,74,105,124,127,142,143] Most hydroxylation occurs on nascent collagen peptides; however, such hydroxylation may occur on collagen chains at any stage of synthesis which are in the random coil but not in the triple helical configuration.[11,135,144] This may be why rat alpha-1 CB2 cyanogen bromide peptide is always hydroxylated less than the theoretical maximum, but to different degrees in skin and tendon.[19,29,68,167] Rapaka et al.[164] suggest that conformational state may determine the extent of hydroxylation of proline and that such hydroxylation occurs within a critical range of conformations. Moreover, the degree of hydroxylation varies greatly between collagen types,[80,124] although each exists as a triple helix.

Although hydroxyproline stabilizes the collagen helix, enzymatic hydroxylation rates may not reflect collagen synthetic rates. The collagen triple helix is stabilized by hydroxyproline.[12,20,29,43,77,89] Trypsin (>10 ng/mℓ) reduces in vitro prolyl hydroxylase activity proportionally.[161] Prolyl hydroxylase activity need not correlate with the rate of collagen synthesis,[93a] suggesting that prolyl hydroxylase may not be limiting in these cases. In contrast, Halme et al.[78] noted substantially increased pulmonary prolyl hydroxylase concentrations before histologic evidence of damage in the lungs of silicotic rats. Prolyl hydroxylase is abundant in lung.[41a] Type I collagen in lung is hydroxylated similarly to that of other tissues.[22,23]

Although several different assays for prolyl hydroxylase have been tried, as reviewed by Cardinale and Udenfriend,[29] the tritium release assay[87] is the most sensitive and can be utilized with the least pure enzyme fractions. Subsequent modifications[10,187] have reduced the amount of substrate and enzyme necessary while still being useful upon crude enzyme preparations. The enzyme is dependent upon cofactors Fe^{++}, atmospheric O_2, alpha-ketoglutarate, and ascorbate.[87, 148, 159, 167] Myllylä et al.[137] indicate that prolylhydroxylase can catalyze hydroxylation of proline for 5 to 10 sec ($\simeq$15 to 30 reaction cycles). However, after this, the rate becomes very low, probably due to oxidation of enzyme bound iron. Ascorbate is then required as a specific reductant to reactivate the enzyme. Cardinale and Udenfriend[29] reviewed possible mechanisms of prolyl hydroxylation, superoxide formation,[109] or the Hamilton[79] mechanism of formation of peroxysuccinic acid with subsequent oxenoid attack on peptidyl proline, but were unable to reach a conclusion on which mechanism was most likely. Concanavilin A binds to purified prolyl hydroxylase and partially inhibits its enzymic activity.[74]

Prolyl hydroxylase is an active dimer or tetramer which has an inactive monomeric precursor. Tudermann et al.[192] and Berg and Prockop[11] purified prolyl hydroxylase to near homogeneity by affinity chromatography. The chick embryo enzyme is estimated to have a molecular weight of 248,000 or 230,000 with two dissimilar subunits of 60,000 and 64,000, suggesting a tetrameric conformation.[11,146,160] Chen-kiang and Udenfriend[33] isolated and characterized a protein which cross-reacts with antiprolyl hydroxylase, but has no enzyme activity. This is called an inactive cross-reacting protein (CRP). It has a molecular weight of 65,000 and may thus be a subunit of the active enzyme. By contrast, the rat enzyme had a molecular weight of 130,000 with subunits of 65,000.[166] The consistently higher molecular weight (250,000 to 300,000) of prolyl hydroxylase determined by molecular sieve chromatography[78] may reflect a high frictional ratio of the native enzyme.[146]

Antibodies against prolyl hydroxylase demonstrated that large amounts of CRP are present as precursors to prolyl hydroxylase. Using purified enzyme preparations,[12, 117, 118] antibodies were prepared against prolyl hydroxylase to study the enzyme's activation.[81a] Using the general method of measuring enzyme precursors,[118, 187] prolyl hydroxylase and a cross-reacting protein were measured in several mammalian tissues. Chichester et al.[34] demonstrated that part of the cross-reacting protein was a precursor to prolyl hydroxylase. Prolyl hydroxylase tended to decrease with increasing age reflecting decreasing growth. However, the proportion which prolyl hydroxylase constituted of total cross-reacting protein in skin, lung, kidney, heart, and liver remained consistent during this period. This proportion differed from a high of 15 to 19% in heart to a low of 2 to 4% in liver. Lung was intermediate with 6 to 9%.

Each tissue indicates considerable ability to increase prolyl hydroxylation without increasing total prolyl hydroxylase.[187] This mechanism would differ biochemically from the case of cellular activation reported by Kao et al.[93] where the addition of procollagen to culture medium increased the proportion of bound ribosomes and the collagen synthetic rate. Either mechanism would be unimportant in cases of fibroblast proliferation or changes in the number of collagen producing cells. A four- to fivefold increase of active and a modest increase of total prolyl hydroxylase in atherosclerotic aortae suggested a cellular activation.[65, 67] In contrast, Kao et al.[93a] reported that ascorbate can increase hydroxyproline synthesis in fibroblasts without activation of prolyl hydroxylase. They suggest a cofactor effect. Kuttan et al.[101] indicated that an enzyme activation which requires all the cofactors is unusual and indicated a common mechanism. Cardinale[29a] has proposed the release of prolyl hydroxylase bound to pro alpha chains which would be activated in the presence of additional ascorbate to explain Kuttan's and Kao's data. Intense study of this area has revealed considerable knowledge about an enzymatic conversion which, although not rate-limiting, is necessary to the formation of stable triple helical collagen. Theoretically, underhydroxylated collagen would be less stable, although such collagen has not been reported in vivo. Presumably, the body either rapidly degrades such collagen because it provides inadequate support, or does not produce it.

2. Lysine

Lysine hydroxylation reviewed by several groups[20,29,80,81,124,195] seems to have similar cofactor requirements and be similar in many ways to proline hydroxylation. Lysine residues preceding glycine in the sequence of nascent pro alpha chains are the natural substrate for hydroxylation by an enzyme located on the non-translating side of the membrane-bound protein translation aggregate.[73, 74] An enzyme separated from prolyl hydroxylase on DEAE cellulose or DEAE sephadex has been designated lysyl hydroxylase.[96, 126, 157] Ryhänen and Kivirikko[171] found enzyme concentration in the chick lung to be lower than that of skin and bone but to approximate that of heart and kidney. Type I and III collagens are known to have less hydroxylation of lysine than types II and IV, although lung collagens[22, 23, 120, 176] have more hydroxylysine than most other tissue collagens. The hydroxylation of lysine can change either in a single type of collagen but in different tissues or as a function of increasing age.[123] Perhaps this is consistent with the inhibition of lysyl hydroxylase by triple helical collagen.[97, 144]

Lysine hydroxylation is important in the formation of cross-links, and in the subsequent glycosylation of hydroxylysine residues. Both lysyl and hydroxylysyl residues are involved in cross-linking of collagen. The nature and stability of the cross-link depends upon lysine hydroxylation. Hydroxylysyl residues are important sites at which carbohydrates are attached, although the function of glycosylation is not determined. The exact function(s) of hydroxylysine remains to be defined. Trypsin in cultured trypsinized cells inhibits lysyl hydroxylase more severely than prolyl hydroxylase.[161]

D. Glycosylation of Hydroxylysine Residues

Certain residues of hydroxylysine undergo glycosylation by two enzymes. The first enzyme, UDP galactosyl transferase, adds galactose, while UDP glucosyl transferase may in some cases add glucose to the galactosylated hydroxylysine.[68,80,81,185] Hydroxylysine-linked galactose and galactosyl glucose have recently been identified on nascent peptide collagen chains,[25] although subsequent glycosylation is not ruled out. The fact that both enzymes can act on triple helical collagen implies activity at several sites.[81] Indeed, additional carbohydrates, including mannose, are added in Golgi apparatus.

High but equitalent amounts of each enzyme were identified in rat lung microsomes.[185] The activity of each enzyme decreased with increasing age, reflecting lowered pulmonary collagen synthetic rates.[80,81]

Although the function of glycosylation has not been elucidated, one must consider the possibility of involvement in either platelet aggregation[91] or in indirectly regulating collagen cross-link formation.[5, 56] The glycosylation may identify collagen as a protein destined for secretion; however, inhibition of prolyl and lysyl hydroxylation and glycosylation fail to abolish procollagen secretion.[163] Spiro[184] suggested the role of glycosylation in fibril formation, since a high degree of glycosylation was associated with a more amorphous structure. Certainly both type II and IV collagen are synthesized more slowly, possibly relating to their higher carbohydrate content.[81, 122]

E. Registration of Pro Alpha Chains

Since Speakman's[183] proposal of the necessity of non-helical extensions, it has become increasingly obvious that aligning the nascent peptides to initiate helix formation (registration) would greatly speed and make easier the formation of triple helical procollagen. Since the discovery of procollagen,[9] a logical candidate for this role has always seemed to be the amino terminal extension, because it is synthesized first and would most logically be in a position to align the three nascent collagen peptides. Fessler and Fessler[64] review evidence that suggests that normal selection (registration) proceeds through the amino propeptides. However, when this is prevented, the carboxyl propeptides can do the job. Veis and Brownell[195] when reviewing collagen biosynthesis speculated that the three chains might be initiated upon free ribosomes which subsequently attached in such a manner that the peptides upon entering the cisternae of the RER might become registered. Gross's[75] observation that triple helical collagen is not synthesized in a cell free system suggests that both the membrane and the amino terminal extension may play a role in registration, agreeing with the concept of Sabatini et al.[172] Hance and Crystal's[81] data concerning cell free synthesis of collagen by lung polysomes would seem to agree with this concept, since they observe some but less translation of collagen message by free ribosomes than by bound ribosomes. Likewise, their observation of rapid intracellular breakdown of new collagen chains suggests that mismatched chains may be destroyed.[14]

Registration probably does not affect formation of the triple helix; its subcellular location is not known. If registration occurs at this early time period, concomitant with prolyl and lysyl hydroxylation and glycosylation, then one must examine the direct effect of membrane-bound ribosomes upon the formation of the collagen triple helix in nascent growing chains. Recent evidence of Brownell and Veis,[26] indicating that membrane-bound polysomes do not inhibit helix formation, is enlightening and agrees with Gross's[75] observation concerning cell free collagen synthesis. Likewise, the kinetics of Fessler et al.[63] suggesting that the amino terminal extension undergoes intracellular or early extracellular excision supports the concept that it is primarily used for registration. Indeed, its retention has grave consequences in fibril formation in dermatosporactic collagen.[20, 21] The amino terminal extensions do not seem to form disulfide linkages between the three respective chains, although some evidence suggests their scission in tandem.[44] The subcellular location of registration which must precede helix formation is the subject of much speculation and future research. Whether the reason for delayed helix formation of type II and IV collagen[81] lies in slower registration or elsewhere remains to be investigated. Likewise the potential for the amino terminal extension of procollagen to have a regulatory function in collagen biosynthesis must be investigated.

F. Disulfide Bonds and Triple Helix

1. Formation of Disulfide Bonds and a Triple Helix

Disulfide bonds stabilize the procollagen helix, necessary for optimal collagen secretion. Efficient secretion of procollagen (possibly P_c collagen; collagen lacking the amino terminl but containing the carboxyterminal non-helical extension; Figure 3) requires that it be in a triple helical form.[89] Jimenez and Yankowski[90] reported that underhydroxylated procollagen was secreted at the same rate at 24;gC as hydroxylated procollagen; both were triple helical. At 37°C hydroxylated triple helical procollagen was secreted much more rapidly than underhydroxylated procollagen in a non-helical formation. Procollagen containing azetidine-2-carboxylic acid (hydroxylated but abnormal configuration) was secreted more slowly than hydroxylated collagen at 37;gC or underhydroxylated collagen at 24°C. The results indicate that the hydroxyproline content of the molecules does not determine their rate of secretion. Proper molecular conformation is essential for optimal secretion.[90] Largely non-helical collagen may be secreted at much lower rates; however, the possibility that this portion may be in a triple helical form exists.[163] Darnell and Rosenbloom[43] used ultracentrifugation to probe conformation of under-hydroxylated procollagen and collagen. They found them to be triple helical below the denaturation temperature. Thus, previous experiments had measured denaturation of true triple helices. Formation of stable triple helical collagen requires hydroxylation of proline.[89, 135] Fessler[57] reviews self-assembly of collagen chains, postulating that disulfide bonds in the carboxyterminal extension determine or improve the correct mutual alignment between chains. This association of the extension peptides proceeds similarly when hydroxylation is inhibited, but this collagen is denatured at body temperature.[62] Moreover, the disulfide bonds are stable to chymotrypsin digestion.[197] As the trimers had stoichiometric composition, [pro α_1, (I)]$_2$ pro α_2, the extension peptides must have the ability to associate this way independently of the helical portion of the collagen molecule.[57]

The subcellular site of formation of the collagen helix and disulfide bonds is not completely determined, although it probably is in or near the cisternae of the RER.[160] Weinstock and Leblond[196] indicate that it passes through the RER cisternae and Golgi. Harwood et al.[82] suggested that most helices are formed prior to entering the Golgi apparatus. Triple helical formation seems delayed in type IV and II collagen.[81, 197] Whether this represents a slowing due to glycosylation or a different mechanism of helix formation is not determined. Schofield and Prockop[175] and Harwood et al.[82] suggest that nascent chains do not form triple helices. However, Brownell and Veis[26] have recently indicated that membrane-bound polysomes do not inhibit the formation of a triple helix. Williams et al.[197] indicate that disulfide bonding is complete enough to resist chymotrypsin at 4 hr but not at 2 hr and that digestion by chymotrypsin can be used as a tool to establish completion of disulfide bonding. The site of helix formation remains somewhat uncertain, but most investigations suggest that disulfide bond formation occurs as a concerted process with helix formation under normal circumstances. Moreover, Lukens[112] suggests that single released pro α-chains are the precursors of disulfide-linked pro α-chains.

The possibility that each event from transcription to helix formation may occur as a concerted series of events, differing minutely for each portion of each molecule, must be considered. Although many possibilities are not inconsistent with existing data, the description of these complex phenomena increases each year. In this series of events are several likely points of either primary or secondary control of collagen synthesis.

2. Procollagen

Procollagen, a precursor to tropocollagen, contains amino and carboxy terminal non-helical extensions from the collagen helix. A precursor with a higher molecular weight than tropocollagen was noted as a possibility by Bellamy and Bornstein.[9] These precursors were separable from alpha chains on CM cellulose chromatography, acrylamide gel electrophoresis, and subsequently by DEAE cellulose chromatography and sedimentation equilibrium centrifugation[37, 37a, 114, 133, 134, 182, 194] indicating differing sizes and charges. Although early studies suggested that procollagen contained only an aminoterminal extension,[20] which lacked disulfide bonds,[28] more systematic studies were consistent with a substantial fraction of the protein containing interchain disulfide bonds.[27, 70, 182] Fessler et al.[60] suggest that interchain disulfide bonds are formed only after the entire procollagen molecule is formed and may assure alignment and stabilize the precursor. When vertebrate collagenase cleaves either procollagen or P_N-collagen, the amino fragments (Figure 3) are not disulfide linked.[64] Sherr et al.,[178] utilizing bacterial collagenase, isolated a collagenase-resistant fragment with disulfide bonds, agreeing closely with Fessler et al.[63] Combining Sherr's[178] findings with earlier ones[132] suggests the presence of both an amino and a carboxy terminal extension.[21, 114] These were subsequently demonstrated by Lichtenstein et al.[108] Hoffman et al.[84] have isolated a COOH terminal fragment and find such fragments different in α_1 and α_2 chains as indicated by tryptic peptides.

Cysteine is incorporated into both non-helical extensions; and procollagen synthesis is amino to carboxy terminal, producing a molecule with increased thermal stability. The kinetics of disulfide incorporation observed by Morris et al.[134] suggested that two such extensions, both containing cysteine, existed but that most such incorporation occurred at the early time and was likely to be carboxy terminal. Merry et al.[121] noted cysteine in the non-helical extensions of type I collagen. In a subsequent paper, Fessler et al.[63] found the center of mass of cysteine incorporation of the carboxy terminal extension to precede that of the aminoterminal one, clearly indicating the collagen helix to lie between two extension peptides. Byers et al.[28] have shown interchain disulfide bonds to be exclusively in the carboxy terminal portion of procollagen. Moreover, this suggests that procollagen is synthesized as a single chain from amino to carboxy terminal with a molecular weight of approximately 150,000. Type III procollagen has disulfide bonds at both extensions.[61a] Kao et al.[93] have recently indicated the ascorbate-mediated increase of procollagen synthesis to be a secondary effect of the accumulation of stable triple helical procollagen, perhaps by binding to the memrane of the cell synthesizing the procollagen. Fessler and Fessler[62] indicate that procollagen has a higher T_m ($\simeq$42°C) than does type I collagen. Although this disagreed with the findings of Byers et al.,[28] the possibility that they had a considerable quantity of alpha chains in their procollagen type III is indicated.

The function of procollagen is still being defined, but Bornstein[20] proposed (1) initiation of triple helix formation, (2) inhibition of intracellular fibrogenesis, (3) facilitation of transmembrane movement of collagen, and (4) a role in extracellular fibrogenesis. Regarding initiation of triple helix formation, Veis et al.[194] reported that "heavy" alpha chains accomplished stable "in-register" renaturation more rapidly than native collagen, indicating a role for the aminoterminal portion of procollagen similar to that proposed by Speakman.[183] These results are confirmed by Fujii et al.[66] Bornstein[21] expresses caution at accepting this since acid-extracted procollagen has no greater rate of renaturation than collgen. However, acid-extracted collagen was probably P_N-collagen, not procollagen (Figure 3). Veis et al.[194] did not define their procollagen molecule, and there is a possibility that it was somewhat different from Bornstein's, now characterized as lacking the COOH terminal extension peptide (P_N-collagen). The markedly enhanced renaturation rate of disulfide bonded procollagen compared to collagen[194] suggests that the carboxy terminal extension peptide may play an important role in extracellular fibrogenesis.[63] Moreover, their finding that ALT procollagen (P_c-collagen; Figure 3) has a long life suggests that this molecule may be important in controlling the rate of procollagen biosynthesis and collagen fibrogenesis. A crucial question is whether P_c-collagen is also a long-lived intermediate and serves such a function in lung.

Little is known concerning procollagen's prevention of intracellular fibrogenesis. If P_c-collagen is ideal for "in-register" fibrogenesis, the intact procollagen molecule should logically be necessary to prevent it. In light of Fessler et al.'s[59] observation that intact procollagen forms fine fibrils, the inhibition of fibrogenesis may be incomplete. Dermatosporaxis in cattle is the result of preventing both intracellular and extracellular fibrogenesis, by retention of the amino terminal but not the carboxy terminal extension.[44] This suggests that the amino terminal extension peptides may be an important factor in the lack of fibrogenesis. Following this reasoning to its logical conclusion would place the amino terminal cleavage of procollagen to ALT procollagen (P_c-collagen) near the time of collagen secretion, either shortly preceding or following it. The kinetic data of Fessler et al.[63] suggests that the time of cleavage (formation of ALT procollagen-P_c-collagen) may precede the time of secretion, although further definitive data relative to this process will be necessary to resolve the site of conversion. Evidence reviewed by Bornstein[20] supports an extracellular cleavage, but does little to resolve the site of both conversions.

Tissues having specific procollagens may respond differently. For instance, in the extreme case of basement membrane collagen, it may escape complete conversion,[20] as indicated by the lack of conversion of procollagen to collagen in parietal yolk sac endoderm.[128] A similar possibility is proposed by Gay et al.[69] for type III procollagen. The possibility that this adaptation is useful in either forming the membrane or maintaining it is an intriguing one to which future attention will be devoted. Procollagen (or possibly its derivative) may not only function as an extracellular structural element, but may be required. Little is known concerning facilitation of the transcellular movement by either non-helical extension of procollagen.

G. Packaging and Secretory Vesicle Formation in the Golgi Apparatus

The role of the Golgi apparatus in collagen secretion is not currently elucidated. Early work concerning the involvement of the Golgi apparatus in collagen secretion was inconclusive.[20, 195] However, Golgi involvement was demonstrated in two tissues secreting mostly collagen, that is, corneal epithelium[83] and odontoblasts,[196] as well as in osteoblasts using ferritin-labelled antibodies.[141] Trelstad[190] noted a change in position of the Golgi apparatus from apical to basilar during laying down of corneal stroma. He further noted[191] that secretory vesicles were formed prior to secretion of aggregated collagen contained within them.

Further sugars are added to procollagen for an undefined reason; they are not retained in deposited collagen. Bornstein[21a] indicated that incorporation of mannose and fucose into collagen in the Golgi was evidence of further processing of the collagen molecule at that point. The presence of these sugars in the glycoprotein but not the collagen component of basement membrane raises a question as to how the collagen is processed and what the function of such processing might be. Whether these carbohydrates are retained and serve the role in structural collagen function that they seem to in basement membranes remains to be demonstrated. The suggestion by Schramm et al. (reviewed by Massaro and Massaro[115]) that secretory vesicles of other proteins may form pseudopodia to aid in the protein secretion is an exciting one which raises a question concerning the operation and possibly the control of a similar process in pulmonary cells synthesizing collagen.

H. Transcellular Movement and Secretion of Collagen and Intracellular Cleavage of the Amino Terminal Procollagen Extension

The newly formed vesicles of collagen must undergo transcellular movement to an appropriate spot for secretion into the surrounding interstitium. Microtubules are involved in transcellular movement or secretion of collagen,[51, 52] although the mechanism is not defined. Colchicine inhibits procollagen secretion and its conversion to collagen. Cells exposed to colchine had dilated Golgi-associated vacuoles and vesicles which contained parallel filamentous aggregates resembling procollagen. Colchine was used at a level which did not affect RER morphology and did not reduce non-collagen protein synthesis. However, collagenous protein synthesis was reduced.[52] Earlier work[51] had indicated colchicine to have a dose-dependent reduction of collagen conversion at a concentration as low as 10^{-6} *M* while non-collagen protein synthesis was unaffected at 10^{-4} M. Olmsted and Borisy[142] reviewed microtubules and indicate that colchicine binds their subunits, disrupting normal microtubular assembly. This binding is often enhanced by GTP, because GTP prevented denaturation (indicated by shifted circular dichroism spectra) of the microtubules in the presence of colchicine. Once formed, the colchicine-microtubule subunit complex seemed reasonably stable, indicating that microtubules are unavailable for their function in secreting collagen. However, Stephens and Edds[188] caution that colchicine has pleiotropic action and that an alternate possibility is that colchicine's effect on microtubules causes an effect upon microfilaments or upon their ability to develop motive force, reducing collagen secretion.

A microtubular organizing center (MTOC) would facilitate this organelle's role in collagen secretion. Olmsted and Borisy[142] indicate existence of such in specialized cells, but that evidence for this center in most cells is conjectural. Osborn and Weber[145a] reported the existence of a MTOC to organize cytoplasmic microtubules in 3T3 fibroblasts which existed as a focal point from which microtubules appeared to radiate. Exposure of cells to microtubule disruptive drugs or low temperatures failed to destroy this MTOC. As cells recovered from such treatment, each MTOC acted as a nucleating center. Microtubules grew toward the plasma membrane, assembling in vivo in an ordered undirectional manner. This avoids assembling unoriented or unwanted microtubules, suggesting regulation in vito. These principles are clearly in agreement with collagen transcellular movement involving microtubules. Microtubules may act as either an active or passive transport conduit along which secretory vesicles move from their point of formation in the Golgi apparatus to their termination in fusion with the plasma membrane.[195]

The exact mechanism by which colchicine inhibits collagen secretion remains undefined. Whether this represents a primary inhibition of microtubules or some other mechanism, the microtubules seem to be involved. If the microfilaments are also involved, their role is not a clear one. Logically, both may be involved and future research will be required to determine not only their respective roles, but also their interrelationships in the transcellular movement of collagen.

Early work of Ehrlich and Bornstein[51] indicated that an energy requirement was present when procollagen was secreted. Inhibition of oxidative phosphorylation reduced conversion of procollagen to collagen. Since the secretory pathway for procollagen involves the Golgi complex,[141,196] associated membrane fission and fusion should be energy-requiring processes. Inhibition of both glycolysis and oxidative phosphorylation decreased cellular ATP and inhibited collagen secretion.[100] Continued protein synthesis was not required since inhibition of such synthesis by cycloheximide or puromycin did not reduce collagen secretion appreciably. These findings are consistent with an active role of microtubules and/or microfilaments in collagen secretion.

Secretion follows transcellular movement of collagen, involving fusion of the secretory vesicles with the plasma membrane and extrusion of collagen into the interstitum,[80,81,195,196] presumably by the merocrine mechanism (glandular secretion in which the secreting cell remains intact). While some data may suggest that hydroxylation of proline is not an absolute requirement for secretion,[62] secretion at a normal rate requires hydroxylation of proline commensurate with the body temperature and collagen type.[20,26] Satir[173] portrays secretory events: approach of the secretory vesicle to the plasma membrane, touching of the membranes, lipids in each membrane moving aside due to enzyme induced fluidity, fusion of the vesicle with the membrane, and extrusion of the contents of the vesicle. He postulates that an equivalent portion of the membrane is removed by phagocytosis at some other point and indicates this as a possible mechanism of membrane renewal. Certainly the observation of continuity and similarity of composition between vesicle and plasma membrane supports this mechanism. Moreover, Massaro and Massaro[115] cite the formation of pseudopods on vesicles as evidence of active assistance of secretion by these vesicles and, thus, a suggestion of possible control. Poorly hydroxylated collagen which is not in the triple helical form can also be secreted but at a slower rate.[62] Whether this represents intracellular degradation,[14] or some other mechanism, or both is not fully defined. Maragoudakis et al.[113] indicate that under-hydroxylated basement membrane collagen (2 to 10% hydroxylation normally found) can be secreted in vitro but was not deposited on Reichert's membrane. The prolyl hydroxylase inhibition did not inhibit production of the glucosamine portion of the basement membrane; it was also deposited.[113] One can see that this would have profound effects on function of basement membrane.

Considerable controversy exists concerning the location at which the first cleavage of non-helical procollagen extensions occurs. Since procollagen prevents or reduces the intracellular formation of fibers, there is no requirement that the initial cleavage of the amino terminal extension be intracellular.[20,21,59] The cleavage occurs in several steps, probably involving two enzymes([44,49] which need not be located together and which have different inhibition properties.[49,50] If ALT procollgen (P_c-collagen) is formed early and is a long-lived intermediate with a presumed structural role,[63] then the formation of P_C-collagen late enough to prevent or reduce intracellulr fibrogenesis but early enough to allow extracellular fiber formation is a definite possibility. The scission of the amino terminal extension at or neap the plasma memrane was regarded as a good possibility.[195] The scission kinetics describing the formation of ALT procollagen (P_c-collagen)[63] are consistent with but do not prove this idea. Finally, Tuderman et al.[192a] assay their partially purified P_N-collagen peptidase (molecular weight 98,000 or 260,000 daltons) using a solule system.[192a] Arginine doesj't inhibit P_N collagen peptidase,[105a] indicating it to prefer soluble substrate, be intracellular, or both. While this does not demonstrate the cleavage to occur as intracellular in the soluble portion of the cell, the evidence is provoking. Cleavage of type II procollagen infers broad specificity. Definition of the site of cleavage of the amino terminal extension will be a major advance. Whether the enzyme is bound in an inactive form to the plasma membrane, to the secretory vesicles, or to the collagen itself must be determined. The isolation of the enzyme should aid in the determination of its site of action.

I. Fibril Formation and Cleavage of the Carboxy Terminal Extension

Fibril formation is thought to occur spontaneously between tropocollagen monomers.[71] The polymerization pattern is proposed as an alternating 5-chain and 4-chain alignment capable of forming the collagen fibrils with a 67 nm (or a multiple of that distance) overlap. Subsequently the fibers which support the various tissues are formed. Final proof of this molecular configuration is yet to be demonstrated.[154]

Collagen tactoids are formed in vitro with high saline concentrations of tropocollagen. Bard and Chapman[7] indicate that the differential equations of collagen molecular association predict the formation of cigar-shaped elongate tactoids (axial ratio ≃45:1). Tactoids of varying sizes and shapes have been formed in vitro in the presence of DNA, following trypsin treatment, following collagen precipitation in cold acetate buffer (pH = 4.2),[7] and in high salt concentrations. However, these differ markedly from the collagen fibrils and fibers formed in various tissues. One potential difference may be the polymerizing monomer. Tropocollagen was used in the previously mentioned in vitro studies.

ALT procollagen (P_c-collagen) may align more readily than tropocollagen and form fibrils in vivo. Fessler et al.[63] indicated ALT procollagen (P_c-collagen) to have a prolonged existence and postulated a role in fibril formation. Thus, the additional carboxy terminal extension may play a role in fibril formation. Interestingly, arginine inhibited the formation of microfibrils from the collagen monomer units. What this says concerning the nature of the initial alignment is unclear. The observations that H-collagen (possibly P_c-collagen) renatures more readily than tropocollagen[194,195] tend to substantiate this idea. The evidence that the amino terminal extension prevents fibril formation has been discussed previously and indicates that this extension must be cleaved for appreciable fibril formation.

Small molecules such as urea allow proper alignment of collagen chains without leading to chain disassociation. Fessler and Tandberg[58] investigated interactions of collagen chains and fiber formation as a function of urea concentration. Urea concentration had a small effect upon disassociation of collagen fibers into monomer units (stability of helical structure). This indicated that ample opportunity was present for any mismatched regions of lower stability to disassociate and reform in proper alignment. However, urea concentrations of 0.1 *M* had a substantial effect upon fiber formation, bringing the temperature of this formation closer to body temperature. Fiber formation is not reversible; the complex factors in helical stability and cross-linking account for this factor. Other materials in the collagen environment may greatly affect fiber formation.[76] This is accomplished by promoting correct association of collagen molecules via a destabilization of incorrect associations so that the correct ones occur at nearer normal body temperature.[58] The concentration of blood urea nitrogen is normally lower by a factor of approximately 10 to 20 times than the concentrations used to produce this effect upon fiber formation. However, in some cases of uremia these concentrations are exceeded. This does not rule out the effect of other materials in collagen's environment in forming aligned fibers.

ALT procollagen (P_c-collagen) monomers align extracellularly, fibrils form, and the carboxy terminal extension of it is trimmed by procollagen peptidease II; the amino terminal extension has already been trimmed by procollagen peptidase I. The carboxy terminal extension of P_c-collagen (ALT procollagen) may be important in initial fibril contact by monomer units. After the fibril is formed, the final cleavage by procollagen peptidase could trim the extension.[195] If true, this enzyme should prefer (as in lysyl oxidase, Siegel[180]) particulate as opposed to soluble substrate. Duksin and Bornstein[50] have suggested that P_c-collagen peptidase (procollagen peptidase II) is a glycoprotein because tunicamycin inhibits its secretion. This seems to be consistent with but does not prove that the enzyme may be membrane bound. If so, this tends to support the concept that P_c-collagen peptidase like lysyl oxidase may prefer particulate substrate. Procollagen peptideases can act on associated procollagen molecules; such associations are not a necessary prerequisite for their action.[105a] Further research should define this concept. Binding to proteoglycan such as dermatan[40a] or fibronectin and as discussed in Chapter 4 could provide the particulization necessary for this enzyme. Whether procollagen peptidase II acts in such a manner awaits further definitive study.

Others[104,189] have reported procollagen peptidase activity, but have not defined its cellular location(s). Davidson et al.[44,45] have shown procollagen peptidase to degrade procollagen to collagen in four or more steps. One step leads to cleavage of the amino terminal extension of collagen either just before[63] or after[20,21] secretion. This step is inhibited by tunicamycin[49,50] and thus presumably different from the remaining three steps catylyzed by a second enzyme. Likewise, the identification of dermatosporatic collagen as P_N-collagen, which lacks a carboxy terminal extension peptide, suggests that there are two enzymes. These steps are most probably extracellular[20,21] and may occur after the fiber has been aligned, although such has neither been demonstrated nor refuted. The stepwise excision of each of two carboxy terminal extension peptides which remain attached by interchain disulfide bonds precedes the final cleavage, yielding the disulfide bonded carboxy terminal fragment, which has been characterized.[136] An important aside is that specialized collagens such as basement membrane collagen may not undergo cleavage of either extension peptide.[128] The finding by Gay et al.[69] of type III procollagen extracellularly suggests that it may also be metabolized differently from type I procollagen. Thus proteolytic removal of propeptides is rapid for procollagens I and II, delayed for type III, and probably does not occur at all for type IV. Both procollagen III and IV have short (5nm) carboxyl extensions removed by pepsin.[64] The influence of the cleaved non-helical carboxy terminal fragment upon structural collagen synthesis is an intriguing problem. The fragment could signal the formation of a functioning collagen fibril. Moreover, it is large enough to interact with the cell membrane or to be phagocytized. This constitutes one possible way in which the cell may be signaled that new fibrillar collagen has been formed, a phenomenon which has puzzled others.[20] By knowing the rate of formation of functional fibrillar collagen, the cell can produce the amount of collagen necessary for support.

J. Intra- and Intermolecular Cross-Linking

Cross-linking occurs as a concerted process; inter- and intramolecular formation cannot be distinguished biochemically. Although cross-linking is unnecessary for fibril formation, the fibers which are formed without cross-linking lack tensile strength[80] and cannot adequately support their respective tissues. Pinto and Bentley[156] showed that the major incorporated activity moves from alpha chains to beta units, with increasing time after proline radiolabel. However, the major peak does not go to a peak they identify as a gamma unit. This gamma unit chromatographed in the area of type III collagen,[36] which, although quite insoluble, may be extractable to the very small extent shown on their carboxymethyl cellulose chromatogram. Their evidence indicates a puzzling lack of progression from alpha to cross-linked gamma units. One possible interpretation may indicate the beta units to be gamma degradation products. This might then indicate that the time of formation of inter- and intramolecular cross-links was indistinguishable in their in vito system. Their proposal that the collagen eluting in 0.5 M NaCh is a "nucleation" factor for fibrogenesis is intriguing. It might be consistent with the previous interpretation if the S peak were a precursor form of triple helical collagen, as some of their evidence indicates. This in vivo study demonstrated some of the same type of kinetics as those shown by Fessler et al.[63] in a more detailed in vitro system.

Lysyl oxidase catalyzes the first step of cross-linking, has a copper cofactor, and has a preference for particulate as opposed to soluble substrate. The oxidation of the epsilon-amino group of lysyl or hydroxylysyl residues on neighboring chains leads to formation of the corresponding delta-semialdehyde, specifically allysine or hydroxyallysine.[68,153,179] This enzymatic process requires lysyl oxidase, a copper requiring enzyme,[55,181] which is inhibited by beta amino proprionitrile[138] and by $5 + 10^{-4}$ M concentrations of Zn^{++}, Cd^{++}, Mn^{++}, Ni^{++}, Ca^{++}, Mg^{++} and Fe^{+++}, but not Co^{++} or Fe^{++}.[181] These findings suggest that the inhibitory ions cannot replace Cu^{++} as a cofactor. In normal situations only Ca^{++} would be present at near that concentration. The relatively high concentration of Cd^{++} and Ni^{++} required suggest that this is not their primary mode of toxicity. Narayanan et al.[139] recovered lysyl oxidase in high yield using purification on DEAE cellulose and subsequently on collagen derivatized sephadex®. This enabled Siegel[180] to determine the K_m (0.95 μm) with precipitated collagen forms and low activity to either soluble or denatured forms, indicating that lysyl oxidase prefers particulate, possibly partially aligned substrate. It is, however, not trapped by the formed cross-link as additional substrate is acted upon with equal efficiency. Misirowski et al.[131] have developed a microassay for lysyl oxidase. Brody et al.[24] identified lung lysyl oxidase; it seems to have properties similar to that in other tissues.

Formation of allysine precedes aldehyde interaction of adjacent chains and rearrangement to a more stable cross-link. Lysyl oxidase catalyzed formation of allysine or hydroxyallysine; then intepaction occurred with other aldehydes on adjacent collagen chains.[5,68,153] This step cah be inhibited by semicarbazide, or by the penicillamine-induced formation of a thiazolidine complex with the aldehyde.[107] Penicillamine has no direct effect on lysyl oxidase.[155,168] After cross-link formation, rearrangement occurs(which presumably results in the formation of more spable cross-links.[6] The disappearance of cross-links with increasing age may suggest that the more stable cross-links have not been completely identified, or cannot be completely quantitated. The contents of measured cross-links vary in different tissues[80,81] suggesting a relation to different functions of the tissues, or alternatively, that different stages of arrangement may be present in proceeding toward the formation of as yet unidentified but more stable cross-links.

Inter- and intrachain disulfide bonds may influence the solubility of pulmonary collagen. The helical portion of both type III and IV collagen contains cysteine residues, [80, 81] suggesting the possibility of intra- or intermolecular disulfide bonds. Investigation of this possibility in type III collagen suggested that intermolecular bonds were not present,[174] raising the intriguing possibility of intrachain disulfide bonds. McLees et al.[120] presented preliminary evidence for such bonds. Sufficient amounts of type IV collagen have not been isolated to perform standard analysis for interchain disulfide bonds. Collagen cross-links are probably important determinants of lung structure. Since inhibitors of cross-linking increase the solubility of lung collagen,[23] interchain cross-links most likely exist. The location amount and changes of cross-links with aging or in lung disease have not been investigated directly. However, Seyer et al.[176] reported greater pepsin digestion efficiency in human lungs with idiopathic pulmonary fibrosis than in controls, although the majority of their lung collagen was not solubilized and even though repeated pepsin solubilization failed to release all the lung collagen. In vivo inhibition of cross-linking, either induced[46, 186] or naturally occurring,[55] resulted in a lack of structural stability and sometimes of elasticity.

II. COLLAGEN SYNTHETIC RATES

Most synthetic rates utilize the incorporation of radiolabelled proline into collagen in vitro[193] or in vivo[149, 152] as indicated by radioactive hydroxyproline using the method of Juva and Prockop,[90a] Diegelmann et al.,[47] or by using separation by ion exchange chromatography. Proline incorporation into imino acids is five times as high as that in non-collagenous protein. Moreover, hydroxylation of proline in vivo and most in vitro systems is probably not rate limiting.[20, 151] Underhydroxylated collagen in such cases is unlikely to exist in quantities sufficient to affect synthetic rates determined experimentally.

Collagen synthesis decreases with increasing age in hamster, rat, and rabbit lungs, reflecting a decreasing instantaneous growth rate. Since collagen is a structural protein, one would expect synthetic rates to parallel organ or body growth rates, assuming an unchanged breakdown rate. Important in this equation is the question of balance. Some types of collagen, specifically type III, may turn over (at least in some form) more rapidly as indicated by their susceptibility to trypsin,[122] although in vivo turnover rates approximate those of type I.[98] Little is known about turnover of basement membrane collagen. Moreover, in injury, lung collagen is produced and broken down more rapidly than in normal animals.[151] Newman and Langner[140] report that lung collagen synthesis decreases as a function of increasing age. Likewise Crystal,[41] Bradley et al.,[22,23] and Hance and Crystal[80,81] report a similar trend in rabbits from birth to nearly a year of age. Our data in Syrian hamster lungs closely parallels these studies. In Figure 4a we compare our fraction of proline incorporated into collagen with the rabbit data of Hance and Crystal[80,81] using an interconversion scale based on the formula of Diegelmann and Peterkofsky.[48] In each case the data compare well, and a certain minimum level of collagen synthesis probably reflects the turnover of lung collagen. The reduction of collagen synthetic rate in the presence of consistent collagen breakdown rates[152b] (Figure 4b) reflects the falling instantaneous growth rate and the maturity of the animals. Whether such trends reflect a change of collagen type, such as that discussed earlier, in vessels and skin, remains to be determined. Likewise, the relative importance of each collagen type in establishing the turnover rate of collagen, especially the progression to a minimal turnover rate, is important. Incorporation of proline into non-collagenous proteins (Figure 4c) and collagen content/unit body weight (Figure 4d) remains constant with increasing age.

Chelating agents, proline analogs, and even hydroxyproline may alter rates of collagen synthesis and lung growth. Proline analogs which reduce collagen synthesis alter growth rates of lung,[4] in chicken embryos and rat tumor granulomas,[88,170] in healing anastomized colon,[42] and tissue cultures of mammalian cells.[81b,95] When these analogs inhibit lung growth and alter collagen and elastin secretion rates, the possibility of intracellular degradation of connective tissue being altered[14] to eliminate imperfect molecules must be considered. Hydroxyproline reduces basement membrane synthesis in isolated renal glomeruli.[16] The significance of this finding is as yet unclear. However, suppression of basement membrane synthesis in vivo would be quite useful in conditions where production was pathologically increased. The rapid clearance of free hydroxyproline via the kidney may preclude in vivo systemic usage. Likewise chelating agents reduced hydroxylation of proline and lysine, but to a greater extent with lysine.[17] This led to reduced glycosylation of hydroxylysine. The mechanism of the differentially severe reduction of lysine hydroxylation is poorly understood, but not unlike the trypsin effect noted by Quinn et al.[161] following trypsinization of cells. Penicillamine seems to decrease lung elastic recoil due to inhibition of lung elastin and collagen cross-linking.[85] Likewise as yet unidentified peptides elicit collagen synthetic increases in synovial cells[31] and in liver.[117] The ability of such molecules to influence collagen synthetic rates is most interesting, but far from resolved. Answers to the question of what underlies or controls such responses are essential to manipulating lung injury.

It is important to demonstrate the relation of each segment of collagen synthesis to each other and to the other connective tissue constituents at the time of rapid collagen metabolism. The relative amounts of various collagen types are of considerable interest. Kawamoto and Nagai[94] indicate that collagen synthesis and deposition in chicken embryo skin is maximized by 16 days, agreeing with Woessner et al.,[198] although heart collagen synthesis continues to hatching. Whether this represents a difference in prolyl hydroxylation[169] remains to be determined. At 16 days, the highest amount of ultra-

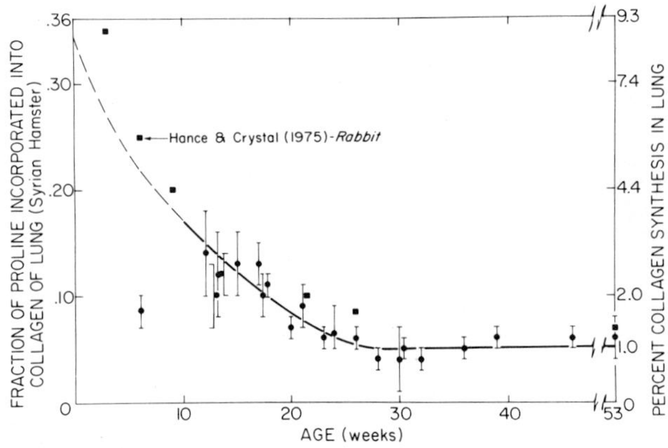

4A

FIGURE 4. (A) Collagen synthesis in hamster lung expressed as either fraction of proline incorporated into collagen of lung or percent collagen synthesis in lung decreased exponentially (least squares fit) in lungs of both hamster and rabbit[80] from 10 to 25 weeks of age (hamster) or birth to 25 weeks of age (rabbits). This probably reflected decreasing instantaneous lung growth rate. Following 25 weeks, synthesis continued at a constant lower rate (eye fit), probably reflecting minimal pulmonary collagen turnover. (B) Collagen breakdown rate expressed as ultrafilterable hydroxyproline peptides varied from one extraction in cold physiological saline to another. However, it was generally quite consistent in a given extraction. Little change with increasing age was noted (least squares fit). (C) Non-collagenous protein synthesis, expressed as non-collagenous incorporation of proline was reasonably consistent among hamsters but had no significant change from 6 to 53 weeks of age (least squares fit). (D) Pulmonary collagen content was modestly variable among hamsters but had no significant change from 6 to 53 weeks of age (least squares fit).

filterable hydroxyproline and collagenase which can be activated by 3 *M* NaSCN treatment was observed.[94] The reduction of chondroitin sulfate and increased dermatan sulfate is interesting. This correlates with dermatan sulfate being the proteoglycan linked to collagen and tends to negate the importance of synthesis of type II (cartilage) collagen in the absence of chondroitin SO_4 increases. Minor et al.[129, 130] find a similar time of peak collagen synthesis in parietal yolk sac. Since it synthesizes only basement membrane collagen,[38, 128-130] the relative rates of this collagen type seem to parallel that of embryo skin, indicating the similarity of these two systems at the time of maximum synthesis. Grant et al.[72] indicate disulfide bonds to be of considerable importance in forming the triple helix. Likewise, Minor et al.[128] indicate the lack of post-translational cleavage in in vitro cultures. Al-Adnani et al.[3] indicated that collagen synthesis by human breast cancer cells (in vivo) occurs in the absence of such activity in stromal cells. He considered this collagen synthesis inappropriate to normal breast tissue. Whether this relates to tumor invasion is undetermined. However, the importance of this mechanism must be considered in light of Langness and Udenfriend's[103] observation that numerous cell lines can synthesize collagen.

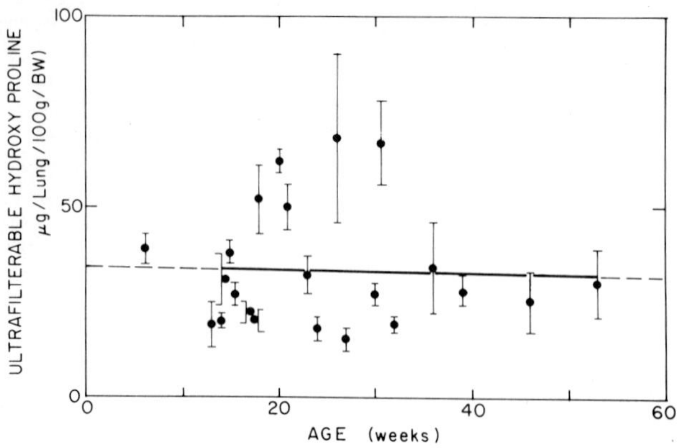

FIGURE 4B

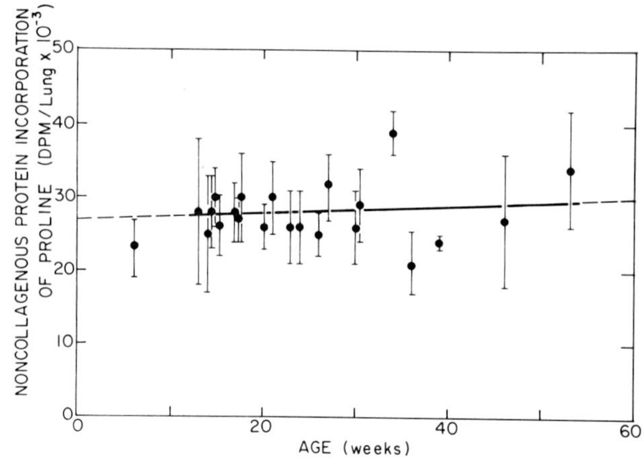

FIGURE 4C

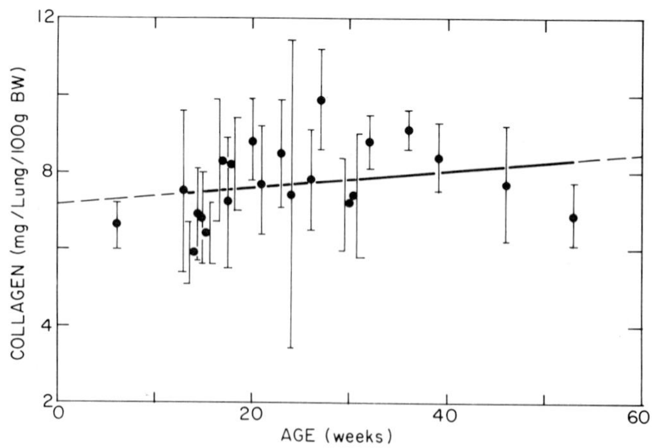

FIGURE 4D

REFERENCES

1. **Adams, S. L., Sobel, M. E., Howard, B. H., Olden, K., Yamada, K. M., de Crombrugshe, B., and Pastan, I.**, Levels of translatable mRNAs for cell surface protein, collagen precursors, and two membrane proteins are altered in Rous sarcoma virus transformed chick embryo fibroblasts, *Proc. Natl. Acad. Sci. U.S.A.*, 74(8), 3399, 1977.
2. **Adli, F. A., Burgeson, R. E., Kaitila, I. I., and Hollister, D. W.**, Identification of two new collagen alpha chains in human fetal membranes, paper presented at meeting of West Coast Connective Tissue Workers, March 5 to 7, 1976, Heber, Utah.
3. **Al-Adnani, M. S., Kirrane, J. A., and McGee, J. O'D.**, Inappropriate production of collagen and prolyl hydroxylase by human breast cancer cells *in vivo*, *Br. J. Cancer*, 31, 653, 1975.
4. **Alescio, T.**, Effect of a proline analogue, azetidine-2-carboxylic acid, on the morphogenesis *in vitro* of mouse embryonic lung, *J. Embryol. Exp. Morphol.*, 29, 439, 1973.
5. **Bailey, A. J., Robins, S. P., and Balian, G.**, Biological significance of intermolecular crosslinks of collagen, *Nature (London)*, 251, 105, 1974.
6. **Bailey, A. J. and Robins, S. P.**, Development and maturation of the crosslinks in the collagen fibres of skin, *Front. Matrix Biol.*, 1, 130, 1973.
7. **Bard, J. B. L. and Chapman, J. A.**, Diameters in collagen fibrils grown *in vitro*, *Nature (London) New Biol.*, 246, 83, 1973.
8. **Baum, B. J., Moss, J., Breul, S. D., and Crystal, R. G.**, Association in normal human fibroblasts of elevated levels of adenosine 3′:5′-monophosphate with a selective decrease in collagen production, *J. Biol. Chem.*, 253(10), 3391, 1978.
9. **Bellamy, G. and Bornstein, P.**, Evidence for procollagen, a biosynthetic precursor of collagen, *Proc. Natl. Acad. Sci. U.S.A.*, 68, 1138, 1971.
10. **Bentley, J. P. and Weiser, K. A.**, A simple microassay of prolyl hydroxylase applicable to skin punch biopsy specimens, *Connect. Tissue Res.*, 4, 255, 1976.
11. **Berg, R. A. and Prockop, D. J.**, Affinity column purification of protocollagen proline hydroxylase from chick embryos and further characterization of the enzyme, *J. Biol. Chem.*, 248, 1175, 1973.
12. **Berg, R. A. and Prockop, D. J.**, Purification of ^{14}C protocollagen and its hydroxylation by prolyl-hydroxylase, *Biochemistry*, 12, 3395, 1973.
13. **Berman, A. E., Oborotova, T. A., and Mazurov, V. I.**, *Biochemistry (USSR)*, 40, 364, 1975; as cited in **Fessler, J. H., and Fessler, L. I.**, *Annu. Rev. Biochem.*, 47, 158, 1978.
14. **Bienkowski, R. S., Cowan, M. J., McDonald, J. A., and Crystal, R. G.**, Degradation of newly synthesized collagen, *J. Biol. Chem.*, 253(12), 4356, 1978.
15. **Blobel, G. and Sabatini, D. D.**, Ribosome-membrane interaction in eukaryotic cells, *Biomembranes*, 2, 193, 1971.
16. **Bloodworth, J. M. B., Jr., Wilken, D. R., and Anderson, P. J.**, Basement membrane (BM) biosynthesis: (1) methodology; (2) suppression by free hydroxyproline (HYP) and its possible therapeutic use in diabetic microangiopathy, *Fed. Proc. Abstr.*, 36, 1055, 1977.
17. **Blumenkrantz, N. and Asboe-Hansen, G.**, Effect of chelating agents on the biosynthesis of collagen, *Acta Derm. Venereol.*, 53, 94, 1973.
18. **Boedtker, H., Crkvenjakov, R. B., Last, J. A., and Doty, P.**, The identification of collagen messenger RNA, *Proc. Natl. Acad. Sci. U.S.A.*, 71, 4208, 1974.
19. **Bornstein, P.**, Comparative sequence studies of rat skin and tendon collagen. I. Evidence for incomplete hydroxylation of individual prolyl residues in the normal proteins, *Biochemistry*, 6, 3082, 1967.
20. **Bornstein, P.**, The biosynthesis of collagen, *Annu. Rev. Biochem.*, 43, 567, 1974.
21. **Bornstein, P.**, The structure and assembly of procollagen — a review, *J. Supramol. Struct.*, 2, 108, 1974.

21a. **Bornstein, P.**, Research communication, 1976.

22. **Bradley, K., McConnell-Breul, S., and Crystal, R. G.**, Lung collagen heterogeneity, *Proc. Natl. Acad. Sci. U.S.A.*, 71, 2828, 1974.
23. **Bradley, K. H., McConnell, S. D., and Crystal, R. G.**, Lung collagen composition and synthesis: characterization and changes with age, *J. Biol. Chem.*, 249, 2674, 1974.
24. **Brody, J. S., Kagan, H. M., Manalo, A. D., Hu, C. A., and Franzblau, C.**, Lung lysyl oxidase and elastin synthesis during compensatory lung growth, *Chest*, 69(2), 271, 1976.
25. **Brownell, A. G. and Veis, A.**, Intracellular location of triple helix formation of collagen: enzyme probe studies, *J. Biol. Chem.*, 251, 7137, 1976.
26. **Brownell, A. G. and Veis, A.**, The intracellular location of the glycosylation of hydroxylysine of collagen, *Biochem. Biophys. Res. Commun.*, 63, 371, 1975.
27. **Burgeson, R. E., Wyke, A. W., and Fessler, J. H.**, Collagen synthesis by cells. II: secretion of a disulfide linked material, *Biochem. Biophys. Res. Commun.*, 48, 892, 1972.

28. **Byers, P. H., McKenney, K. H., Lichtenstein, J. R. and Martin, G. R.,** Preparation of type III procollagen and collagen from rat skin, *Biochemistry,* 13, 5243, 1974.
29. **Cardinale, G. J. and Udenfriend, S.,** Prolyl hydroxylase, *Adv. Enzymol.,* 41, 245, 1975.
29a. **Cardinale, G.,** Research communication, 1976.
30. **Carpousis, A., Christner, P., and Rosenbloom, J.,** Preferential usage of tRNA isoaccepting species in collagen synthesis, *J. Biol. Chem.,* 252(22), 8023, 1977.
31. **Castor, C. W., Smith, S. F., Ritchie, J. C., and Scott, M. E.,** Connective tissue activation: mechanism and significance, in *Biology of Fibroblast,* Academic Press, New York, 1973, 483.
32. **Chan, S. J., Keim, P., Steiner, D. F.,** Cell-free synthesis of rat preproinsulins: characterization and partial amino acid sequence determination, *Proc. Natl. Acad. Sci. U.S.A.,* 73, 1964, 1976.
33. **Chen-Kiang, S. and Udenfriend, S.,** Isolation of a prolyl hydroxylase related antigen from rat skin, *Fed. Proc. Abstr.,* 36, 753, 1977.
34. **Chichester, C. O., Fuller, G. C., and Cardinale, G. J.,** *In vivo* labeling and turnover of prolyl hydroxylase and a related immunoreactive protein, *Biochem. Biophys. Res. Commun.,* 73, 1056, 1976.
35. **Christner, P. J. and Rosenbloom, J.,** Possible control of collagen synthesis by specific isoaccepting tRNA species, in *Extracellular Matrix Influences on Gene Expression,* Slavkin, H. C. and Greulich, R. C., Eds., Academic Press, New York, 1975, 111.
36. **Chung, E. and Miller, E. J.,** Collagen polymorphism: characterization of molecules with the chain composition $[\alpha 1\ (III)]_3$ in human tissues, *Science,* 183, 1200, 1974.
37. **Church, R. L., Pfeiffer, S. E., and Tanzer, M. L.,** Collagen biosynthesis: synthesis and secretion of a high molecular weight collagen precursor (procollagen), *Proc. Natl. Acad. Sci. U.S.A.,* 68, 2638, 1971.
37a. **Church, R. L., Tanzer, M. L., and Lapiere, C. M.,** Identification of two distinct species of procollagen synthesized by a clonal line of calf dermatosparactic cells, *Nature (London) New Biol.,* 244, 188, 1973.
38. **Clark, C. C., Minor, R. R., Koszalka, T. R., Brent, R. L., and Kefalides, N. A.,** The embryonic rat parietal yolk sac; changes in the morphology and composition of its basement membrane during development, *Dev. Biol.,* 46, 243, 1975.
39. **Collins, J. F. and Crystal, R. G.,** Characterization of cell-free synthesis of collagen by lung polysomes in a heterologous system, *J. Biol. Chem.,* 250, 7332, 1975.
40. **Collins, J. F. and Crystal, R. G.,** Protein synthesis, in *The Biochemical Basis of Pulmonary Function,* Crystal, R. G., Ed., Marcel Dekker, New York, 1976, 171.
40a. **Comper, W. D. and Laurent, T. C.,** Physiological function of connective tissue polysaccharides, *Physiol. Rev.,* 58(1), 255, 1978.
40b. **Crystal, R.,** Post-translational control of collagen production by intracellular degradation. Presented at the Western Connective Tissue Society Meeting, February 9 to 11, 1979, Seattle, Wash.
41. **Crystal, R. G.,** Lung collagen: definition, diversity and development, *Fed. Proc.,* 33, 2248, 1974.
41a. **Cutroneo, K. R., Guzman, N. A., and Sharawy, M. M.,** Evidence for a subcellular vesicular site of collagen prolyl hydroxylation, *J. Biol. Chem.,* 249, 5989, 1974.
42. **Daly, J. M., Steiger, E., Prockop, D. J., and Dudrick, S. J.,** Inhibition of collagen synthesis by the proline analogue *cis*-4-hydroxyproline, *J. Surg. Res.,* 14, 551, 1973.
43. **Darnell, J. and Rosenbloom, J.,** Ultracentrifugation as a probe of conformation of unhydroxylated procollagen and collagen, *Biochem. Biophys. Res. Commun.,* 57, 910, 1974.
44. **Davidson, J. M., McEneany, L. S. G., and Bornstein, P.,** Intermediates in the limited proteolytic conversion of procollagen to collagen, *Biochemistry,* 14, 5188, 1975.
45. **Davidson, J. M., McEneany, L. S. G., and Bornstein, P.,** Intermediates in the conversion of procollagen to collagen: evidence for stepwise limited proteolysis of the COOH-terminal peptide extensions, *Eur. J. Biochem.,* 81, 349, 1977.
46. **Deshmukh, K., Just, M., and Nimni, M. E.,** A defect in the intramolecular and intermolecular cross-linking of collagen caused by penicillamine. III. Accumulation of acid soluble collagen with a high hydroxylysine content in bone, *Clin. Orthop. Relat. Res.,* 91, 186, 1973.
47. **Diegelmann, R. F., Bernstein, L., and Peterkofsky, B.,** Cell-free collagen synthesis on membrane-bound polysomes of chick embryo connective tissue and the localization of prolyl hydroxylase on the polysome-membrane complex, *J. Biol. Chem.,* 248, 6514, 1973.
48. **Diegelmann, R. F. and Peterkofsky, B.,** Collagen biosynthesis during connective tissue development in chick embryo, *Dev. Biol.,* 28, 443, 1972.
49. **Duksin, D. and Bornstein, P.,** Impaired conversion of procollagen to collagen by fibroblasts and bone treated with tunicamycin, an inhibitor of protein glycosylation, *J. Biol. Chem.,* 252, 955, 1977.
50. **Duksin, D. and Bornstein, P.,** Impaired conversion of procollagen caused by tunicamycin, an inhibitor of protein glycosylation, *Fed. Proc. Abstr.,* 35, 1739, 1976.

51. **Ehrlich, H. P. and Bornstein, P.**, Microtubules in transcellular movement of procollagen, *Nature (London) New Biol.*, 238, 257, 1972.
52. **Ehrlich, H. P., Ross, R., and Bornstein, P.**, Effects of antimicrotubular agents on the secretion of collagen, *J. Cell Biol.*, 62, 390, 1974.
53. **Ehrlich, H. P., Tarver, H., and Hunt, T. K.**, Effects of vitamin A and glucocorticoids upon inflammation and collagen synthesis, *Ann. Surg.*, 177, 222, 1973.
54. **Etherington, D. J.**, The dissolution of insoluble bovine collagens by cathepsin B1, collagenolytic cathepsin and pepsin, *Connect. Tissue Res.*, 5, 135, 1977.
55. **Eyre, D. R.**, Collagen defects in genetic disorders of connective tissue, *Dev. Med. Child Neurol.*, 16, 531, 1974.
56. **Eyre, D. R. and Glimcher, M. J.**, Analysis of a crosslinked peptide from calf bone collagen: evidence that hydroxylysyl glycoside participates in the crosslink, *Biochem. Biophys. Res. Commun.*, 52, 663, 1973.
57. **Fessler, J. H.**, Self-assembly of collagen, *J. Supramol. Struct.*, 2, 99, 1974.
58. **Fessler, J. H. and Tandberg, W. D.**, Interactions between collagen chains and fiber formation, *J. Supramol. Struct.*, 3, 17, 1975.
59. **Fessler, J. H., Doege, K. J., Siegel, R. C., and Fessler, L. I.**, Procollagen associations into supramolecular structures, *Fed. Proc. Abstr.*, 36, 680, 1977.
60. **Fessler, L. I., Burgeson, R. E., Morris, N. P., and Fessler, J. H.**, Collagen synthesis: a disulfide-linked collagen precursor in chick bone, *Proc. Natl. Acad. Sci. U.S.A.*, 70, 2993, 1973.
61. **Fessler, J. H., Morris, N. P., Greenberg, G. M., and Fessler, L. I.**, Assembly and processing of procollagen, in *Extracellular Matrix Influence on Gene Expression*, Slavkin, H. C., and Greulich, R. C., Eds., Academic Press, New York, 1975, 101.
61a. **Fessler, L. I. and Fessler, J. H.**, Characterization of type III procollagen from chick embryo blood vessels, *J. Biol. Chem.*, 254, 233, 1979.
62. **Fessler, L. I. and Fessler, J. H.**, Protein assembly of procollagen and effects of hydroxylation, *J. Biol. Chem.*, 249, 7637, 1974.
63. **Fessler, L. I., Morris, N. P., and Fessler, J. H.**, Procollagen: biological scission of amino and carboxyl extension peptides, *Proc. Natl. Acad. Sci. U.S.A.*, 72, 4905, 1975.
64. **Fessler, J. H. and Fessler, L. I.**, Biosynthesis of procollagen, *Annu. Rev. Biochem.*, 47, 129, 1978.
65. **Fisher, D. O., Matoney, A. L., and Fuller, G. C.**, Parameters of aortic and liver collagen synthesis in rabbits with experimental arteriosclerosis, *Fed. Proc. Abstr.*, 34, 697, 1975.
66. **Fujii, K., Tanzer, M. L., and Cooke, P. H.**, Collagen fibrogenesis and the formation of complex crosslinks, *J. Mol. Biol.*, 106, 223, 1976.
67. **Fuller, G. C., Matoney, A. L., Fisher, D. O., Fausto, N., and Cardinale, G. J.**, Increased collagen synthesis and the kinetic characteristics of prolyl hydroxylase in tissues of rabbits with experimental atherosclerosis, *Atherosclerosis*, 24, 483, 1976.
68. **Gallop, P. M., Blumenfeld, O. O., and Seifter, S.**, Structure and metabolism of connective tissue proteins, *Annu. Rev. Bioch.*, 41, 617, 1972.
69. **Gay, S., Martin, G. R., Müller, P. K., Timpl, R., and Kühn, K.**, Simultaneous synthesis of types I and III collagen by fibroblasts in culture, *Proc. Natl. Acad. Sci. U.S.A.*, 73, 4037, 1976.
69a. **Gerter, M.**, DNA replication, *Ann. Rev. Bioch.*, 44, 45, 1975.
70. **Goldberg, B. and Sherr, C. J.**, Secretion and extracellular processing of procollagen by cultured human fibroblasts, *Proc. Natl. Acad. Sci. U.S.A.*, 70, 361, 1973.
71. **Grant, M. E. and Prockop, D. J.**, The biosynthesis of collagen (I, II and III), *N. Engl. J. Med.*, 286, 194, 242, 291, 1972.
72. **Grant, M. E., Schoefield, J. D., Kefalides, N. A., and Prockop, D. J.**, The biosynthesis of basement membrane collagen in embryonic chick lens. III. Intracellular formation of the triple helix and the formation of aggregates through disulfide bonds, *J. Biol. Chem.*, 248, 7432, 1973.
73. **Guzman, N. A., Sharawy, M. M., and Cutroneo, K. R.**, Localization of collagen lysyl hydroxylation on the non-ribosomal side of collagen microsomes, *Fed. Proc. Abstr.*, 34(3), 563, 1975.
74. **Guzman, N. A., Berg, R. A., and Prockop, D. J.**, Concanavalin A binds to purified prolyl hydroxylase and partially inhibits its enzymic activity, *Biochem. Biophys. Res. Commun.*, 73, 279, 1976.
74a. **Guzman, N. A., Rojas, F. J., and Cutroneo, K. R.**, Collagen lysyl hydroxylation occurs within the cisternae of the rough endoplasmic reticulum, *Arch. Biochem. Biophys.*, 172, 449, 1976.
75. **Gross, J.**, Collagen biology: structure, degradation and disease, *Harvey Lect.*, 68, 351, 1974.
76. **Gross, J.**, Thermal denaturation of collagen in the dispersed and solid state, *Science*, 143, 960, 1964.
77. **Gustavson, K. H.**, The function of hydroxyproline in collagens, *Nature (London)*, 175, 70, 1955.
78. **Halme, J., Uitto, J., Kahanpää, K., Karhunen, P., and Lindy, S.**, Protocollagen proline hydroxylase activity in experimental pulmonary fibrosis of rats, *J. Lab. Clin. Med.*, 75, 535, 1970.
79. **Hamilton, G. A.**, The proton in biological redox reactions, in *Progress in Bioorganic Chemistry, Vol. 1*, Kaiser, E. T., and Kezdy, F. J., Eds., Wiley Interscience, New York, 1971, 83.

80. **Hance, A. J. and Crystal, R. G.,** The connective tissue of lung, *Am. Rev. Respir. Dis.,* 112, 657, 1975.

81. **Hance, A. J. and Crystal, R. G.,** Collagen, in *The Biochemical Basis of Pulmonary Function,* Crystal, R. G., Ed., Marcel Dekker, New York, 1976, 215.

81a. **Hartman, B. K. and Udenfriend, S.,** A method for immediate visualization of proteins in acrylamide gels and its use for preparation of antibodies to enzymes, *Anal. Biochem.,* 30, 391, 1969.

81b. **Harsch, M., Murphy, L., and Rosenbloom, J.,** Metabolism by isolated fibroblasts of abnormal collagens containing analogues of proline or lysine, *FEBS Lett.,* 26, 48, 1972.

82. **Harwood, R., Grant, M. E., and Jackson, D. S.,** The sub-cellular location of interchain disulfide bond formation during procollagen biosynthesis by embryonic chick tendon cells, *Biochem. Biophys. Res. Commun.,* 55, 1188, 1973.

83. **Hay, E. D. and Dodson, J. W.,** Secretion of collagen by corneal epithelium. I. Morphology of the collagenous products produced by isolated epithelia grown on frozen-killed lens, *J. Cell Biol.,* 57, 190, 1973.

84. **Hoffman, H. P., Olsen, B. R., Chen, H. T., and Prockop, D. J.,** Segment-long-spacing aggregates and isolation of COOH-terminal peptides from type I procollagen, *Proc. Natl. Acad. Sci. U.S.A.,* 73, 4304, 1976.

85. **Hoffman, L., Mondshine, R. B., and Park, S. S.,** Effect of DL-penicillamine on elastic properties of rat lung, *J. Appl. Physiol.,* 30, 508, 1971.

86. **Horwitz, A. L., Elson, N. A., and Crystal, R. G.,** Proteoglycans and elastic fibers, in *The Biochemical Basis of Pulmonary Function,* Crystal, R. G., Ed., Marcel Dekker, New York, 1976, 273.

87. **Hutton, J. J., Tappel, A. L., and Udenfriend, S.,** A rapid assay for collagen proline hydroxylase, *Anal. Biochem.,* 16, 384, 1966.

88. **Jimenez, S. A. and Prockop, D. J.,** Specific inhibition of collagen synthesis in rat granulomas by incorporation of the proline analog *cis*-4-hydroxyproline into intracellular collagen, *J. Clin. Invest.,* 50, 49A, 1971.

89. **Jimenez, S., Harsch, M., and Rosenbloom, J.,** Hydroxyproline stabilizes the triple helix of chick tendon collagen, *Biochem. Biophys. Res. Commun.,* 52, 106, 1973.

90. **Jimenez, S. A. and Yankowski, R.,** Role of molecular conformation on secretion of chick tendon procollagen, *J. Biol. Chem.,* 253(5), 1420, 1978.

90a. **Juva, K. and Prockop, D. J.,** Modified procedure for the assay of H^3 or C^{14}-labeled hydroxyproline, *Anal. Biochem.,* 15, 77, 1966.

91. **Kang, A. H., Beachey, E. H., and Katzman, R. L.,** Interaction of an active glycopeptide from chick skin collagen (α1-CB5) with human platelets, *J. Biol. Chem.,* 249, 1054, 1974.

92. **Kao, W., Berg, R. A., Flaks, J. G., and Prockop, D. J.,** Ascorbate can increase hydroxyproline synthesis in cultured fibroblasts without activation of prolyl hydroxylase, *Fed. Proc. Abstr.,* 34, 562, 1975.

93. **Kao, W. W. Y., Flaks, J. G., and Prockop, D. J.,** Primary and secondary effects of ascorbate on procollagen synthesis and protein synthesis by primary cultures of tendon fibroblasts, *Arch. Biochem. Biophys.,* 173, 638, 1976.

94. **Kawamoto, T. and Nagai, Y.,** Developmental changes in glycosaminoglycans, collagen and collagenase activity in embryonic chick skin, *Biochim. Biophys. Acta,* 437, 190, 1976.

95. **Kerwar, S. S. and Felix, A. M.,** Effect of L-3,4-dehydroproline on collagen synthesis and prolyl hydroxylase activity in mammalian cell cultures, *J. Biol. Chem.,* 251, 503, 1976.

96. **Kivirikko, K. I. and Prockop, D. J.,** Partial purification and characterization of protocollagen lysine hydroxylase from chick embryos, *Biochim. Biophys. Acta,* 258, 366, 1972.

97. **Kivirikko, K. I., Ryhanen, L., Anttinen, H., Bornstein, P., and Prockop, D. J.,** Further hydroxylation of lysyl residues in collagen by protocollagen lysyl hydroxylase *in vitro, Biochemistry,* 12, 4966, 1973.

98. **Klein, L. and Chandrarajan, J.,** Comparison of collagen turnover (types I versus III) in skin and intestine during rapid growth in rats, *Fed. Proc. Abstr.,* 36, 677, 1977.

99. **Kleinman, H. K., McGoodwin, E. B., Martin, G. R., and Klebe, R. J.,** Binding of cell attachment protein to collagen: effects of chemical modification, *Ann. N.Y. Acad. Sci.,* 312, 436, 1978.

100. **Kruse, N. J. and Bornstein, P.,** The metabolic requirements for transcellular movement and secretion of collagen, *J. Biol. Chem.,* 250, 4841, 1975.

101. **Kuttan, R., Cardinale, G. J., and Udenfriend, S.,** *In vitro* activation of prolyl hydroxylase, *Fed. Proc.,* 34, 562, 1975.

102. **Lande, M. A., Adesmik, M., Sumida, M., Tashiro, Y., and Sabatini, D. D.,** Direct association of messenger RNA with microsomal membranes in human diploid fibroblasts, *J. Cell Biol.,* 65, 513, 1975.

103. **Langness, U. and Udenfriend, S.,** Collagen biosynthesis in nonfibroblastic cell lines, *Proc. Natl. Acad. Sci. U.S.A.,* 71, 50, 1974.

104. **Layman, D. L. and Ross, R.**, The production and secretion of procollagen peptidase by human fibroblasts in culture, *Arch. Biochem. Biophys.*, 157, 451, 1973.

105. **Lazarides, E. and Lukens, L. N.**, Collagen synthesis on polysomes *in vivo* and *in vitro, Nature (London) New Biol.*, 232, 37, 1971.

105a. **Leung, M. K. K., Fessler, L. I., Greenberg, D. R., and Fessler, J. H.**, Separate amino and carboxyl procollagen peptidases in chick embryo tendon, *J. Biol. Chem.*, 254, 224, 1979.

106. **Levene, C. I. and Bates, C. J.**, Ascorbic acid and collagen synthesis, in *Biology of Fibroblast*, Kulonen, E., and Pikkarainen, J., Eds., Academic Press, New York, 1973, 397.

107. **Levene, C. I.**, Lathyrism, in *Molecular Pathology of Connective Tissues*, Vol. 3, Pérez-Tamayo, R., and Rojkind, M., Eds., Marcel Dekker, New York, 1973, 175.

108. **Lichtenstein, J. R., Bauer, E. A., and Uitto, J.**, Cleavage of human fibroblast type I procollagen by mammalian collagenase: demonstration of amino- and carboxy-terminal extension peptides, *Biochem. Biophys. Res. Commun.*, 73, 665, 1976.

109. **Liu, T. Z. and Bhatnagar, R. S.**, Mechanism of hydroxylation of proline, *Fed. Proc. Abstr.*, 32, 613, 1973.

110. **Lodish, H. F.**, Translational control of protein synthesis, *Annu. Rev. Biochem.*, 45, 39, 1976.

111. **London, I. M., Clemens, M. J., Ranu, R. S., Levin, D. H., Cherbas, L. F., and Ernst, V.**, *Fed. Proc.*, 35, 2218, 1976.

112. **Lukens, L. N.**, Time of occurrence of disulfide linking between procollagen chains, *J. Biol. Chem.*, 251, 3530, 1976.

113. **Maragoudakis, M. E., Kalinsky, H. J., and Wasvary, J.**, Basement membrane biosynthesis: secretion without deposition of underhydroxylated basement membrane collagen by parietal yolk sacs, *Biochim. Biophys. Acta*, 538, 139, 1978.

114. **Martin, G. R., Byers, P. H., and Piez, K. A.**, Procollagen, in *Advances in Enzymology*, Vol. 42, Meister, A., Ed., John Wiley & Sons, New York, 1975, 167.

115. **Massaro, D. and Massaro, G. D.**, Synthesis, intracellular transport, and secretion of macromolecules by the lung, in *The Biochemical Basis of Pulmonary Function*, Crystal, R. G., Ed., Marcel Dekker, New York, 1976, 389.

116. **McGee, J. O'D., Langness, U., and Udenfriend, S.**, Immunological evidence for an inactive precursor of collagen proline hydroxylase in cultured fibroblasts, *Proc. Natl. Acad. Sci. U.S.A.*, 68, 1585, 1971.

117. **McGee, J. O'D., O'Hare, R. P., and Patrick, R. S.**, Stimulation of the collagen biosynthetic pathway by factors isolated from experimentally-injured liver, *Nature (London) New Biol.*, 243, 121, 1973.

118. **McGee, J. O'D. and Udenfriend, S.**, A general method for the rapid measure of enzyme precursors by the displacement of enzyme from antibody: the measurement of collagen proline hydroxylase precursor in cultured fibroblasts, *Biochem. Biophys. Res. Commun.*, 46, 1646, 1972.

119. **McGee, J. O.'D. and Udenfriend, S.**, Partial purification and characterization of peptidyl proline hydroxylase precursor from mouse fibroblasts, *Arch. Biochem. Biophys.*, 152, 216, 1972.

120. **McLees, B. D., Schleiter, G., and Pinnell, S. R.**, Isolation of type III collagen from human adult parenchymal lung, *Biochemistry*, 16, 185, 1977.

121. **Merry, A. H., Harwood, R., Woolley, D. E., Grant, M. E., and Jackson, D. S.**, Identification and partial characterization of the non-collagenous amino- and carboxyl-terminal extension peptides of cartilage procollagen, *Biochem. Biophys. Res. Commun.*, 71, 83, 1976.

122. **Miller, E. J., Finch, J. E., Jr., Chung, E., and Butler, W. T.**, Specific cleavage of the native type III collagen molecule with trypsin, *Arch. Biochem. Biophys.*, 173, 631, 1976.

123. **Miller, E. J., Martin, G. R., Piez, K. A., and Powers, M. J.**, Characterization of chick bone collagen and compositional changes associated with maturation, *J. Biol. Chem.*, 242, 5481, 1967.

124. **Miller, E. J. and Matukas, V. J.**, Biosynthesis of collagen — the biochemist's view, *Fed. Proc.*, 33, 1197, 1974.

125. **Miller, E. J., Woodall, D. L., and Vail, M. S.**, Biosynthesis of cartilage collagen: use of pulse labeling to order the cyanogen bromide peptides in the $\alpha 1$ (II) chain, *J. Biol. Chem.*, 248, 1666, 1973.

126. **Miller, R. L.**, Chromatographic separation of the enzymes required for hydroxylation of lysine and proline residues of protocollagen, *Arch. Biochem. Biophys.*, 147, 339, 1971.

127. **Miller, R. L. and Udenfriend S.**, Hydroxylation of proline residues in collagen nascent chains, *Arch. Biochem. Biophys.*, 139, 104, 1970.

128. **Minor, R. R., Clark, C. C., Strause, E. L., Koszalka, T. R., Brent, R. L., and Kefalides, N. A.**, Basement membrane procollagen is not converted to collagen in organ cultures of parietal yolk sac endoderm, *J. Biol. Chem.*, 251, 1789, 1976.

129. **Minor, R. R., Hoch, P. S., Koszalka, T. R., Brent, R. L., and Kefalides, N. A.,** Organ cultures of the embryonic rat parietal yolk sac. I. Morphologic and autoradiographic studies of the deposition of the collagen and the noncollagen glycoprotein components of basement membrane, *Dev. Biol.*, 48, 344, 1976.
130. **Minor, R. R., Strause, E. L., Koszalka, T. R., Brent, R. L., and Kefalides, N. A.,** Organ cultures of the embryonic rat parietal yolk sac. II. Synthesis, accumulation, and turnover of collagen and noncollagen basement membrane glycoproteins, *Dev. Biol.*, 48, 365, 1976.
131. **Misirowski, R. L., Ulreich, J. B., and Chvapil, M.,** A microassay for lysyl oxidase activity, *Anal. Biochem.*, 71, 186, 1976.
132. **Monson, J. M. and Bornstein, P.,** Identification of a disulfide-linked procollagen as the biosynthetic precursor of chick-bone collagen, *Proc. Natl. Acad. Sci. U.S.A.*, 70, 3521, 1973.
133. **Monson, J. M., Click, E. M., and Bornstein, P.,** Further characterization of procollagen. Purification and analysis of pro $\alpha 1$ chain of chick bone procollagen, *Biochemistry*, 14, 4088, 1975.
134. **Morris, N. P., Fessler, L. I., Weinstock, A., and Fessler, J. H.,** Procollagen assembly and secretion in embryonic chick bone, *J. Biol. Chem.*, 250, 5719, 1975.
135. **Murphy, L. and Rosenbloom, J.,** Evidence that chick tendon procollagen must be denatured to serve as substrate for proline hydroxylase, *Biochem. J.*, 135, 249, 1973.
136. **Murphy, W. H., von der Mark, K., McEneany, L. S. G., and Bornstein, P.,** Characterization of procollagen-derived peptides unique to the precursor molecule, *Biochemistry*, 14, 3243, 1975.
137. **Myllylä, R., Kuutti-Savolainen, E.-R., and Kivirikko, K. I.,** The role of ascorbate in the prolyl hydroxylase reaction, *Biochem. Biophys. Res. Commun.*, 83(2), 441, 1978.
138. **Narayanan, A. S., Siegel, R. C., and Martin, G. R.,** On the inhibition of lysyl oxidase by β-aminopropionitrile, *Biochem. Biophys. Res. Commun.*, 46, 745, 1972.
139. **Narayanan, A. S., Siegel, R. C., and Martin, G. R.,** Stability and purification of lysyl oxidase, *Arch. Biochem. Biophys.*, 162, 231, 1974.
140. **Newman, R. A. and Langner, R. O.,** Age related changes in the synthesis of connective tissues in the rabbit, *Connect. Tissue Res.*, 3, 231, 1975.
141. **Nist, C., von der Mark, K., Hay, E. D., Olsen, B. R., Bornstein, P., Ross, R., and Dehm, P.,** Location of procollagen in chick corneal and tendon fibroblasts with ferritin-conjugated antibodies, *J. Cell Biol.*, 65, 75, 1975.
142. **Olmsted, J. B. and Borisy, G. G.,** Microtubules, *Annu. Rev. Biochem.*, 42, 507, 1973.
143. **Olsen, B. R., Berg, R. A., Kishida, Y., and Prockop, D. J.,** Further characterization of embryonic tendon fibroblasts and the use of immunoferritin techniques to study collagen biosynthesis, *J. Cell Biol.*, 64, 340, 1975.
144. **Oppenheim, B. and Englard, S.,** Inhibition by collagen chains of lysyl hydroxylase of chick embryo and of WI-38 human lung fibroblasts, *Biochem. Biophys. Res. Commun.*, 70, 248, 1976.
145. **Oppenheim, B. and Englard, S.,** Inhibition of prolyl hydroxylase by collagen, *Biochem. Biophys. Res. Commun.*, 59, 710, 1974.

145a. **Osborn, M. and Weber, K.,** Cytoplasmic microtubules in tissue culture cells appear to grow from an organizing structure towards the plasma membrane, *Proc. Natl. Acad. Sci. U.S.A.*, 73, 867, 1976.

146. **Pänkäläinen, M., Aro, H., Simons, K., and Kivirikko, K. I.,** Protocollagen proline hydroxylase: molecular weight, subunits and isoelectric point, *Biochim. Biophys. Acta*, 221, 559, 1970.
147. **Pawlowski, P. J., Gillette, M. T., Martinelli, J., and Lukens, L. N.,** Identification and purification of collagen - synthesizing polysomes with anti-collagen antibodies, *J. Biol. Chem.*, 250, 2135, 1975.
148. **Peterkofsky, B. and Udenfriend, S.,** Conversion of proline to collagen hydroxyproline in a cell-free system from chick embryo, *J. Biol. Chem.*, 238, 3966, 1963.
149. **Pickrell, J. A., Harris, D. V., Benjamin, S. A., Cuddihy, R. G., Pfleger, R. C., and Mauderly, J. L.,** Pulmonary collagen metabolism after lung injury from inhaled ^{90}Y in fused clay particles, *Exp. Mol. Pathol.*, 25, 70, 1976.
150. **Pickrell, J. A., Harris, D. V., Hahn, F. F., Belasich, J. J., and Jones, R. K.,** Biological alterations resulting from chronic lung irradiation. III. Effect of partial ^{60}Co thoracic irradiation upon pulmonary collagen metabolism and fractionation in Syrian hamsters, *Radiat. Res.*, 62, 133, 1975.
151. **Pickrell, J. A., Harris, D. V., Mauderly, J. L., and Hahn, F. F.,** Altered collagen metabolism in radiation-induced interstitial pulmonary fibrosis, *Chest*, 69, 311, 1976.
152. **Pickrell, J. A., Harris, D. V., Pfleger, R. C., Benjamin, S. A., Belasich, J. J., Jones, R. K., and McClellan, R. O.,** Biological alterations resulting from chronic lung irradiation. II. Connective tissue alterations following inhalation of ^{144}Ce fused clay aerosol in Beagle dogs, *Radiat. Res.*, 63, 299, 1975.

152a. **Pickrell, J. A. and Rodriquez, R.,** Research communication, 1977.

152b. **Pickrell, J. A., Straus, F. C., and Harris, D. V.,** Research communication, 1976.

153. **Piez, K. A.**, Cross-linking of collagen and elastin, *Annu. Rev. Biochem.*, 37, 547, 1968.

154. **Piez, K. A. and Miller, A.**, The structure of collagen fibrils, *J. Supramol. Struct.*, 2, 121, 1974.

155. **Pinnel, S. R. and Martin, G. R.**, The crosslinking of collagen and elastin: enzymatic conversion of lysine in peptide linkage to α-aminoadipic-δ-semi-aldehyde (allysine) by an extract of bone, *Proc. Natl. Acad. Sci. U.S.A.*, 61, 708, 1968.

156. **Pinto, J. S. and Bentley, J. P.**, The timecourse of collagen cross-linking, *Biochim. Biophys. Acta*, 354, 254, 1974.

157. **Popenoe, E. A. and Aronson, R. B.**, Partial purification and properties of collagen lysine hydroxylase from chick embryos, *Biochim. Biophys. Acta*, 258, 380, 1972.

158. **Pritchard, P. M., Staton, G. W., Jr., and Cutroneo, K. R.**, *In vitro* synthesis of collagen peptides on fetal and neonatal rat skin polysomes by rabbit reticulocyte initiation factors, *Arch. Biochem. Biophys.*, 163, 178, 1974.

159. **Prockop, D. J. and Juva, K.**, Synthesis of hydroxyproline *in vitro* by the hydroxylation of proline in a precursor of collagen, *Proc. Natl. Acad. Sci. U.S.A.*, 53, 661, 1965.

160. **Prockop, D. J., Berg, R. A., Kivirikko, K. I., and Uitto, J.**, Intracellular steps in the biosynthesis of collagen, in *Biochemistry of Collagen*, Ramachandran, G. N. and Reddi, A. H., Eds., Plenum Press, New York, 1976, 163.

161. **Quinn, R. S., Rosenblatt, M., and Krane, S. M.**, Proteolytic activity in human skin fibroblasts harvested with trypsin and its effect on measurements of collagen hydroxylase activities, *Biochem. Biophys. Res. Commun.*, 71, 300, 1976.

162. **Raj, C. V. S., Church, R. L., Creagan, R. P., and Ruddle, F. H.**, *J. Cell Biol.*, 70, A78, 1976; as cited in **Fessler, J. H., and Fessler, L. I.**, Biosynthesis of procollagen, *Annu. Rev. Biochem.*, 47, 129, 1978.

163. **Ramaley, P. B., Jimenez, S. A., and Rosenbloom, J.**, Conformation of underhydroxylated collagen synthesized by 3T6 fibroblasts in culture, *FEBS Lett.*, 33, 187, 1973.

164. **Rapaka, R. S., Renugopalakrishnan, V., Urry, D. W., and Bhatnagar, R. S.**, Hydroxylation of proline in polytripeptide models of collagen: stereochemistry of polytripeptide-prolyl hydroxylase interaction, *Biochemistry*, 17(14), 2892, 1978.

165. **Revel, M. and Groner, Y.**, Post-transcriptional and translational controls of gene expression in eukaryotes, *Annu. Rev. Biochem.*, 47, 1079, 1978.

166. **Rhoads, R. E. and Udenfriend, S.**, Purification and properties of collagen proline hydroxylase from newborn rat skin, *Arch. Biochem. Biophys.*, 139, 329, 1970.

167. **Rhoads, R. E., Udenfriend, S., and Bornstein, P.**, *In vitro* enzymatic hydroxylation of prolyl residues in the α1-CB2 fragment of rat collagen, *J. Biol. Chem.*, 246, 4138, 1971.

168. **Rojkind, M. and Zeichner, M.**, Maturation of collagen and elastin, in *Molecular Pathology of Connective Tissues*, Vol. 3 of *The Biochemistry of Disease*, Pérez-Tamayo, R., and Rojkind, M., Eds., Marcel Dekker, New York, 1973, 135.

169. **Rokosova, B. and Chvapil, M.**, Relationship between the dose of ascorbic acid and its structural analogs and proline hydroxylation in various biological systems, *Connect. Tissue Res.*, 2, 215, 1974.

170. **Rosenbloom, J. and Prockop, D. J.**, Incorporation of cis-hydroxyproline into protocollagen and collagen. Collagen containing cis-hydroxyproline in place of proline and trans-hydroxyproline is not extruded at a normal rate, *J. Biol. Chem.*, Σ 46, 1549, 1971.

171. **Ryhänen, L. and Kivirikko, K. I.**, Developmental changes in protocollagen lysyl hydroxylase activity in chick embryo, *Biochim. Biophys. Acta*, 343, 121, 1974.

172. **Sabatini, D. D., Ojakian, G., Lande, M. A., Lewis, J., Mok, W., Adesnik, M., and Kreibich, G.**, Structural and functional aspects of the protein synthesizing apparatus in the rough endoplasmic reticulum, *Adv. Exp. Med. Biol.*, 62, 151, 1974.

173. **Satir, B.**, The final steps in secretion, *Sci. Am.*, 233(4), 29, 1975.

174. **Schneir, M. and Miller, E.**, The absence of sulfhydryl group reactivity in type III collagen, paper presented at meeting of West Coast Connective Tissue Society, Heber, Utah, March 5 to 7, 1976.

175. **Schofield, J. D. and Prockop, D. J.**, Procollagen — a precursor form of collagen, *Clin. Orthop.*, 97, 175, 1973.

176. **Seyer, J. M., Hutcheson, E. T., and Kang, A. H.**, Collagen polymorphism in idiopathic chronic pulmonary fibrosis, *J. Clin. Invest.*, 57, 1498, 1976.

177. **Shatkin, A. J., Banerjee, A. K., Both, G. W., Furuichi, Y., and Muthukrishnan, S.**, Dependence of translation on 5′-terminal methylation of mRNA, *Fed. Proc.*, 35, 2214, 1976.

178. **Sherr, C. J., Taubman, M. B., and Goldberg, B.**, Isolation of a disulfide-stabilized, three-chain polypeptide fragment unique to the precursor of human collagen, *J. Biol. Chem.*, 248, 7033, 1973.

179. **Siegel, R. C.**, Collagen cross-linking, synthesis of collagen cross-links *in vitro* with highly purified lysyl oxidase, *J. Biol. Chem.*, 251, 5786, 1976.

179a. **Siegel, R. C. and Fu, J. C. C.**, Collagen cross-linking; purification and substrate specificity by lysyl oxidase, *J. Biol. Chem.*, 251, 5779, 1976.

180. **Siegel, R. C.,** Biosynthesis of collagen cross-links: increased activity of purified lysyl oxidase with reconstituted collagen fibrils, *Proc. Natl. Acad. Sci. U.S.A.,* 71, 4826, 1974.
181. **Siegel, R. C., Pinnell, S. R., and Martin, G. R.,** Cross-linking of collagen and elastin. Properties of lysyl oxidase, *Biochemistry,* 9, 4486, 1970.
182. **Smith, B. D., Byers, P. H., and Martin, G. R.,** Production of procollagen by human fibroblasts in culture, *Proc. Natl. Acad. Sci. U.S.A.,* 69, 3260, 1972.
183. **Speakman, P. T.,** Proposed mechanism for the biological assembly of the collagen triple helix, *Nature (London),* 229, 241, 1971.
184. **Spiro, R. G.,** Characterization and quantitative determination of the hydroxylysine-linked carbohydrate units of several collagens, *J. Biol. Chem.,* 244, 602, 1969.
185. **Spiro, R. G. and Spiro, M. J.,** Studies on the biosynthesis of the hydroxylysine-linked disaccharide unit of basement membranes and collagens. III. Tissue and subcellular distribution of glycosyltransferases and the effect of various conditions on the enzyme levels, *J. Biol. Chem.,* 246, 4919, 1971.
186. **Stanley, N. N., Alper, R., Cunningham, E. L., Cherniack, N. S., and Kefalides, N. A.,** Effects of a molecular change in collagen on lung structure and mechanical function, *J. Clin. Invest.,* 55, 1195, 1975.
187. **Stassen, F. L. H., Cardinale, G. J., McGee, J. O'D., and Udenfriend, S.,** Prolyl hydroxylase and an immunologically related protein in mammalian tissues, *Arch. Biochem. Biophys.,* 160, 340, 1974.
188. **Stephens, R. E. and Edds, K. T.,** Microtubules: structure, chemistry, and function, *Physiol. Rev.,* 56, 709, 1976.
189. **Taubman, M. B. and Goldberg, B.,** The processing of procollagen in cultures of human and mouse fibroblasts, *Arch. Biochem. Biophys.,* 173, 490, 1976.
190. **Trelstad, R. L.,** The Golgi apparatus in chick corneal epithelium: changes in intracellular position during development, *J. Cell Biol.,* 45, 34, 1970.
191. **Trelstad, R. L.,** Vacuoles in the embryonic chick corneal epithelium, an epithelium which produces collagen, *J. Cell Biol.,* 48, 689, 1971.
192. **Tuderman, L., Kuutti, E. R., and Kivirikko, K. I.,** An affinity-column procedure using poly(L-proline) for the purification of prolyl hydroxylase. Purification of the enzyme from chick embryos, *Eur. J. Biochem.,* 52, 9, 1975.
192a. **Tuderman, L., Kivirikko, K. I., and Prockop, D. J.,** Partial purification and characterization of a neutral protease which cleaves the N-terminal propeptides from procollagen, *Biochemistry,* 17, 2948, 1978.
193. **Uitto, J.,** A method for studying collagen biosynthesis in human skin biopsies *in vitro, Biochim. Biophys. Acta,* 201, 438, 1970.
194. **Veis, A., Anesey, J., Yuan, L., and Levy, S. J.,** Evidence for an amino-terminal extension in high-molecular-weight collagens from mature bovine skin, *Proc. Natl. Acad. Sci. U.S.A.,* 70, 1464, 1973.
195. **Veis, A. and Brownell, A. G.,** Collagen biosynthesis, *Crit. Rev. Biochem.,* 2, 417, 1975.
195a. **Vuust, J. and Piez, K. A.,** A kinetic study of collagen biosynthesis, *J. Biol. Chem.,* 247, 856, 1972.
195b. **Vuust, J. and Piez, K. A.,** Biosynthesis of the α chains of collagen studied by pulse-labeling in culture, *J. Biol. Chem.,* 245, 6201, 1970.
196. **Weinstock, M. and Leblond, C. P.,** Formation of collagen, *Fed. Proc.,* 33, 1205, 1974.
197. **Williams, I. F., Harwood, R., and Grant, M. E.,** Triple helix formation and disulphide bonding during the biosynthesis of glomerular basement membrane collagen, *Biochem. Biophys. Res. Commun.,* 70, 200, 1976.
198. **Woessner, J. F., Jr., Bashey, R. I., and Boucek, R.,** Collagen development in heart and skin of the chick embryo, *Biochim. Biophys. Acta,* 140, 329, 1967.

Chapter 6

COLLAGEN DEGRADATION

J. A. Pickrell

TABLE OF CONTENTS

I. GENERAL

Continual synthesis of collagen in adult lungs whose collagen concentration is unchanged suggests that considerable collagen degradation occurs. Native collagen is resistant to degradation by non-specific proteases at neutral pH. As late as 1959[27] collagen was believed to be resistant to degradation at this pH. However, the discovery of tadpole and subsequently of mammalian collagenase[22] led to the characterization of vertebrate collagenase.

Collagenase cleaves native collagen extracellularly and at neutral pH into two fragments by splitting a specific gly-ile bond. The reduced susceptibility of type II collagen is currently undefined. This enzyme attacks native collagen in either neutral solution or in native or reconstituted fibrillar form making a single cleavage through triple helical collagen. Gelatin is a poor collagenase substrate,[44] indicating the influence of conformation upon collagenase activity, probably by collagenase binding to collagen.[74] Several reviews[22,24,27,47,48] indicate that vertebrate collagenase cleaves collagen into two tropocollagen (TC) fragments (TC^A three fourths and TC^B one fourth of the original length). These are further digested into small fragments by proteases. In several specific instances[22] collagenase cleaves one or two fragments, leaving TC^A at 67 or 62% of the original length, similar to that observed by Wahl et al.[68] in macrophage collagenase. A specific gly-ile bond is split in the sequence gly-x-gly-ile-ala-gly-x-y.[23a,48] These enzymes are secreted and attack collagen in the extracellular space.[24] Miller[45] reviewed the cleavage site in various collagen chains and reached the conclusion that it is highly conserved. Pulmonary alveolar macrophages,[30,31] platelets,[13] and polymorphonuclear leucocytes[52] have demonstrable collagenolytic activity at neutral pH, as have fibroblasts in culture.[7,46,53,72,91] Collagenases from a variety of sources are immunologically similar. Bauer et al.,[4] using immunofluorescence, indicated collagenase to be located at the peripheral edge of the alveolar septa and in the interstitum, in each case delineating delicate collagen fibrils. The lack of susceptibility of type II collagen to collagenase[22,25,47,56] may indicate an effect of either binding or catalysis. Such effect may relate to the carbohydrate attachments of cartilage. However, the low molecular weight collagenase inhibitor (11,000 daltons) isolated from cartilage[37] may contribute to this reduced susceptibility.

Increased levels of collagenase are associated with dividing cells and with rapid collagen synthesis. Colchicine, which inhibits these, is also associated with higher collagenase levels than expected. Collagenase is associated with rapidly dividing cells in wound healing, in epithelial cells, and in rheumatoid nodules.[27] Wirl[73,73a] measured extractable collagenase on mouse skin after 3-methylcholanthrene application. This finding tends to support that made by Harris and Krane.[27] Bosmann et al.[11] report that aging WI-38 cells lack a critical neutral protease. Strauch[64] and Mazzucco[43] indicate collagenolytic activity to be qualitatively associated with tumor invasiveness. Pérez-Tamayo[53] reviews findings that suggest collagenase levels may even correlate with clinical outcome of some neoplasms and that collagenase is elevated in experimental wound healing. The site of rabbit V_2-carcinoma apparently influences collagenolytic activity.[9] Kuettner et al.[39] note that both osteosarcoma and mammary carcinoma produce collagenase when cultured. The association of cultured dividing cells with collagenolytic activity lends support to this idea. Colchicine (0.1 $\mu g/m\ell$) increases collagenase 10 times in cultures of rheumatoid synovium. Increased collagenase may reflect an attempt of cells to divide at an increased rate to offset reduced collagen secretion,[23] although colchicine inhibits mitosis. The meaning is unclear. At the same time that collagen deposition in chick embryo skin became maximal, collagenolysis (as measured by ultrafilterable hydroxyproline) and collagenase activity by 3 *M* NaSCN were likewise maximal,[35] indicating a relation to rapidly synthesizing and presumably rapidly dividing connective tissue cells. Proteases can induce the secretion of collagenase and plasminogen activator in rabbit synovial fibroblasts.[70] Pickrell et al.[55] observed increased collagenolysis (ultrafilterable hydroxyproline) in irradiated lungs from Syrian hamsters prior to increased synthesis and accumulation of collagen, or to increased lysosomal activity (acid phosphatase). These findings suggest that lung collagenase may be of importance in the regenerating, injured lung. Although collagenase has been primarily observed in alveolar macrophages,[30] collagenases from other sources may be present in the complex pulmonary parenchyma.

II. INHIBITION

Collagenase is inhibited by serum, but albumin, the major serum protein, is not a collagenase inhibitor. Collagenase is inhibited by EDTA, dithiothreitol, phenylmethyl sulfonyl fluoride, cysteine, and serum (human, sheep, calf, and fetal calf) histones and egg white lysozyme, but not by other protease inhibitors such as *n*-ethylmaleimide (NEM), parachloromercuribenzoate (PCMB), soybean trypsin inhibitor, Tos-lys-Ch_2Cl, tos-phe-CH_2Cl, Ac-$(Ala)_3$ Ala CH_2Cl, Ac-$(Ala)_2$ pro ala CH_2Cl, pepstatin, and bovine serum albumin.[23,30,71] Both $alpha_1$ antitrypsin, and $alpha_2$ macroglobulin inhibit collagenase. The nature of this inhibitor has intrigued numerous workers. Nagai et al.[48] review his earlier work[1,2] leading to the discovery that α_2 macroglobulin binds tenaciously to collagenase, inactivating it. The α_2-macroglobulin-collagenase complex is partially disassociated by 3 *M* NaSCN. In vivo importance of regulation of collagenase activity is apparent, considering work of Abe and Nagai,[1] Nagai,[47] and Abe et al.,[3] in which latent collagenase was isolated from rheumatoid synovial fluid. This latent collagenase could be activated by 3 *M* NaSCN and was much higher in rheumatoid than in normal synovial fluid. Moreover, both α_2 macroglobulin and α_1 antitrypsin were also increased, suggesting attempts at biological compensation. Bauer et al.[5,6] noted that both α_2 macroglobulin and α_1 antitrypsin (AAT) inhibit collagenase, although AAT binds collagenase less tenaciously.[48] Wahl[67] has shown that collagenase increases following inducement of endotoxin shock. This response is not present in pregnant animals. Moreover, Jeffrey et al.[34] have shown that progesterone inhibits the production of active collagenase by uterine culture.

An α-globulin is present in sera and inhibits collagenase. The presence of an α-macroglobulin in the sera of normal pregnant women and pregnant women with cancer was observed.[59,60,62] This was characterized[62] as an α_2-globulin peculiar to the maternal circulation and with a molecular weight of 507,000, containing glucose, galactose, mannose, sialic acid, and glucosamine. Whether this has the same role as the α_2 macroglobulin elucidated by Nagai et al.[48] is the subject of considerable interest. Likewise the ability of human leucocytes to synthesize this pregnancy associated α-macroglobulin[61] raises important questions relating to its role in injury, since it can be synthesized locally by leucocytes. Measurement of this constituent by radioimmunoassay[63] provides the tool to follow such relationships. The increase of α_1 antitrypsin in pregnancy[20,41] is likewise interesting. The relationship of these constituents to the blockage of collagenase increases in pregnant rats[67] may be quite revealing when characterized.

The role of low molecular weight inhibitors of collagenase is somewhat less definitively elucidated. However, they may migrate from plasma to tissue; they may be associated with neoplasia resistance. Jeffrey, in discussing the results presented by Nagai et al.,[48] indicates that although α_1 antitrypsin (AAT) will inhibit collagenase,[5] it binds much less tenaciously on a molar basis than does α_2 macroglobulin. This is not surprising, because there is much more AAT than α_2 macroglobulin. Moreover, the reversible binding would be of more use as a modulator than would the stronger macroglobulin binding. The suggestion that collagenase action might be modulated in vivo by more than one substance is an intriguing one. Certainly the low molecular weight compounds which can escape the bloodstream provide a means of passive regulation of collagenase at sites distant from its production. The vasodilation of inflammation would tend to provide more of this antiprotease, offsetting the increased proteolysis. The close correlation between in vivo degradation rates and lysosomal activity[57] indicates not only the tools to study such proteolysis, but also the value of determining lysosomal activity. This mechanism would be a useful adjunct to other regulatory mechanisms. Kuettner et al.[37,38] who isolated low molecular weight inhibitors (11,000 daltons) from aorta and cartilage indicate the presence of inhibitors of collagenolytic action which are distinct from either AAT or α_2 macroglobulin. These low molecular weight cationic proteins can be extracted from cartilage and aorta.[37] Platelet factor IV is also a low molecular weight collagenase inhibitor,[29] probably to maintain collagen for attachment in platelet adhesion. As will be discussed in Chapter 9, platelet attachment also requires cold insoluble globulin. These inhibitors are especially interesting in light of the ability of cartilage or aorta extracts to suppress tumor growth,[16,19] the relationship of collagenase to this tumor growth,[9,27,64] and the suppression of tumor collagenase by a low molecular weight inhibitor of collagenase isolated from cartilage.[37-39]

III. PROPERTIES AND ASSAY

Active collagenase has a variable size and requires calcium. Molecular weight of rheumatoid synovial collagenase ≃25,000 or ≃50,000 daltons is within the range of bone and gingiva (41,000) and cornea (65,000), although higher values (≃80,000 to 160,000) have been observed in cornea, mouse bone, and tadpole skin.[47] Seltzer et al.[58] have shown that calcium is essential for thermostabilization of collagenase between 30 and 40°C, whether collagen is present or not. Ba^{++} and Sr^{++} may serve as effective substitutes in human skin but not in rat uterus or skin. The concentration of Ca^{++} necessary to achieve half-maximal activation was 0.5 m*M*. However, calcium seems to play no role in the binding of collagen to collagenase.

Pérez-Tamayo[53] in his excellent review on collagen degradation indicates that collagenase is most frequently measured by explanting the tissue in question and culturing it in a medium without serum. The medium is changed every 1 to 2 days, collected, precipitated with 40 to 60% ammonium sulfate, redissolved in 0.05 *M* TRIS buffer, pH 7.4, 0.005 *M* $CaCl_2$, and extensively dialyzed against that buffer. It may be activated by limited proteolysis with trypsin[53,72] or with 3.0 *M* NaSCN or NaI.[1] Some workers measure collagenase from direct tissue extracts and claim recovery of 60 to 70%.[69] These methods use the 6000 g pellet followed by either heating at 60°C for short time periods or exposure to 5.0 *M* urea. They seem to be extracting collagen-bound collagenase. Collagenase is normally bound to structural forms of collagen.[46] This collagenase may be separated from collagen after denaturation by acrylamide gel electrophoresis. The collagenase is in the lower one half of the gel but is recovered with a low yield. Alternatively, prolonged digestion with trypsin (5 days) will release collagenase in extremely low yield.[53] High yields of collagenase have been obtained by serum free cultures of fibroblasts from human skin, polymorphonuclear leucocytes,[51] and platelets.[13] Collagenase has not been extracted directly from pulmonary tissue, but is present in pulmonary macrophages.[30,31,53]

Most collagenase assays[22,27] are based upon the solubilization of labelled peptides from collagen fibrils and the quantification of such released peptides. Lysis of collagen gels with tissue fragments is a more graphic but less sensitive procedure. Levenson[42] has developed a collagen film microassay using collagenolysis of film and subsequent staining with Coomasie Blue. Recently, others[33,40] utilized an extremely high specific activity tritiated collagen fibril in a peptide release assay and achieved substantial increase of apparent sensitivity. Further work with these assays may reveal subtle facets of the collagenase mechanisms.

IV. CLEAVAGE

The steps of neutral collagenolytic cleavage are reviewed by Harris and Krane.[27] Collagenase initially cleaves all three α-chains into TC^A (three fourths) and TC^B (one fourth) fragments. The triple helix facilitates enzyme recognition, cleavage, or both. Since the melting temperatures of TC^A (32°C) and TC^B (29°C) are less than body temperature, these fragments are immediately solubilized and denatured if not bound to other molecules by intermolecular cross-links. Finally, the solubilized and denatured fragments may be degraded by proteases either intra- or extracellularly, often at acid but occasionally at neutral pH. The fate of cross-linked fragments is poorly understood, but cross-links make collagen more resistant to digestion with collagenase, and purified cartilage collagen fibrils have been shown to be 100 times more resistant to rheumatoid synovial collagenase than are non-cross-linked fibrils.[26,27,53] Some of this may be due to the presence of low molecular weight inhibitor of collagenase present in cartilage;[37-39] however, collagen degradation in vivo is simply not comparable to that measured in vitro. Collagenase acts considerably more slowly on cross-linked fibrils. However, in inflamed synovium the temperature is considerably higher, and collagenase increased 10 times in activity when incubated at 36 instead of 30°C. Recently synthesized collagen is more susceptible to degradation.[23b,36] An intriguing possibility[27] that during enhanced collagen resorption, fragments consisting of many molecules may be split from a collagen fiber, endocytized and degraded within phagolysosomes should be considered. This agrees well with the electron microscopic data reviewed by TenCate and DePorter[65] in fibroblasts and with preliminary data from Weinstock which they cite. The method of intracellular degradation is generally thought to be by lysosomal proteases at acid pH.[24] However, TenCate and DePorter[65] raise the possibility that collagenase may act intracellularly. If so, this must be at a neutral pH since Werb and Burleigh[71] have shown collagenase to be active at neutral pH. Coffey et al.[14] have shown lysosomal proteases which are collagenolytic to be active at acid pH. Further work is required to elucidate this interesting area.

V. PROCOLLAGENASE

Material which is probably procollagenase has been noted in tadpole tails, skin fibroblasts, bone culture medium, leucocyte homogenates, macrophages, and lymphocytes. Tadpole collagenase has been shown to be secreted as inactive procollagenase which is subsequently activated to collagenase.[28] This procollagenase is incapable of binding to collagen; incubation with collagenase free tail fin medium but not trypsin or chymotrypsin will activate the collagenase, freeing a portion which is heat labile and nondialyzable. The γG fraction of anticollagenase antisera blocked the activated collagenase as well as the purified tadpole collagenase. Neurath and Walsh[49] indicated several other zymogens which are activated by limited proteolysis. Bauer et al.[7] reported that collagenase can be activated after brief incubation with trypsin or by autoactivation. The inhibitor secreted by human skin fibroblasts is probably produced by the cells, and is not a residual of serum, and not α_1 antitrypsin. Materials which may be procollagenases have also been found in bone culture medium[66] and in leukocyte homogenates.[52] However, the presumptive zymogens have not been isolated and characterized.[23] It is obviously difficult to distinguish the cleavage of a fragment of procollagenase from the removal of a low molecular weight inhibitor of approximately equal size such as that isolated by Kvettner et al.[37-39] The possibility that both factors control collagenase in the same or different systems must be considered.[23] However, Horwitz et al.[32] have isolated a neutral protease which is secreted by and activates collagenase from alveolar macrophages. Lymphocytes stimulated by phytohemagglutinin A or concanavilin A secrete a 12,000-dalton compound and affect the product of rheumatoid synovial collagenase up to 400-fold.[15] The nature of this effect is undefined. Future investigations will define this problem more completely.

VI. CATHEPSINS

Cathepsins degrade collagen fragments intracellularly and at low pH, probably releasing collagen molecules. Cathepsin B-1 has been described in rat liver lysosomes.[12,27] It is capable of degrading collagen fibrils at acid pH. In contrast to vertebrate collagenases, it is activated by cysteine and EDTA, cleaving at multiple helical sites. Most other cathepsins do not attack collagen.[17] However, Etherington[17] proposes a collagenolytic cathepsin having many features of cathepsin B-1, but which chromatographs differently on DEAE Sephadex®. This enzyme may be different from cathepsin B-1. This enzyme had maximum activity at pH 3.5. It attacked cross-linked regions of collagen, not helical regions, indicating a potential role in degradation of endocytized collagen fragments. In a later paper Etherington[18] reported that collagenolytic cathepsin and cathepsin B-1 gave approximately equal collagen solubilization. These were less than or nearly equal to pepsin. The number and location of the intramolecular cross-links and the type and quantity of proteoglycans were important in determining the degree of resistance of the collagen to enzymatic dissolution.[18] Genetic type of collagen would seem to be of little importance in determining the extent of dissolution by these enzymes.[8] The cathepsins may act as a "cross-linkase" in vivo. Alternatively or additionally, they may play an important role of freeing underlying connective tissue by a mechanism analogous to that proposed by Goldstein et al.[21] for elastase. The susceptibility of fibronectin, an important protein in the extracellular matrix[10] to cathepsin has not been documented. However, a breakdown of fibronectin would surely free the intertwined collagen, break the cell-matrix association, and provide a stimulus for cell division. This will be discussed in some detail in Chapters 9 and 10.

Other lysosomal enzymes may degrade collagen (presumably freed from the matrix) at acid pH to form ultrafilterable hydroxyproline. Coffey et al.[14] report that lysosomes contain a mixture of proteinases and peptideases capable, at acid pH, of degrading collagen to amino acids and small peptides. Thus collagen molecules or fragments of collagen molecules incorporated by endocytosis into secondary lysosomes,[27,65] whose pH may be as low as 4, would be degraded, presumably within the lysosomes, to a mixture of amino acids and small peptides. The product of these processes might be represented by ultrafilterable hydroxyproline.

VII. INTRACELLULAR COLLAGEN BREAKDOWN

Intracellular breakdown of collagen can also occur on newly synthesized collagen chains and by enzymes other than cathepsins or external collagenase. Bienkowski et al.[8] demonstrated that 20 to 40% of the newly synthesized pulmonary collagen α-chains were destroyed within minutes of being synthesized and long before such chains would normally be extruded from the cell producing it. The percentage of newly synthesized collagen did not increase with time, occurred when no collagenase could be detected, even with activation, was independent of the addition of serum, inhibitors of proteolysis, sodium dodecyl sulfate, or boiling, was age invariant, and was noted to a similar extent in vivo four hr post injection with radiolabelled proline.[8] Four hr post injection was considered to be an optimal labelling period by numerous investigators. Pickrell et al.[54] noted that most radioactive CO_2 from a proline label had been exhaled by 3 to 5 hr post injection. Bienkowski et al.[8] obtained similar results in vitro using a radiolysine label. Radiolabelled hydroxyproline was found mostly in proteins >90,000 daltons and in peptides $\leqslant$200 daltons.[8] Pickrell and Straus[55a] have noted a significant fraction ($\sim$10%) of radiolabelled hydroxyproline present as ultrafilterable hydroxyproline peptides in normal hamster lungs when the hamsters were sacrificed 24 hr post injection of labelled proline and between 6 and 53 weeks of age. Obviously, clearance of the ultrafilterable hydroxyproline peptides is rapid. In this instance, they would seem to have a biological half-life of $\leqslant$1 day, comparing our data with that of Bienkowski et al.,[8] although such comparisons may not be completely valid. Thus, the quantity of ultrafilterable hydroxyproline peptides present reflected the very recent history of collagen breakdown. Degradation of newly synthesized collagen is probably a normal process independent of collagenase or phagocytosis, by which tissues may modulate the quantity, quality, or both of collagen being secreted from the cell. R. Crystal[14a] has reported that this response is modulated by β-adrenergic receptors in lung, constituting a rapid way of modulating collagen synthesis of some lung cells. Lungs of animals exposed to radioactive aerosols to produce pulmonary fibrosis had $\leqslant$60% as much label in low molecular weight hydroxyproline. This indicated that collagen breakdown was occurring more rapidly in these animals, correlating with the increased ultrafilterable hydroxyproline. This could most likely have been due to either extracellular breakdown or phagocytosis. Likewise the ultrafilterable hydroxyproline probably represents a modest underestimate in exposed animals, indicating that increases observed by this method may represent slight underestimates.

REFERENCES

1. **Abe, S. and Nagai, Y.**, Evidence for the presence of a latent form of collagenase in human rheumatoid synovial fluid, *J. Biochem.*, 71, 919, 1972.
2. **Abe, S. and Nagai, Y.**, Evidence for the presence of a complex of collagenase with α_2-macroglobulin in human rheumatoid synovial fluid: a possible regulatory mechanism of collagenase activity *in vivo*, *J. Biochem.*, 73 , 897, 1973.
3. **Abe, S., Shinmei, M., and Nagai, Y.**, Synovial collagenase and joint diseases: the significance of latent collagenase with special reference to rheumatoid arthritis, *J. Biochem.*, 73, 1007, 1973.
4. **Bauer, E. A., Eisen, A. Z., and Jeffery, J. J.**, Immunologic relationship of a purified human skin collagenase to other human and animal collagenases, *Biochim. Biophys. Acta*, 206, 152, 1970.
5. **Bauer, E. A., Eisen, A. Z., and Jeffrey, J. J.**, Studies on purified rheumatoid synovial collagenase *in vitro* and *in vivo*, *J. Clin. Invest.*, 50, 2056, 1971.
6. **Bauer, E. A., Jeffrey, J. J., and Eisen, A. Z.**, Preparation of three vertebrate collagenases in pure form, *Biochem. Biophys. Res. Commun.*, 44, 813, 1971.
7. **Bauer, E. A., Stricklin, G. P., Jeffrey, J. J., and Eisen, A. Z.**, Collagenase production by human skin fibroblasts, *Biochem. Biophys. Res. Commun.*, 64, 232, 1975.
8. **Bienkowski, R. S., Cowan, M. J., McDonald, J. A., and Crystal, R. G.**, Degradation of newly synthesized collagen, *J. Biol. Chem.*, 253(12), 4356, 1978.
9. **Biswas, C., Moran, W. P., Bloch, K. J., and Gross, J.**, Collagenolytic activity of rabbit V_2-carcinoma growing at multiple sites, *Biochem. Biophys. Res. Commun.*, 80(1), 33, 1978.
10. **Bornstein, P., Duksin, D., Balian, G., Davidson, J. M., and Crouch, E.**, Organization of extracellular proteins on the connective tissue cell surface: relevance to cell-matrix interactions *in vitro* and *in vivo*, *Ann. N.Y. Acad. Sci.*, 312, 93, 1978.

11. **Bosmann, H. B., Gutheil, R. L., Jr., and Case, K. R.,** Loss of a critical neutral protease in ageing WI-38 cells, *Nature (London),* 261, 499, 1976.
12. **Burleigh, P. M. C. and Poole, A. R., Eds.,** Dynamics of Connective Tissue Macromolecules, American Elsevier, New York, 1975.
13. **Chesney, C. M., Harper, E., and Colman, R. W.,** Human platelet collagenase, *J. Clin. Invest.,* 53, 1647, 1974.
14. **Coffey, J. W., Fiedler-Nagy, C., Georgiadis, A. G., and Salvador, R. S.,** Digestion of native collagen, denatured collagen, and collagen fragments by extracts of rat liver lysosomes, *J. Biol. Chem.,* 251, 5280, 1976.
14a. **Crystal, R.,** Post-translational control of collagen production by intracellular degradation, presented at the Western Connective Tissue Society Meeting, Seattle, Wash., February 9 to 11, 1979.
15. **Dayer, J. M., Russel, R. G. G., and Krane, S. M.,** Collagenase production by rheumatoid synovial cells: stimulation by a human lymphocyte factor, *Science,* 195, 181, 1977.
16. **Eisenstein, R., Schumacher, B., Meineke, C., Matijevitch, B., and Kuettner, K. E.,** Growth regulators in connective tissue. Systemic administration of an aortic extract inhibits tumor growth in mice, *Am. J. Pathol.,* 91(1), 1, 1978.
17. **Etherington, D. J.,** The nature of the collagenolytic cathepsin of rat liver and its distribution in other rat tissues, *Biochem. J.,* 127, 685, 1972.
18. **Etherington, D. J.,** The dissolution of insoluble bovine collagens by cathepsin B1, collagenolytic cathepsin and pepsin, *Connect. Tissue Res.,* 5, 135, 1977.
19. **Folkman, J.,** The vascularization of tumors, *Sci. Am.,* 234(5), 59, 1976.
20. **Ganrot, P. O. and Bjerre, B.,** Alpha$_1$-antitrypsin and alpha$_2$-macroglobulin concentration in serum during pregnancy, *Acta Obstet. Gynecol. Scand.,* 46, 126, 1967.
21. **Goldstein, R. H., Faris, B., Hu, C. L., Snider, G. L., and Franzblau, C.,** The fate of newly synthesized lung collagen after endotracheal administration of ^{14}C-proline to hamsters, *Am. Rev. Respir. Dis.,* 117, 281, 1978.
22. **Gross, J.,** Collagen biology: structure, degradation and disease, *Harvey Lect.,* 68, 351, 1974.
23. **Gross, J.,** Aspects of the animal collagenases, in *Biochemistry of Collagen,* Ramachandran, G. N. and Reddi, A. H., Eds., Plenum Press, New York, 1976, 275.
23a. **Gross, J., Harper, E., Harris, E. D., Jr., McCroskery, P., Highberger, J. H., Corbett, C., and Kang, A. H.,** Animal collagenases: specificity of action and structures of the substrate cleavage site, *Biochem. Biophys. Res. Commun.,* 61, 605, 1974.
23b. **Gross, J. and Bruschi, A. B.,** The pattern of collagen degradation in cultured tadpole tissues, *Dev. Biol.,* 26, 36, 1971.
24. **Hance, A. J. and Crystal, R. G.,** The connective tissue of lung, *Am. Rev. Respir. Dis.,* 112, 657, 1975.
25. **Harris, E. D. and Krane, S. M.,** An endopeptidase from rheumatoid synovial culture, *Biochim. Biophys. Acta,* 258, 566, 1972.
26. **Harris, E. D. and Krane, S. M.,** Cartilage collagen: substrate in soluble and fibrillar form for rheumatoid collagenase, *Trans. Assoc. Am. Physicians,* 86, 82, 1973.
27. **Harris, E. D. and Krane, S. M.,** Collagenases (I, II, III), *N. Engl. J. Med.,* 291, 557, 605, 652, 1974.
28. **Harper, E., Bloch, K. J., and Gross, J.,** The zymogen of tadpole collagenase, *Biochemistry,* 10, 3035, 1971.
29. **Hiti-Harper, J., Wohl, H., and Harper, E.,** Platelet factor 4: an inhibitor of collagenase, *Science,* 199, 991, 1978.
30. **Horwitz, A. L. and Crystal, R. G.,** Collagenase from rabbit pulmonary alveolar macrophages, *Biochem. Biophys. Res. Commun.,* 69, 296, 1976.
31. **Horwitz, A. L., Kelman, J. A., Brin, S. C., and Crystal, R. G.,** Collagenase production by lung cells in culture, *Fed. Proc. Abstr.,* 35, 1740, 1976.
32. **Horwitz, A. L., Kelman, J. A., and Crystal, R. G.,** Activation of alveolar macrophage collagenase by a neutral protease secreted by the same cell, *Nature (London),* 264, 772, 1976.
33. **Hu, C. L., Crombie, G., and Franzblau, C.,** A new assay for collagenolytic activity, *Anal. Biochem.,* 88(2), 638, 1978.
34. **Jeffrey, J. J., Coffey, R. J., and Eisen, A. Z.,** Studies of uterine collagenase in tissue culture. I. Relationship of enzyme production to collagen metabolism, *Biochim. Biophys. Acta,* 252, 136, 1971.
35. **Kawamoto, T. and Nagai, Y.,** Developmental changes in glycosaminoglycans, collagen and collagenase activity in embryonic chick skin, *Biochim. Biophys. Acta,* 437, 190, 1976.
36. **Krane, S. M., Munoz, A. J., and Harris, E. D.,** Urinary polypeptides related to collagen synthesis, *J. Clin. Invest.,* 49, 716, 1970.
37. **Kuettner, K. E., Hiti, J., Eisenstein, R., and Harper, E.,** Collagenase inhibition by cationic proteins derived from cartilage and aorta, *Biochem. Biophys. Res. Commun.,* 72, 40, 1976.

38. **Kuettner, K. E., Soble, L., Croxen, R. L., Marczynska, B., Hiti, J., and Harper, E.,** Tumor cell collagenase and its inhibition by a cartilage-derived protease inhibitor, *Science,* 196, 653, 1977.
39. **Kuettner, K. E., Soble, L., Croxen, R., Hiti, J., Harper, E., and Paul, B.,** Inhibition of tumor collagenases by a cartilage-derived inhibitor, *Fed. Proc. Abstr.,* 36, 677, 1977.
40. **LaBrosse, K. R., Liener, I. E., and Hargrave, P. A.,** A sensitive assay for collagenolytic activity using tritiated collagen, *Anal. Biochem.,* 70, 218, 1976.
41. **Laurell, C.-B., Kullander, S., and Thorell, J.,** Effect of administration of a combined estrogen-progestin contraceptive on the level of individual plasma proteins, *Scand. J. Clin. Lab. Invest.,* 21, 337, 1968.
42. **Levenson, R.,** A collagen film microassay for tissue collagenase, *Anal. Biochem.,* 76, 579, 1976.
43. **Mazzucco, K.,** The role of collagen in tissue interactions during carcinogenesis in mouse skin, in *Tissue Interactions in Carcinogenesis,* Tarin, D., Ed., Academic Press, New York, 1972, 377.
44. **McCroskery, P. A., Wood, S., Jr., and Harris, E. D.,** Gelatin: a poor substrate for a mammalian collagenase, *Science,* 182, 70, 1973.
45. **Miller, A.,** Molecular packing in collagen fibrils, in *Biochemistry of Collagen,* Ramachandran, G. N., and Reddi, A. H., Eds., Plenum Press, New York, 1976, 85.
46. **Montfort, I. and Pérez-Tamayo, R.,** The distribution of collagenase in normal rat tissues, *J. Histochem. Cytochem.,* 23, 910, 1975.
47. **Nagai, Y.,** Vertebrate collagenase: further characterization and the significance of its latent form *in vivo, Mol. Cell. Biochem.,* 1, 137, 1973.
48. **Nagai, Y., Hori, H., Kawamoto, T., and Komiya, M.,** A regulation mechanism of collagenase activity *in vitro* and *vivo,* in *Dynamics of Connective Tissue Macromolecules,* Burleigh, P. M. C. and Poole, A. R., Eds., North-Holland, Amsterdam, 1975, 171.
49. **Neurath, H. and Walsh, K. A.,** Role of protelytic enzymes in biological regulation, a review, *Proc. Natl. Acad. Sci. U.S.A.,* 73, 3825, 1976.
50. **Ohlsson, K.,** Interaction between endogenous proteases and plasma protease inhibitors *in vitro* and *in vivo, Bayer Symposium V, Proteinase Inhibitors,* Springer-Verlag, Basel, 1974, 96.
51. **Ohlsson, K. and Olsson, I.,** The neutral proteases of human granulocytes. Isolation and partial characterization of granulocyte elastases, *Eur. J. Biochem.,* 42, 519, 1974.
52. **Oronsky, A. L., Perper, R. J., and Schroder, H. C.,** Phagocytic release and activation of human leukocyte procollagenase, *Nature (London),* 246, 417, 1973.
53. **Pérez-Tamayo, R.,** Pathology of collagen degradation, a review, *Am. J. Pathol.,* 92, 509, 1978.
54. **Pickrell, J. A., Harris, D. V., Hahn, F. F., Belasich, J. J., and Jones, R. K.,** Biological alterations resulting from chronic lung irradiation. III. Effect of partial ^{60}Co thoracic irradiation upon pulmonary collagen metabolism and fractionation in Syrian hamsters, *Radiat. Res.,* 62, 133, 1975.
55. **Pickrell, J. A., Harris, D. V., Mauderly, J. L., and Hahn, F. F.,** Altered collagen metabolism in radiation-induced interstitial pulmonary fibrosis, *Chest,* 69, 311, 1976.

55a. **Pickrell, J. A. and Straus, F. C.,** Research communication, 1978.

56. **Robertson, P. B. and Miller, E. J.,** Cartilage collagen: inability to serve as a substrate for collagenases active against skin and bone collagen, *Biochim. Biophys. Acta,* 289, 247, 1972.
57. **Segal, H. T., Winkler, J. R., and Miyagi, M. P.,** Relationship between degradation rates of proteins *in vivo* and their susceptibility to lysosomal proteases, *J. Biol. Chem.,* 249, 6364, 1974.
58. **Seltzer, J. L., Welgus, H. G., Jeffrey, J. J., and Eisen, A. Z.,** The function of Ca^{2+} in the action of mammalian collagenases, *Arch. Biochem. Biophys.,* 173, 355, 1976.
59. **Stimson, W. H.,** Correlation of the blood-level of a pregnancy-associated α-macroglobulin with the clinical course of cancer patients, *Lancet,* 1975(1), 777, 1975.
60. **Stimson, W. H.,** Variations in the level of a pregnancy-associated α-macroglobulin in patients with cancer, *J. Clin. Pathol.,* 28, 868, 1975.
61. **Stimson, W. H. and Blackstock, J. C.,** Synthesis of a pregnancy-associated α-macroglobulin by human leucocytes, *Experientia,* 31, 371, 1975.
62. **Stimson, W. H. and Eubank-Scott, L.,** The isolation and partial characterization of a new α-macroglobulin from human pregnancy serum, *FEBS Lett.,* 23, 298, 1972.
63. **Stimson, W. H. and Sinclair, J. M.,** An immunoassay for a pregnancy-associated α macroglobulin using antibody-enzyme conjugates, *FEBS Lett.,* 47, 190, 1974.
64. **Strauch, L.,** The role of collagenases in tumour invasion, in *Tissue Interactions in Carcinogenesis,* Tarin, D., Ed., Academic Press, New York, 1972, 399.
65. **TenCate, A. R. and Deporter, D. A.,** The degradative role of the fibroblast in the remodelling and turnover of collagen in soft connective tissue, *Anat. Rec.,* 182, 1, 1975.
66. **Vaes, G.,** Multiple steps in the activation of the inactive precursor of bone collagenase by trypsin, *FEBS Lett.,* 28, 198, 1972.
67. **Wahl, L. M.,** Hormonal regulation of macrophage collagenase activity, *Fed. Proc. Abstr.,* 35, 280, 1976.

68. **Wahl, L. M., Wahl, S. M., Mergenhagen, S. E., and Martin, G. R.,** Collagen production by lymphokine-activated macrophages, *Science,* 187, 261, 1975.
69. **Weeks, J. G., Halme, J., and Woessner, J. F., Jr.,** Extraction of collagenase from the involuting rat uterus, *Biochim. Biophys. Acta,* 445, 205, 1976.
70. **Werb, Z. and Aggeler, J.,** Proteases induce secretion of collagenase and plasminogen activator by fibroblasts, *Proc. Natl. Acad. Sci. U.S.A.,* 75, 1839, 1978.
71. **Werb, Z. and Burleigh, M. C.,** A specific collagenase from rabbit fibroblasts in monolayer culture, *Biochem. J.,* 137, 373, 1974.
72. **Werb, Z. and Reynolds, J. J.,** Purification and properties of a specific collagenase from rabbit synovial fibroblasts, *Biochem. J.,* 151, 645, 1975.
73. **Wirl, G.,** Extraction of collagenase from the 6000 × G sediment of uterine and skin tissues of mice: a comparative study, *Hoppe Seyler's Z. Physiol. Chem.,* 356, 1289, 1975.
73a. **Wirl, G.,** Extractable collagenase and carcinogenesis of the mouse skin, *Connect. Tissue Res.,* 5, 171, 1977.

Chapter 7

ELASTIN METABOLISM

J. A. Pickrell

TABLE OF CONTENTS

I. GENERAL

Elastin biosynthesis encompasses events between transcription and the formation of elastic fibers capable of providing support and elasticity to various tissues including the bronchii, bronchioles, vasculature, and alveolar networks. Although the sequence of events is incompletely elucidated, it presumably includes (1) transcription of DNA and translation of m-RNA leading to production of amorphous and microfibrillar elastin; (2) processing of amorphous and microfibrillar elastin; (3) transcellular movement and secretion; (4) cleavage of amorphous elastin to the polymerizing unit; (5) combination with microfibrillar elastin; (6) cross-linking amorphous elastin; and (7) elastolysis (Figure 1). These are discussed speculatively in light of recent findings. They are analogized to the more completely elucidated collagen biosynthesis because of similarities. However, no such analogy has been demonstrated, nor is one necessarily required.

Fibroblasts, smooth muscle cells, and possibly alveolar contracile cells produce elastin. Hance and Crystal[8] indicate that the fibroblast and smooth muscle cell produce elastin. This is consistent with Uitto et al.[27] and Foster et al.[6] who report isolation of "precursor" forms of amorphous elastin from chick aortae. In light of their resemblance to smooth muscle cells and fibroblasts, the possibility that alveolar contractile cells and myofibroblasts synthesize elastin must be explored.

Soluble precursor forms of elastin have been isolated, providing information concerning the biosynthesis of elastin. Since cross-linked elastin is a complex insoluble polymer, progress toward elucidating its biosynthetic sequence was hampered. Progressive improvements in isolating various forms of elastin resulted in the isolation of a soluble form of elastin generally called tropoelastin.[19,20] Recently, Foster et al.[6] reported the isolation of a high molecular weight ($\simeq$135,000 daltons) soluble elastin which they call proelastin. Rucker et al.[17b,17c] reported isolation of a 90,000 to 100,000-dalton soluble elastin which was precursor to tropoelastin. Although it is doubtful that the molecule represented an initial product of elastin translation, it may represent a truncated form of proelastin. Although quite promising, the significance of this data is unclear in light of several laboratories' difficulties in isolating high molecular weight precursor of tropoelastin.[17a] Future work in this area should prove exciting and enlightening. Schein et al.[22] report that tropoelastin is in a random coil, based on prolylhydroxylation and on centrifugation data. Schein et al.[23] indicate that 3,4-dehydroproline causes an inhibition of tropoelastin secretion, while 4-*cis*-hydroxy-L-proline has no effect. They propose that 3,4-dehydroproline but not 4-*cis*-hydroxy-L-proline alters the structure (in light of the random coil[22]) of tropoelastin in such a way as to inhibit tropoelastin secretion. Whether this is accompanied by an increased intracellular degradation as in the case of procollagen[2] needs to be investigated. Christner et al.[4] have immunologically identified an intracellular soluble elastin which they call tropoelastin. The antiserum did not cross-react with chick procollagen. This enables them to identify soluble elastin in biological systems in which other methods of characterization were difficult or impossible. One should be able to detect considerably less than 50 ng of soluble elastin. The investigation of heterogeneity of elastin awaits development of methods capable of solubilizing but not significantly degrading native amorphous elastin. The equivalent of pepsin digestion of insoluble collagen has not yet been perfected for elastin. Further work on the function of microfibrillar elastin is vital to the understanding of such heterogeneity.

II. TRANSCRIPTION AND TRANSLATION

Little concerning transcription of elastin DNA is known. Precursors of microfibril-

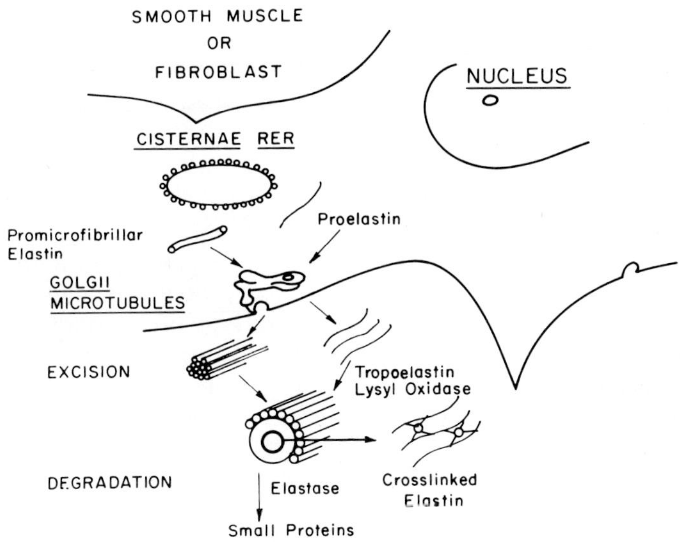

FIGURE 1. Elastin synthesis has several features which seem to resemble collagen synthesis. Cells producing elastin may be the same or very similar to mesenchymal cells in lung.[8] A high molecular weight species of soluble elastin termed proelastin[6] probably represents the precursor of amorphous elastin. It is most likely synthesized by the rough endoplasmic reticulum and released into its cisternae. Presumably there is a counterpart high molecular weight species which may be termed promicrofibrillar elastin.[8] Both are probably secreted by separate but similar routes, presumably undergo limited excision, and are combined into an elastic fiber. The microfibrillar component probably forms a scaffolding upon which amorphous tropoelastin monomers attach and are cross-linked by lysyl oxidase. Elastic fibers, especially amorphous elastin, may be degraded to small proteins by elastase.

lar and amorphous elastin are synthesized by translation of m-RNAs on ribosomes which, like other proteins destined for export, attach to membranes of the rough endoplasmic reticulum (RER). Presumably, while the chains are being translated, both amorphous and microfibrillar elastin chain are vectorially secreted into the cisternae of the RER.[18] Prolyl hydroxylase (PH) is probably bound to the RER since a variable degree of prolyl hydroxylation occurs (usually $\simeq$ 10 residues/1000 but sometimes higher). This hydroxylation can be forced higher with more PH.[27] This is consistent with proline hydroxylation being unimportant to elastin secretion, since conformational change would most likely inhibit further hydroxylation as it does after the formation of triple helical collagen. For this reason Uitto et al.[27] postulate that hydroxylation of proline is unimportant to the structural integrity or the secretion of soluble precursors of amorphous elastin. Urry et al.[27a] indicate that excess hydroxylation of proline in elastin may inhibit association of elastin chains and alignment into configurations optimal for cross-linking. Poorly cross-linked elastin is more rapidly degraded. So hydroxylation of proline may be more important than indicated by Uitto.[27]

III. PROCESSING

Both proelastin[6,17b] and the precursor of microfibrillar elastin indicated by Hance and Crystal[8] to be a non-collagenous glycoprotein (or group), are presumably packaged into secretory vesicles in the Golgi. At this point they may well be in the form in which they are secreted into the interstitum. Since microfibrillar elastin is probably a glycoprotein, carbohydrate moieties are most likely added in the Golgi apparatus prior to vesicle formation. Likewise, the highly polar nature of microfibrillar elastin[8] suggests that it may be packaged in such a form that these polar amino acids and the cysteine residues are covered or buried.

IV. TRANSCELLULAR MOVEMENT AND SECRETION

The inhibition of secretion of elastin by colchicine[27] indicates a similarity to the intracellular events of collagen and other secreted proteins. The concentration was appropriately low; thus, microtubules are probably involved and energy (ATP) required for transcellular movement of either proelastin or precursor to microfibrillar elastin. The observation[15] that a microtubular organizing center (MTOC) in the cytoplasm of 3T3 fibroblasts induced microtubules to grow peripherally toward the plasma membrane was discussed under collagen biosynthesis (transcellular movement).

Veis and Brownell[28] speculated that microtubules act as either an active or passive transport conduit along which collagenous secretory vesicles move from their point of origin to their termination in fusion with the plasma membrane. This speculation seems appropriate for elastin. Following fusion with the plasma membrane, elastin is presumably extruded in the manner described by Satir.[29]

V. CLEAVAGE

Once microfibrillar elastin and proelastin are secreted, cleavage probably takes place. Foster et al.[6] demonstrated spontaneous cleavage of lyophilized proelastin to numerous fragments, one of which is 72,000 daltons, and similar to tropoelastin. Rucker et al.[17b] chased the label in proelastin to a 100,000 P-elastin and to a 72,000 tropoelastin. Some label was removed by alcoholic extraction of non-elastin protein in the case of proelastin and tropoelastin. The association of proelastin with an inactive cleavage enzyme was considered a possibility. Subsequent activation of this enzyme by mild or specific proteolysis would lead to cleavage of tropoelastin. However, further characterization is necessary to define this process.

VI. COMBINATION OF AMORPHOUS AND MICROFIBRILLAR ELASTIN

Microfibrillar and amorphous elastin combine (probably extracellularly) to form an elastic fiber. The important question concerning when microfibrillar elastin associates with precursors of amorphous elastin must be subordinate to the question concerning the function of microfibrillar elastin. The function of microfibrillar elastin is not defined. However, the possibility that it forms a scaffold upon which elastin may be cross-linked should be considered. This is consistent with Siegel's[24] observation that lysyl oxidase prefers particulate rather than soluble substrate. Thus, it is clear that the combination of microfibrillar and elastin components must occur prior to cross-linking of elastin. Hance and Crystal[8] note that microfibrils are isolated from elastic fibers by use of dithiothreitol, suggesting that a disulfide linkage exists between amorphous and microfibrillar elastin. Neither Sandberg et al.,[19] Foster et al.,[6] nor Narayanam and Page[13] needed to use this reagent to extract soluble precursors of amorphous elastin. Thus, the disulfide linkage probably occurred later than the formation of such soluble precursors. Hance and Crystal[8] cite unpublished data of Muir, Ross, and Bornstein indicating the isolation of a 270,000-dalton cysteine containing protein (reduced) which may be a precursor of microfibrillar elastin. These data are consistent with the combination of microfibrillar and amorphous elastin occurring extracellularly.

VII. CROSS-LINKING

A conformational change of precursor microfibrillar elastin exposing the polar amino acids presumably leads to rapid adherence to membranous surfaces and presumably to each other. This then forms a scaffold onto which a polymerizing unit of tropoelastin adheres with disulfide bonds. Alternatively, disulfide bonds may maintain the structure of microfibrillar elastin necessary for amorphous elastin to combine. At this point the tropoelastin is presumably a particulate substrate, which lysyl oxidase prefers.[24] It becomes cross-linked into amorphous elastin and elastic fibers form.

Lysine of soluble tropoelastin is cross-linked into insoluble elastin to form desmosine. Narayanan and Page[13] have used pulse-chase experiments to demonstrate a precursor-product relationship between soluble (tropoelastin) and cross-linked elastin. They have chased labeled precursor lysine into desmosines in vitro and in a cell free system. They note that while BAPN completely inhibits cross-linking (desmosine formation), it does not affect the insolubilization of elastin. This supports binding to the microfibrillar component, although prior aldehyde binding was not ruled out. Furthermore, the time course of cross-linking is such that one must consider other enzymes besides lysyl oxidase as modulating and possibly controlling the formation of desmosines. Eleven years earlier Miller et al.[12] noted a progression from labelled lysine to desmosine in chick aortas. This response was also blocked by BAPN. It probably represented a sequence of events similar to that reported by Narayanan and Page.[13] Francis et al.[7] proposed a series of reactions leading from lysine to lysinonorleucine, merodesmosine, desmosine, and isodesmosine. Approximately one third of the lysine residues present in tropoelastin cannot be accounted for in desmosines of mature elastin. Narayanan and Page[13] experienced a similar phenomena although they interpreted this as requiring additional conversions rather than the lysines going into unidentified cross-links.

VIII. ELASTOLYSIS

Elastolysis is a natural mechanism for modulating location and amount of elastic fibers. Present assays, even if related to disease, may not reflect true elastolytic rate. Elastin is synthesized actively,[11,17] although mature elastin turns over slowly, especially in lung.[16] Elastin does not accumulate continually in adult lungs. Continued breakdown of newly synthesized and incompletely cross-linked elastin is consistent with these data.[8] Christner et al.[5] have recently shown that tropoelastin is rapidly cleaved by a variety of proteases, including leucocytic elastase at physiologic pH and ionic strength. The data support the hypothesis of Hance and Crystal.[8] Likewise, these results suggest the possibility that degradation of tropoelastin and other synthetic intermediates may play a role in development of emphysema. Mature elastin is resistant but tropoelastin susceptible to trypsin,[6] suggesting that nonspecific proteolysis may be an important mechanism in some forms of emphysema or lung injury. Immune response is very low to peptides produced by digestion of either microfibrils or amorphous elastin.[5a] However, Kuhn and Starcher[11] intensified developing elastase-induced emphysema by inhibiting connective tissue cross-linking, suggesting that turnover of mature elastin may also be represented. "Elastase" degrades mature elastin and has been found in pancreas, leucocytes, macrophages, and possibly platelets, although these may represent different enzymes.[9] Elastase is not specific for elastin, but must be considered a protease possessing broad specificity. Moreover, for convenience, substrates[9] other than purified elastin (congo red or orcein elastin, remazol-brilliant-blue elastin)[3] and several *N*-blocked alanine methyl esters are used to measure elastase activity. None may represent true breakdown of native elastic fibers.[25]

Pancreatic elastase has an inactive precursor and may be activated or inhibited. Pancreatic elastase amino acid analysis suggested it to be a 25,000-dalton globular protein with 240 amino acids. Pancreatic proelastase is an inactive precursor of elastase which will bind but not break down elastin. Tryptic cleavage of a single peptide bond near the amino terminus activates proelastase.[9] Sodium chloride (50 m*M*) reduced elastase activity to one half of the uninhibited level. Since extracellular sodium concentrations are much higher, this suggests most elastase to operate intracellularly in vivo. Serum α globulin (α_1 antitrypsin) also inhibits elastolytic activity[14] by binding with a 1:1 stoichiometry to elastase.[26] Granulocytic cytosol contains an elastolytic inhibitor distinct from α_1 antitrypsin;[10] granulocyte elastase is inhibited by unsaturated fatty acids.[1] Kagan[10a] indicated that detergent bile salts would activate elastolysis and that amidation of glutamic acid in the early portion of the sequence makes elastin a better substrate. Whether this represents only a substrate effect or not is unclear; however, it may have interesting implications in elastin metabolism. Factors concerning the division of cells thought to synthesize elastin will be discussed in Chapter 9.

REFERENCES

1. **Ashe, B. M. and Zimmerman, M.,** Specific inhibition of human granulocyte elastase by unsaturated fatty acids, *Fed. Proc. Abstr.,* 36, 678, 1977.
2. **Bienkowski, R. S., Cowan, M. J., McDonald, J. A., and Crystal, R. G.,** Degradation of newly synthesized collagen, *J. Biol. Chem.,* 253(12), 4356, 1977.
3. **Bieth, J., Pichoir, M., and Metais, P.,** Pseudo-zero order solubilization of remazol-brilliant-blue elastin by elastase, *Anal. Biochem.,* 70(2), 430, 1976.
4. **Christner, P., Dixon, M., Cywinski, A., and Rosenbloom, J.,** Radioimmunological identification of tropoelastin, *Biochem. J.,* 157, 525, 1976.
5. **Christner, P., Weinbaum, G., Sloan, B., and Rosenbloom, J.,** Degradation of tropoelastin by proteases, *Anal. Biochem.,* 88, 682, 1978.

5a. **Darnule, T. V., Likhite, V., Turino, G. M., and Mandl, I.,** Immune response to peptides produced by enzymatic digestion of microfibrils and elastin of human lung parenchyma, *Connect. Tissue Res.,* 5, 67, 1977.

6. **Foster, J. A., Mecham, R. P., and Franzblau, C.,** A high molecular weight species of soluble elastin, *Biochem. Biophys. Res. Commun.,* 72, 1399, 1976.
7. **Francis, G., John, R., and Thomas, J.,** Biosynthetic pathway of desmosines in elastin, *Biochem. J.,* 136, 45, 1973.
8. **Hance, A. J. and Crystal, R. G.,** The connective tissue of lung, *Am. Rev. Respir. Dis.,* 112, 657, 1975.
9. **Hartley, B. S. and Shotton, D. M.,** Pancreatic elastase, in *The Enzymes. III. Hydrolysis: Peptide Bonds,* Boyer, P. D., Ed., Academic Press, New York, 1971, 323.
10. **Janoff, A.,** Human granulocyte elastase. Further delineation of its role in connective tissue damage, *Am. J. Pathol.,* 68, 579, 1972.

10a. **Kagan, H.,** Research communication, 1976.

11. **Kuhn, C. and Starcher, B.,** The significance of connective tissue repair in elastase-induced emphysema, *Am. Rev. Respir. Dis.,* 113 (abstr.), 209, 1976.
12. **Miller, E. J., Martin, G. R., Mecca, C. E., and Piez, K. A.,** The biosynthesis of elastin cross-links: the effect of copper deficiency and a lathyrogen, *J. Biol. Chem.,* 240, 3623, 1965.
13. **Narayanan, A. S. and Page, R. C.,** Demonstration of a precursor-product relationship between soluble and cross-linked elastin, and the biosynthesis of the desmosines *in vitro, J. Biol. Chem.,* 251, 1125, 1976.

14. **Ohlsson, K. and Olsson, I.**, The neutral proteases of human granulocytes. Isolation and partial characterization of granulocyte elastases, *Eur. J. Biochem.*, 42, 519, 1974.
15. **Osborn, M. and Weber, K.**, Cytoplasmic microtubules in tissue culture cells appear to grow from an organizing structure towards the plasma membrane, *Proc. Natl. Acad. Sci. U.S.A.*, 73, 867, 1976.
16. **Pierce, J. A., Resnick, H., and Henry, P. H.**, Collagen and elastin metabolism in the lungs, skin, and bones of adult rats, *J. Lab. Clin. Med.*, 69, 485, 1967.
17. **Robert, L., Moczar, M., and Robert, M.**, Biogenesis, maturation and aging of elastic tissue, *Experientia*, 30, 211, 1974.
17a. **Rosenbloom, J.**, Research communication, 1979.
17b. **Rucker, R. B., Heng, C. S., Murray, J., and Buckingham, K.**, Putative forms of soluble elastin and their relationship to the synthesis of fibrous elastin paper, presented at meeting of West Coast Connective Tissue Society, Gleneden Beach, Ore., February 25 to 27, 1977.
17c. **Rucker, R. B., Heng-Khoo, C. S., Dubrick, M., Lefevre, M., and Cross, C. E.**, Partial characterization of a tropoelastin precursor isolated from chick aorta, *Biochemistry*, 18(18), 3854, 1979.
18. **Sabatini, D. D., Ojakian, G., Lande, M. A., Lewis, J., Mok, W., Adesnik, M., and Kreibich, G.**, Structural and functional aspects of the protein synthesizing apparatus in the rough endoplasmic reticulum, *Adv. Exp. Med. Biol.*, 62, 151, 1974.
19. **Sandberg, L. B., Bruenger, E., and Cleary, E. G.**, Tropoelastin purification: improvements using enzyme inhibitors, *Anal. Biochem.*, 64, 249, 1975.
20. **Sandberg, L. B., Weissman, N., and Smith, D. W.**, The purification and partial characterization of a soluble elastin-like protein from copper-deficient porcine aorta, *Biochemistry*, 8, 2940, 1969.
21. **Satir, B.**, The final steps in secretion, *Sci. Am.*, 233(4), 29, 1975.
22. **Schein, J., Carpousis, A., and Rosenbloom, J.**, Evidence that tropoelastin exists as a random coil, in *Elastin and Elastic Tissue*, Sandberg, L. B., Gray, W. R., and Franzblau, C., Eds., Plenum Press, New York, 1977.
23. **Schein, J., Frankel, L., and Rosenbloom, J.**, Inhibition of tropoelastin secretion by incorporation of DL-3,4-dehydroproline, *Arch. Biochem. Biophys.*, 183, 416, 1977.
24. **Siegel, R. C.**, Biosynthesis of collagen cross-links: increased activity of purified lysyl oxidase with reconstituted collagen fibrils, *Proc. Natl. Acad. Sci. U.S.A.*, 71, 4826, 1974.
25. **Snider, G. L., Hayes, J. A., Franzblau, C., Kagan, H. M., Stone, P. S., and Korthy, A. L.**, Relationship between elastolytic activity and experimental emphysema-inducing properties of papain preparations, *Am. Rev. Respir. Dis.*, 110, 254, 1974.
26. **Tyndall, M., Largman, C., Brodrich, J. W., and Geokas, M. C.**, The stoichiometry of inhibition of human pancreatic elastase 2 by human alpha$_1$-antitrypsin, *Biochem. Biophys. Res. Commun.*, 74, 857, 1977.
27. **Uitto, J., Hoffman, H. P., and Prockop, D. J.**, Synthesis of elastin and procollagen by cells from embryonic aorta: differences in the role of hydroxyproline and the effects of proline analogs on the secretion of the two proteins, *Arch. Biochem. Biophys.*, 173, 187, 1976.
27a. **Urry, D. W., Bhatnager, R. S., Suzano, H., and Prasad, K. U.**, A molecular basis for defective elastic tissue in environmentally induced lung disease, in *The Molecular Basis of Environmental Toxicity*, Bhatnager, R. S., Ed., Ann Arbor Scientific, Ann Arbor, Mich., in press, 1979.
28. **Veis, A. and Brownell, A. G.**, Collagen biosynthesis, *Crit. Rev. Biochem.*, 2, 417, 1975.

Chapter 8

METABOLISM OF PROTEOGLYCANS AND MUCOPROTEINS

J. A. Pickrell

TABLE OF CONTENTS

Metabolism of proteoglycans and mucoproteins (glycoprotein secretory products of pulmonary goblet cells and mucus glands) includes synthesis and breakdown. Biosynthesis includes each event leading to the production of a functioning proteoglycan or mucoprotein. Many of the ideas proposed in this section are speculative in nature. However, they form a series of concepts useful to the understanding not only of proteoglycan and mucoprotein metabolism, but also of their role in pulmonary injury and its resulting damage. Several excellent reviews[6,8,19,20] cover this area in some depth.

I. PROTEOGLYCAN SYNTHESIS

There is a distinct separation between enzymes of precursor production, protein synthesis, and macromolecular assembly. Enzymes producing precursors or 3′phosphoadenosine 5′phosphosulfate (PAPS) are found in the high speed supernatant fraction, indicating their cytoplasmic origin. UDPG-4′-epimerase is located in the same fraction of cornea and epiphyseal-plate cartilage as UDPG dehydrogenase.[3] Canine respiratory glycosyl transferases were isolated in good quantity from the soluble fraction of homogenates of canine pulmonary tissue.[12] Chicken embryo glycosyl transferases were located in the crude microsomal fraction (10,000 g supernate, 100,000 g precipitate).[17] Activities involved in synthesis of the protein part of proteoglycans are ribosomal. Macromolecular assembly occurs in the crude microsomal fraction. For example, heparan sulphotransferase[4] was isolated in the freeze dried 25,000 g supernatant of ox lung homogenate. Maximum transfer of sulfate is found using the same microsomal fraction promoting polysaccharide polymerization,[18-21] although some soluble activity was present. Sulfation and probably polymerization take place in the Golgi apparatus.[11,16]

Further separations into rough and smooth endoplasmic reticulum[7] suggest that the protein is synthesized on the rough ER, the polysaccharide is linked on the smooth ER, and then polymerization and sulfation take place. Polymerization occurs on individual chains, not continuously on one chain. Since sulfation increases with increasing time, it can be considered an all-or-none event. Moreover, a microsomal primer is necessary to form the oligosaccharide link.[21a] When synthesizing chondroitin sulfate, the attachment of galactose to xylose required phospholipid, since it could be abolished with phospholipase C or A.[17] However, the attachment of xylose to core protein, glucuronic acid to galactose, or the alternating *N*-acetyl galactosamine — glucuronic acid polymer to glucuronic acid required no phospholipid. The relation of primer to protein remains poorly defined.

A. Sugar Nucleotide

Biosynthesis of sugar nucleotide precursors should be considered. These precursors are (1) UDP glucuronic acid and UDP—*N*-acetyl glucosamino for hyal uronic acid; (2) UDP glucuronic acid and UDP-*N*-acetyl galactosamine for chondroitin sulfate (associated with cartilage); (3) presumably UDP glucuronic acid or UDP Iduronic acid and UDP-*N*-acetyl galactosamine for dermatan sulfate (associated with collagen); (4) probably UDP glucuronic acid, UDP-*N*-acetyl glucosamine (even though heparin is sulfated), and UDP Iduronic acid for heparin.[6,19,20] The approximate number of disaccharide units in each of 30 to 100 identical chains ranges from 500 to 2500 for hyaluronic acid, to 60 for chondroitin sulfate, 40 to 60 for dermatan sulfate, and 10 to 20 for heparin and heparan sulfate. Structures are reviewed by Hance and Crystal.[6] The overall structure is depicted by Horwitz et al.[8] (Chapter 4, Figure 1) as having a protein backbone with polymerized glycosaminoglycans extending off it. These are attached to the OH radical of the serine group via xylose - galactose - glucuronic acid.

Sugar nucleotides are formed by a uridine pyrophosphorylase type of reaction, or by conversion from some other sugar nucleotide. Key intermediates are UDP glucose and UDP-*N*-acetyl glucosamine which can be formed by the reaction of UTP and a sugar-1-P. Then interconversion occurs. UDP glucose can be oxidized to UDP glucuronic acid which can be decarboxylated to UDP xylose. UDP glucuronic acid can undergo C-5 epimerization to form iduronic acid. Recent studies suggest that this epimerization may occur after incorporation in dermatan SO_4 and heparin.[12] Both UDP glucose and UDP-*N*-acetyl glucosamine can undergo C-4 epimerization to form UDP galactose and UDP-*N*-acetyl galactosamine. Probably cells synthesizing proteoglycans contain the machinery for synthesizing the precursors; sugar nucleotides and phosphorylated sugars do not readily enter cells.[8,19,20] Thus, the presence of all proteoglycans except keratan SO_4 in lung parenchyma implies operation of these processes. Intracellular conversion of sulfate to adenyl sulfate and then to PAPS requires two ATP molecules and probably represents a cytoplasmic process.

B. Location in the Cell

Proteoglycans are synthesized and processed in several sites within the cell. The protein backbone of proteoglycans is presumably synthesized by translation of the appropriate m-RNA on ribosomes which attach to the RER and vectorially secrete the protein into its cisternae.[16] The protein attaches to a primer in the SER. Polymerization utilizing the UDP-sugar bases and sulfation with PAPS occur as concerted processes, which are as yet incompletely defined. Some final synthesis takes place at the Golgi, i.e., probable partial sulfation of the polymerized *N*-acetyl glucosamine moieties of heparin and possibly some other minor modifications such as C-5 epimerization of polymerized glucuronic acid to iduronic acid in dermatan SO_4 and heparin.[12] The location and process remain presumptive. After processing is complete, intracellular granules are formed which can presumably be extruded on demand.[19,20]

C. Control

Control of these processes is apparently mediated through availability of the UDP sugar bases, through whatever poorly understood protein transcriptional or translational controls may be affected and through the poorly understood lipid requirement to attach galactose to xylose in the primer. The latter two are not defined sufficiently to be considered in this review. With regard to the UDP sugar bases, considerable definition exists and has been reviewed by Silbert[19,20] and Stadtman.[22] UDP-*N*-acetyl glucosamine inhibits the formation of glucosamine-1P from fructose-1-P and glutamine (L-glutamine-D-fructose-6-phosphate aminotransferase). Thus, excess unpolymerized UDP *N*-acetyl glucosamine, an end product, inhibits the first step in its synthesis. UDP-xylose, another end product, inhibits the first step of the conversion of UDP glucose to UDP glucuronic acid. Thus, excess production of unpolymerized glucuronic acids is inhibited by the end product UDP-xylose. The production of UDP glucose is likewise interesting. It is inhibited by UDP glucose at a lower K_I for UDP glucose than the K_m for UTP, suggesting allosteric modulation as opposed to product inhibition. Orthophosphate inhibits UDP glucose production but favors its metabolism. UTP activates the reaction and 5′AMP reduces the K_m for UTP. Inhibition by galactose-1-P probably represents a product inhibition.[22] If glycolysis were activated by an increased intracellular orthophosphate[5] the presence of high UTP (transphosphorylation of ATP) could favor the formation of UDP glucose. The rapid metabolism of this to UDP gluconic acid would be induced by low formation of UDP xylose and possibly by orthophosphate. This would favor formation of UDP glucose and might occur in the formation of hyaluronic acid, which has long chains of glycosaminoglycans (GAG), and, therefore, a lower proportion of UDP xylose formed. This could account for the active formation of hyaluronic acid when glucose consumption is increased and glycolysis activated. Presumably the UDP sugar bases are rapidly polymerized so that no excess inhibits their formation.

D. Synthesis in Lung at Different Ages

The different proteoglycans predominating at different ages probably relate to lung growth and differentiation. Hyaluronic acid (HA) is the most prevalently synthesized proteoglycan in fetal life.[6,8] As birth approaches, only modest reductions of HA are seen. They are made up by increased heparin. Increased heparin SO_4 (HS) and HA six weeks after birth reflect rapid synthesis of GAG and probably represent proliferation of new cells. Collagen synthesis per cell has already fallen, suggesting that a critical connective tissue density has been reached. By six months, hyaluronic acid synthesis has fallen, relative to total GAG synthesis and absolutely. The relative increase in dermatan sulfate actually allows it to remain constant in amount/cell paralleling collagen synthesis for that period. This agrees with the association of Kawamoto and Nagai[10] who see similar events in chicken embryo skin.

II. BREAKDOWN

Proteoglycan degradation is elegantly reviewed by Silbert[19,20] and Neufeld et al.[14] This involves sequential lysosomal degradation of the polysaccharide portion involving, among others, hyaluronidase. Neufeld et al.[14] outline this sequence and the defects which may occur in it. Essentially, the enzymes necessary for such degradation have a small piece of peptide extension which allows them to be concentrated and retained by lysosomes. If they lack this piece or extension, they are not retained intracellularly and large secondary lysosomes form. Hyaluronidase has been noted in rat lung; probably other enzymes will be isolated. Secondly, papain which attacks the protein portion of proteoglycans can mobilize large portions quickly. Lysosomal hydrolases may be involved at this level as well. Macrophage enzymes will degrade chondromucoprotein.[9]

The effect of proteoglycans on the density dependence of fibroblasts was reported by Norrby.[14] Human fetal lung cells formed multilayered tissue-like sheets; 3T3 cells formed confluent monolayers. Heparin caused stimulation of cell multiplication over a wide range of concentrations in dense 3T3 cells; results were variable in human lung fibroblasts. Histamine and serotonin could induce stimulation but only over a much narrower range. Whether heparin's alteration of surface properties or charge elicit a PI response leading to DNA synthesis and cell division has not been determined.

III. MUCOPROTEINS

Even less information exists concerning the synthesis of mucoproteins (mucinglycoproteins) than that for proteoglycans. However, Horwitz et al.[8] and Hance and Crystal[6] indicate that the uronic acids are not incorporated into mucus glycoproteins. Moreover, mucus glycoproteins are apparently produced by goblet cells or submucosal glands, although which is predominant must be defined by future work. Mucoproteins have much shorter carbohydrate side chains than do proteoglycans. Although some mucin glycoproteins are acidic because of the presence of sialic acid, most are neutral relative to proteoglycans. Newly synthesized tracheal glycoproteins are apparently resistant to hyaluronidase, indicating a different conformation.

We can assume that protein portion is synthesized by translating an m-RNA on ribosomes which bind to the RER and vectorially secrete the protein into the cisternae.[16] Probably, in the Golgi, the carbohydrate moiety is attached (or modified if attached in the SER), although this remains to be established. One may postulate that production and control of UDP-*N*-acetyl glucosamine is similar to that of proteoglycans. Likewise, it may be subject to the same epimerizations. UDP glucuronic acid is not present in this pathway. Sialic acid represents a constitutent not present in proteoglycans. Kornfeld cited in Stadtman[22] reports that UDP-*N*-acetyl glucosamine can undergo C-2 epimerization to *N* acetyl mannoseamine (NAM), followed by phosphorylation to NAM-6-P which combines with PEP to form *N*-acetyl neuraminic acid-9-P (NAN-9-P). This undergoes phosphorolysis to NAN and reacts with CTP to form CMP-NAN which is incorporated into glycoprotein as sialic acid. CMP-NAN (an end product) will sigmoidally inhibit UDP-*N*-acetyl glucosamine C-2 epimerization (the first step after a branch point). The observed inhibition reflected the reduced V_{max} of the enzyme. However, the binding of CMP-NAN decreased the apparent K_m. Thus, at low levels of CMP-NAN, the effect on V_{max} is minimized, while at high levels it is important. This allows a relatively slow and complexly controlled incorporation of sialic acid into glycoproteins. At the cellular level, alterations may occur in quantity of rheologic properties of mucus glycoproteins, suggesting that not only mucus production but hydration and, thus, viscosity may be controlled. Breakdown is probably similar to most proteins.

REFERENCES

1. **Baker, A. P., Chakrin, L. W., Sawyer, J. L., Munro, J. R., Hillegass, L. M., and Giannone, E.,** Glycosyltransferases in canine respiratory tissue. Alterations in an experimentally induced hypersecretory state, *Biochem. Med.,* 10, 387, 1974.
2. **Baker, A. P., Chakrin, L. W., and Wardell, J. R.,** Chronic cholinergic stimulation of canine respiratory tissue, *Am. Rev. Respir. Dis.,* 111, 423, 1975.
3. **DeLuca, G., Speziale, P., Balduini, C., and Castellani, A. A.,** Biosynthesis of glycosaminoglycans: uridine diphosphate glucose 4′-epimerase from cornea and epiphysial-plate cartilage, *Connect. Tissue Res.,* 3, 39, 1975.
4. **Foley, T. and Baker, J. R.,** Heparan sulphate sulphotransferase. Properties of an enzyme from ox lung, *Biochem. J.,* 135, 187, 1973.
5. **Gray, P. N., Cullum, M. E., and Griffin, M. J.,** Population density and regulation of cell division in 3T3 cells, *J. Cell. Physiol.,* 89, 225, 1976.
6. **Hance, A. J. and Crystal, R. G.,** The connective tissue of lung, *Am. Rev. Respir. Dis.,* 112, 657, 1975.
7. **Horwitz, A. L. and Dorfman, A.,** Subcellular sites for synthesis of chondromucoprotein of cartilage, *J. Cell Biol.,* 38, 358, 1968.
8. **Horwitz, A. L., Elson, N. A., and Crystal, R. G.,** Proteoglycans and elastic fibers, in *The Biochemical Basis of Pulmonary Function,* Crystal, R. G., Ed., Marcel Dekker, New York, 1976, 273.
9. **Huffer, W. E.,** Degradation of chondromucoprotein by macrophage enzymes, *Lab. Invest.,* 29, 304, 1973.
10. **Kawamoto, T. and Nagai, Y.,** Developmental changes in glycosaminoglycans, collagen and collagenase activity in embryonic chick skin, *Biochim. Biophys. Acta,* 437, 190, 1976.
11. **Lane, N., Caro, L., Otero-Vilardebo, L. R., and Godman, G. C.,** On the site of sulfation in colonic goblet cells, *J. Cell Biol.,* 21, 339, 1964.
12. **Lindahl, U., Backstrom, G., Jansson, L., and Hallén, A.,** Biosynthesis of heparin. II. Formation of sulfamino groups, *J. Biol. Chem.,* 248, 7234, 1973.
13. **Neufeld, E. F., Lim, T. W., and Shapiro, L. J.,** Inherited disorders of lysosomal metabolism, *Annu. Rev. Biochem.,* 44, 357, 1975.
14. **Norrby, K.,** Effect of heparin, histamine and serotonin on the density-dependent inhibition of replication in two fibroblastic cell lines, *Virchows Arch. B,* 15, 75, 1973.

15. **Peterson, M. and Leblond, C. P.,** Synthesis of complex carbohydrates in the Golgi region, as shown by radioautography after injection of labeled glucose, *J. Cell Biol.,* 21, 143, 1964.
16. **Sabatini, D. D., Ojakian, G., Lande, M. A., Lewis, J., Mok, W., Adesnik, M., and Kreibich, G.,** Structural and functional aspects of the protein synthesizing apparatus in the rough endoplasmic reticulum, *Adv. Exp. Med. Biol.,* 62, 151, 1974.
17. **Schwarz, N. B.,** Biosynthesis of chondroitin sulfate. Role of phospholipids in the activity of UDP-D-galactose: D-xylose galactosyltransferase, *J. Biol. Chem.,* 251, 285, 1976.
18. **Silbert, J. E.,** Biosynthesis of heparin. 3. Formation of a sulfated glycosaminoglycan with a microsomal preparation from mast cell tumors, *J. Biol. Chem.,* 242, 5146, 1967.
19. **Silbert, J. E.,** Biosynthesis of mucopolysaccharides and protein-polysaccharides, in *Molecular Pathology of Connective Tissues,* Vol. 3 of *The Biochemistry of Disease,* Peréz-Tamayo, R. and Rojkind, M., Eds., Marcel Dekker, New York, 1973, 323.
20. **Silbert, J. E.,** Catabolism of mucopolysaccharides and protein-polysaccharides. In *Molecular Pathology of Connective Tissues,* Vol. 3 of *The Biochemistry of Disease,* Peréz-Tamayo, R. and Rojkind, M., Eds., Marcel Dekker, New York, 1973, 355.
21. **Silbert, J. E. and DeLuca, S.,** Biosynthesis of chondroitin sulfate. 3. Formation of a sulfated glycosaminoglycan with a microsomal preparation from chick embryo cartilage, *J. Biol. Chem.,* 244, 876, 1969.
21a. **Silbert, J. E.,** Research communication, 1975.
22. **Stadtman, E. R.,** Allosteric regulation of enzyme activity, *Adv. Enzymol.,* 28, 41, 1966.

Chapter 9

LUNG CELL TYPES AND THEIR KINETICS

J. A. Pickrell

TABLE OF CONTENTS

I. GENERAL

The lung is an extremely complex mixture of cells uniquely supported on a connective tissue framework. This organ develops sequentially.[14,88] As reviewed,[17,59] lung cells include several forms of epithelial cells: basal, mucus, ciliated, neuroepithelial brush, special type cells (columnar), mucus gland, bronchiolar, Clara, myoepithelial and cells of the alveolar epithelium, type I and II cells. These cells perform many complex functions indicated by Kuhn[59] and by Fishman and Pietra[33] in reviews of non-respiratory functions of lung. The mucus or Goblet cell produces mucus containing mucoproteins; the type I alveolar epithelium covers the large alveolar surface area; and the type II alveolar epithelium secretes pulmonary surfactant, which aids in maintaining alveolar patency and type I integrity by reducing surface tension. Lymphoid cells, macrophages, and other cells are present and may be affected by lung disease. The composition of pulmonary surface active material has been reviewed by Clements and King;[23] phospholipid metabolism of lungs has been reviewed by van Golde.[90] Airway surface epithelium has a lower mitotic index as one proceeds peripherally in 30- to 50-day-old rats, but not 105-day-old ones.[9] Clara cells become heavily labelled after injection of ^{3}H leucine, indicating their secretion of protein.[28]

Lymphoid cells, macrophages, and other cells are present and may be affected by lung disease. Immunocompetent cells of the lymphoreticular system in the bronchiolar wall of man contain the major classes of immunoglobulins (IgG, IgM, IgA, IgE, and IgD). These cells can be obtained by bronchopulmonary lavage, although the percentage varies from 15 to 25%[34] to 6% in humans,[25] and 0 to 5% in Syrian hamsters[76] and in Beagle dogs.[70a] These cells presumably originate from or relate to cells of the draining nodes which respond to immunologic stimuli.[7] They are increased in human diffuse interstitial lung disease[24,25] and in some cases of radiation-induced pulmonary fibrosis.[76] Characterization of cells recoverable in endobronchial washings may provide considerable information concerning the progress of the pulmonary disease. Likewise, macrophages are present in the lung and pulmonary lavage fluid.[59] Cells of nervous tissue are present, as are mesothelial cells lining the visceral pleura. Scanning electron microscopy revealed considerable regional variation in the length and density of the long slender microvilli which were covered by glycocalyx.

II. CELLS PRODUCING CONNECTIVE TISSUE

Several cells apparently produce connective tissue,[74] the endothelial cell which lines arteries, veins, and the alveolar capillary bed, the fibroblast, and the contractile cell.[48] It is important to understand the physiology of the cells which produce the connective tissue skeleton which gives the lung form and provides the stability necessary to maintain the integrity of the lung.

The presence of proteoglycans necessary to specifically interact with collagen and elastin in the areas supporting the bronchiolar or vascular smooth muscle is considered a good possibility. The smooth muscle cell can make collagen[65] and probably elastin.[35] Both of these connective tissue constituents are produced to support the smooth muscle cells of bronchioles and blood vessels and may be necessary to maintaining their integrity. Proteoglycans specific for collagen (dermatan sulfate) increase differentially as collagen synthesis increases in rapidly growing chick dermis.[49]

The alveolus represents a highly specialized increase in surface area which contains a basement membrane, interstitial collagen,[91,93] elastin,[36,78,83,84] and presumably the specifically interacting proteoglycans necessary to support this unique structure. Basement membrane collagen may be made by endothelial cells as they are in other systems.[45] Preliminary data[21a,79a] revealed certain resemblances between lung basement membrane collagen and that of other systems.[21] Interstitial collagen (type I and III) is produced by the mesenchymal cell with numerous characteristics of a fibroblast, and by an epithelial cell resembling the alveolar type II cell.[42] Our isolation of small amounts of hydroxyproline in a cell fraction enriched in type II cells agreed with this observation. However, the possibility of contamination from other cells or extracellular adherence must be ruled out before our results can support their data.[75a] Since type II cells are apparently not phagocytic,[63,64,75] internal hydroxyproline would probably represent collagen and not degradation products.

Contractile cells synthesize collagen, may provide an alveolar contractile system, and may be important responders to stimuli for cell division. The alveolar contractile cell is reported by Kapanci et al.[48] to resemble the fibroblast but contain actin. They may provide an alveolar contractile system and replace the function of the bronchial and arterial smooth muscle, which are not present to any extent at the alveolar level. These cells resemble the myofibroblasts characterized by Gabbiani et al.[38] which secrete collagen, contain actin, and have contractile properties. Gabbiani et al.[37] report that myofibroblasts of granulation tissue synthesize mostly type III collagen and speculate that they represent differentiated fibroblasts, although this must be more completely elucidated. Whether this cell makes elastin must still be determined, although they have some characteristics of smooth muscle cells which make elastin.[35] Presumably, these cells make the appropriate proteoglycans. How such cells respond to or result from stimuli for cell division has not been completely characterized.

III. FIBROBLAST GROWTH

Fibroblast growth patterns differ, depending upon substrata for growth. Fetal lung fibroblasts grow into multilayered arrays in tissue culture unless the cells and substrata are treated with collagenase.[32] Attempts to grow fibroblasts in agar, which produced only small clones, suggested that these cells cannot satisfy their substrate requirements by mutual contact alone. Such cells grew at a reduced rate on a hydrated collagen lattice; the trend was reversed in the presence of collagenase.[30,31] These findings suggest that collagen substrata inhibit fibroblast proliferation; the mechanism is unclear. Secondly, the findings suggest that when collagenase (probably bacterial), whose mammalian equivalent is associated with fibroblast proliferation, removes the collagen surrounding the fibroblast, a higher rate of proliferation occurs. This suggestion is supported by a similar finding if the collagen is gelatinized. The role of collagen fibrils in development and maintenance of stable parallel arrays in tissue culture is unclear. These cells seem to pass through orthoganal multilayers which will not be formed if cell motility is inhibited by 2% agar stiffened medium. Perhaps collagen provides anchorage for the fibroblast.[30,31] Indeed, some cells producing connective tissue are dependent upon anchorage to divide.[10]

The mechanism for stimulation of proliferation of connective tissue cells may involve platelet or T-lymphocyte factors or mediators of inflammation. In the pulmonary alveolus, the fibroblast must interact with type I and type II epithelial cells. Elsdale and Bard[29] report that the free surface of attached and spreading epithelium is invariably non-adhesive for either fibroblasts or epithelial cells, indicating that fibroblasts will not proliferate over growing epithelium. Vracko[91] indicated that epithelial cells will regenerate in lung injured with oleic acid as long as the basement membrane remains intact. One potential interpretation of his and Elsdale and Bard's data,[29-31] and consistent with the presence of scars, is that fibroblasts proliferate to fill an existing void elicited by the reduction of epithelial proliferation due to continued injury. Harker et al.[43] propose a mechanism similar to this, but involving a platelet released mitogenic factor to smooth muscle cells. Whether a similar factor operates at the alveolar level is an intriguing question. Kravis et al.[57] and Stuart et al.[87] report that T-lymphocytes from patients with pulmonary fibrosis take part in a recognition process resulting in the secretion of lymphokines. The lymphokines are cytolytic to collagen coated cells, red cells, and especially platelets, as indicated by Miller et al.[67] Bradykinin, often elevated in injury, activates T-lymphocytes.[85]

A second epithelial void may be created when the basement membrane is interrupted. In either case, it is conceivable that conditions might well exist which would dissolve sufficient amounts of the normal collagen substrate so that the growth characteristics of the fibroblast might be altered and fibroblast proliferation would result. These facts may account for the puzzlingly good association of fibrinolysis with fibrosis in many pulmonary conditions.[82] Certainly the close association of fibrin and connective tissue has been noted.[15,41a] Steroid interference with fibrinolysis in primary hepatic culture indirectly suggests the mechanism by which therapeutic manipulation of scarring conditions may occur, i.e., interference with fibrinolysis and collagenolysis, inhibiting fibroblast proliferation. The steroid inhibition of fibroblast proliferation in vitro[44,77] supports this concept although other mechanisms may be involved.

A. Cell Division

Serum concentration, cell density, and cellular PO_2 influence growth patterns. Increasing serum concentration increases the relative numbers of WI-38 diploid lung fibroblasts which enter the cell division process in tissue culture, although increasing cell numbers reduce the effect and thus the number of dividing cells. However, this is not a serum/cell density ratio, and suggests that cell density alone can regulate the proportion of cells sensitive to serum and thus the proportion entering the cell cycle.[6] WI-38 fibroblasts incubated at high (291 mmHg) or low (8 mmHg) PO_2 grow more slowly, use more glucose and produce more lactate, suggesting a shift to anerobic glycolysis due to a poorly functioning aerobic metabolism.[3] This is understandable at low PO_2 and consistent with the clinical picture of O_2 toxicity.[50] Although the mechanism at higher PO_2 is unclear, oxidation and possible sulfhydryl depletion and the effect of high oxygen upon the cytochromes, quinones, and enzymes of oxidative phosphorylation are possible mechanisms.

Gray et al.[40] report a relationship between orthophosphate and rate of density-dependent 3T3 fibroblast division. Prior to intercellular contact, intracellular phosphate is 10 m*M*, during critical intercellular contact this phosphate is reduced to 2 m*M*. After confluent 3T3 cells are released from contact inhibition, phosphate must increase several fold before DNA synthesis begins. Gray et al.[40] suggest that this change may regulate glycolytic activity. They further speculate that coordinate counterion changes in calcium may regulate mitochondrial activity, although little definition is provided. The involvement of mitochondria in generating ATP necessary to secrete the collagen matrix[58] ties this regulation to that of cell division. Calcium results in stable aggregation in other cells, while lectins, noted proliferative agents, block the formation of such stable aggregates.[60]

The mechanisms by which this regulation leads to cell division are intriguing. Increased inorganic phosphate[62,94] might stimulate glycolysis by activating hexokinase and phosphofructokinase. This would presumably make more substrate available for the alternate pentose pathway and inhibit the methyl glycoxylate shunt. The pentose pathway is stimulated by the increased NADP/NADPH ratio[53] which results from increased nucleic acid synthesis and is reinforced by positive feedback from pathway intermediates and glucosamine-6-phosphate.[41,72] This would make more NADPH and pentoses available for necessary nucleic acid synthesis. Increased phosphate would activate phosphorylase, making more substrate available for glycolysis. Likewise, it would favor metabolism of UDP glucose,[56] possibly to UDP glucuronic acid.[94] Although high phosphate may moderately inhibit nucleotide pyrophosphorylase,[71a] producing UDPG, the high ATP/AMP ratio from glycolysis might drive the reaction.[56] Certainly the metabolism of UDPG would favor the reaction explaining the confusingly low KI relative to KM. This rather intriguing conversion is then consistent with increased production of hyaluronic acid in dividing fibroblasts as reviewed by Davison[26] and as reported by Castor et al.[19] in response to their connective tissue activating peptide. Why the high ATP/AMP ratio would not inhibit glycolysis remains undefined, unless the ATP is promptly used. Likewise, the relationship of phosphate, glycolysis, and protelytic conditions to fibroblast proliferation remains a mystery.

B. Phosphatidyl Inositol

Mitchell[68] reviewed the relation of inositol phospholipids to cell surface receptor function. He noted an enhanced turnover of the phosphoryl group of phosphatidylinositol without changing the amount of PI. It was accomplished by cycling sequentially through 1,2 diacyl glycerol, phosphatidic acid, CDP diacyl glycerol to phosphatidyl inositol. This cycle requires Ca^{++} and a high ATP/AMP and CTP/CMP ratio (three high energy phosphate bonds) to produce it. Cyclic GMP is often increased with increased PI turnover, while cyclic AMP is reciprocally reduced. The PI response precedes phagocytosis of macrophages or polymorphonuclear leukocytes, degranulation of platelets, and cell division in lymphocytes after lectin stimulation and in fibroblasts after addition of serum to the medium. The PI response may be important in transmitting extracellular information into the cell, in grouping and orienting vectorially directed enzyme systems, in the packaging and translocation of macromolecules, and in selection and control of ion movement. The cyclic nature of this response may alter membrane charge and topological charge configuration.

Pasternak[73] reports that phosphatidyl inositol turnover is stimulated when 3T3 fibroblasts are released from contact inhibition by the addition of serum to the media. Since the biochemical and morphologic changes occur equally rapidly, the theory that the PI response is associated with movement of membrane was supported. Koch and Diringer[55a] report that the PI response is associated with division of STU fibroblasts but not with SV-40 transformed fibroblasts. Koch and Diringer[55] report the isolation of cyclic inositol-1,2 phosphate from SV-40 transformed fibroblasts, and postulate that it may serve as a messenger of cell surface events.

Cyclic nucleotide concentrations influence cell division. Addition of fresh serum to confluent 3T3 cells leads to a decrease in cyclic AMP and an initiation of DNA synthesis. Cyclic AMP also decreases after addition of insulin or trypsin, which stimulate DNA synthesis and cell growth.[71] Baum et al.[5] indicate that as very low levels of cyclic AMP in transformed fibroblasts increase, the fibroblast "normalizes" its shape and differentiated properties, including the proportion of protein synthesis devoted to collagen. However, in normal fibroblasts, increased intracellular cyclic AMP caused an average 47% reduction in the percentage of total protein synthesis represented by collagen. In the absence of detectable collagenase, the authors suggest that cyclic AMP may modulate the differentiated state of normal fibroblasts with respect to collagen production.[5] This change may be important, because when interaction with the extracellular matrix[11] tells the cells they are confluent they may begin to make collagen in response to a specific level of cyclic AMP. Rudland et al.[79] report that the cAMP/cGMP ratio decreases in growing or activated cells relative to rested cells. Addition of PGE and increased cAMP suppressed the rise in cGMP and reduced the induction of DNA synthesis by one third. The changes in cyclic nucleotide concentration are largely lost when cells are transformed.

Microvilli formed in proliferating cells may relate to cyclic nucleotides and ultimate cellular arrangement. Willingham and Pastan[95] report that trypsin, which induces fibroblast division, causes the formation of microvilli which can agglutinate or clump 3T3 fibroblasts. Increased cAMP will reduce these microvilli. They propose that neoplastic cells agglutinate because of low cAMP levels. The function of such surface microvilli is unclear, although they seem to be associated with fibroblast proliferation from protelytic enzymes such as trypsin. Dulbecco and Elkington[27] report that increased levels of calcium lead to increased DNA synthesis and division of Balb/c 3T3 fibroblasts, which mimic the serum effect, but require no serum. Although the mechanism is not clear, increased transport rate of substances into cells and alteration of the cGMP/cAMP ratio are suggested. These proposals are consistent with Mitchell's[68] proposal that calcium influences events which follow the PI response, that is, the effector responses, in this case, of cell division. Finally, Ciechanover and Hershko[22] report that addition of serum to 3T3 fibroblasts caused an accelerated turnover of phosphatidyl inositol, possibly related to increased mobility of membrane constituents. They postulated that this may be related to the commencement of cellular movement or some rearrangement of membrane structure required for initiation of cellular growth.

C. Summary (Fibroblast Proliferation)

The responses of fibroblasts to trypsin and the PI responses of fibroblasts suggest that motility or rearrangement of cell membrane structure is important to fibroblast proliferation.[22] Thus, reduced fibroblast division observed[29-32] in agar or on a hydrated collagen lattice might indicate that collagen's influence on fibroblast proliferation is to impede this molecular rearrangement. Induced fibrinolysis or collagenolysis effectively remove this impedance and proliferation can occur. It is likely that the removal of contact of fibroblasts with cells or substrate would trigger a PI response and raise intracellular phosphate while consuming ATP. This increased phosphate and reduced ATP/AMP would activate glycolysis and increase pentose pathway activity, providing the pentoses and NADPH required for nucleic acid production and the ATP and other factors necessary for protein and lipid synthesis prior to membrane assembly. Are mitogens necessary for fibroblast proliferation? Do they relate to the protein factor of McGee et al.[66] or the connective tissue activating peptides of Castor et al.?[19] How do they fit into the previously elaborated mechanism? An additional intriguing question concerns the stimuli provoking cell division in the other cells producing collagen and perhaps elastin. These cells may be the alveolar type II cell, the alveolar contractile cell of Kapanci et al.,[48] the endothelial cell, and the bronchial or vascular smooth muscle cell. McCullagh and Balian[65] report that vascular media smooth muscle cells synthesize primarily type III collagen. However, when such cells migrate to the intima as in gross intimal thickening, they undergo anatomic change and begin to produce mostly type I collagen. Do different environments of connective tissue producing cells lead to a different response with respect to pulmonary collagen molecular heterogeneity? The relation of Kapanci's et al.[48] contractile cell, the myofibroblast and the smooth muscle cell make interesting speculation regarding this response and its effect on pulmonary physiology. Research is only beginning in this fascinating but complex segment of connective tissue metabolism.

IV. FIBRONECTIN — COLD INSOLUBLE GLOBULIN — LETS PROTEIN: INTERACTION BETWEEN CONNECTIVE TISSUE AND THE CELL SURFACE

Fibronectin, a protease-sensitive protein, is present on the surface of cells and often associated with connective tissue. It is likewise involved in cell-matrix interactions. Little attention has been devoted to interactions of the extracellular matrix with the connective tissue-producing cell. The implications of this interaction relate to adherence to surfaces, ability of the cell to organize and maintain a complex matrix, directed motility, and secretion and response of the cell surface in processes such as tissue differentiation and most especially in tissue injury. Fibronectin is present on the surface of numerous cells, including fibroblasts, endothelial cells, epithelial cells, smooth muscle cells, and pulmonary cells.[5,11,12,16,96] Some properties are reviewed by Bornstein et al.[12] It exists as a dimer with monomer weight of ≃ 220,000 daltons; the dimer is notably sensitive to trypsin and some proteases. It is reduced on surfaces of many malignant or transformed mesenchymal cells. Cultured connective tissue cells elaborate a "microexudate carpet or glycocalyx" which contains collagen, proteoglycans, notably hyaluronic acid, and several glycoproteins. One such glycoprotein has a molecular weight similar to fibronectin. Fibronectin can be isolated from embryonic chick, NIL hamster, or human embryonic fibroblasts.[4,11] Endothelial cells elaborate fibronectin (LETS protein) only on the matrix side, exhibiting directed secretion.[96] Fibronectin and cold insoluble globulin (CIG) are extremely similar with respect to immunologic properties and amino acid composition.[92] This similarity raises the possibility that plasma CIG may be a natural product of endothelial cell turnover and a degradation product of fibronectin.[13] However, fibronectin can be released from cell surface into the medium of cultured lung fibroblasts while retaining the same size.[4] If endothelial cell turnover constitutes a major source of plasma CIG, pulmonary injury with its attendant endothelial and type I epithelial injury[54a,76a] and proteolysis[39] should release CIG into the vascular and airway space. This would indicate accelerated cell-matrix interaction, turnover, and possibly death. This evidence clearly indicates that fibronectin, present on the surface of connective tissue-producing cells, is often involved with cell matrix interactions.

Fibronectin is often distributed in a similar fashion to collagen on the surface of connective tissue cells. It is a protein which determines the matrix, although collagen may form a second matrix or simply bind to the fibronectin. Fibronectin binding to the cell surface has been shown by immunofluorescence.[11,90] Moreover, antifibronectin serum is cytotoxic to fibroblasts in the presence of complement.[81] Fibronectin binds to collagen or gelatin, and to α-chains and α_1(I)-CB-7.[54,80] Recently, Bornstein and Ash[11] have demonstrated that collagen, procollagen, or both are localized on the surface of fibroblasts. A similar pattern was observed for fibronectin. In confluent cultures, type I and III collagen showed extensive codistribution with fibronectin. These proteins were arrayed in a reticular fashion such that the possibility of them forming a meshwork was considered.[11,12,89] Digestion of pericellular collagen or procollagen with collagenase did not affect the fibrillar distribution of the fibronectin matrix. This finding suggests that collagen or procollagen is not necessary to maintain the extracellular matrix and raises the possibility that fibronectin may have an organizing role in matrix formation.[89] Collagen may bind to fibronectin or form a second matrix.[20] However, fibronectin would seem to play a determining role in the organization of the extracellular matrix.

Collagen, procollagen, and fibrin may cross-link to fibronectin. The cross-linking of a major fibroblast-associated glycoprotein, fibronectin, was shown to be catalyzed by factor XIIIa.[52,69] Fibrin, which is known to bind the catalytic subunit of XIIIa, inhibits the cross-linking reaction. Cross-linking of labeled cell surface fibronectin to fibrin could not be demonstrated.[52] However, Ruoslahti and Engvall[80] indicated that fibronectin could bind to both fibrin and fibrinogen. Kleinman et al.[54,54a] have localized the binding site of fibronectin to collagen as being in a region of the α_1(I)-CB-7, less helical than the other regions of the molecule. Binding integrity depends on retention of this structure. Binding of collagen to fibronectin is also inhibited by anions, specifically proteoglycans.[54a] Fibrinogen inhibits binding to collagen, but is not very active. Collagen inhibits binding of fibronectin to fibrinogen.[80] Thus, it would seem that fibronectin might mediate the attachment of collagen extracellular matrix to cells in normal tissue, or fibrin to cells in a healing wound. This could serve an important role in localizing fibroblasts in this healing wound.[12,80] Since stationary fibroblasts make collagen but proliferating ones do not, localizing fibroblasts in the healing process would limit the extent of fibroblast proliferation and possibly initiate elaboration of collagen. These properties are important determinants of the extent, shape, and effectiveness of scar formation.

Fibronectin binds to the cytoskeleton. Hunt and Brown[46] report that a high molecular weight L cell surface protein (fibronectin) binds poorly to transformed cells which have a poorly developed cytoskeleton. A high molecular weight protein has been associated with ridges of chick embryo fibroblasts. Underlying these ridges are bundles of actin containing microfilaments. This high molecular weight protein is associated with actin. These data suggest more than a casual indirect relationship of external protein with cytoskeleton.[46] Ash et al.[2] report that antibody-induced linkage of cultured fibroblast plasma membrane proteins (such as β_2 microglobulin, aminopeptides and Na^+-K^+ ATPase) to intracellular actomyosin-containing microfilaments resulted in stabilizing these proteins on the cell surface. Presumably actin is associated with the cytoplasmic side of the plasma membrane by attachment to a link protein. When other proteins form clusters, they bind to actin filaments.[2] Kurkinen et al.[61] have shown that treatment of cultured fibroblasts with cytochalasin B results in disappearance of microfilaments and the release of fibronectin from the cell surface.[61] These data suggest that fibronectin binds to microfilaments. This provides a way in which the cell can realize that it is "confluent" in vitro or the in vivo equivalent. Since confluent cells in vitro make collagen, but dividing cells do not (but merely divide), it is especially important for the cells in a healing wound to realize when they should begin to make collagen, although Baum et al.[5] indicated that intracellular c-AMP might also play a role. Contact with cytoskeleton (microfilaments) provides a basis by which the cell is notified of reaching contact inhibition. The extent to which these microfilaments interact with collagen production is unclear. Likewise the control points of this process (if any) were undefined. The number of fibroblasts in this healing wound or injury may well determine approximately the quantity of connective tissue production.

Finally, one may well ask the question, "Are fibroblasts alone in this interaction?" Bornstein et al.[12] review data indicating that in addition to fibroblasts, smooth muscle cells, glial cells, endothelial cells, and some epithelial cells have fibronectin present on their surfaces. Possibly a cell in lung such as type II epithelial cells which do not form tight junctions would require an extracellular matrix and undergo a similar interaction. If so, the matrix interaction would have to be on the tissue side only. Zetter et al.[96] and Birdwell et al.[8] report elaboration of fibronectin only on the tissue side, indicating that this phenomenon occurs in endothelial cells. This suggests that at least fibroblasts (mesenchymal cells) and endothelial cells may well be controlled by an extracellular pulmonary alveolar matrix. Moreover, type II epithelial cells fulfill many of the criteria for such interaction. Type I epithelial cells in the pulmonary alveolus are cells specialized for covering large surface areas. Moreover, they do form tight junctions and would be much less likely to undergo such interaction. Likewise there is little need for them to do so since type I cells do not divide. If type II epithelial cells are subject to contact inhibition or control by fibronectin in the extracellular matrix, one can begin to understand the interactions which initiate type II cell proliferation. Although quite common in most lung injuries, this phenomenon had received almost no attention beyond recording its presence. Indeed, some believed proliferation to be tied closely, if not inseparably, to the other function of these cells, secretion of surfactant. This secretion has been elegantly described by Clements and King.[23] An understanding of conditions under which type II pulmonary alveolar epithelial cells proliferate is vital to understanding the course of lung injury. For instance, degree of proliferation may infer the extent and intensity of lung injury. Elsdale and Bard[29] indicate that fibroblasts will not proliferate on viable and growing epithelium. Thus, again, understanding of the nature of proliferation of type II cells (or lack of it) relates to an understanding of pulmonary fibrosis and other changes relating to connective tissue of the lung.

Proteolysis degrades fibronectin, releasing a smaller protein, cold-insoluble globulin. Cold-insoluble globulin functions to enhance platelet adherence to the endothelial surface. Some proteolytic enzymes can induce cell division in quiescent chick embryo fibroblasts.[18] The specificity of a protease for the cell surface would probably determine cellular response to that enzyme. For instance, both trypsin and thrombin induce thymidine incorporation, but trypsin alone removes LETS protein (fibronectin). With several other proteases equal difficulty was experienced correlating quantity of surface LETS protein with the growth state of the cells. Surprisingly, a 205,000-dalton protein was removed in each case.[18] The significance is far from clear. The small difference in molecular weight between plasma (CIG) and cell surface fibronectin suggests that plasma fibronectin may arise from a specific proteolytic cleavage. The additional 20,000-dalton piece may bind fibronectin to the cell surface.[69] This may be complicated by the observation of Hynes et al.[47] that platelets recruit CIG from the plasma to bind to collagen. Thus, CIG in plasma serves a useful role and is probably essential to platelet attachment. The observation of Hiti-Harper et al.[44a] that platelet factor IV is a low molecular weight collagenase inhibitor takes on more meaning in this process. In an injury destroying endothelial cells by proteolysis, one could envision a removal of the actin-fibronectin attachment and a release of cold-insoluble globulin. This could result in endothelial or mesenchymal cell proliferation, depending on how severe the conditions were. The more severe conditions might prevent endothelial proliferation and lead to fibroblast proliferation. In addition, more platelets would recruit cold-insoluble globulin, initiating platelet attachment and leading to reduced platelet life in circulation, and either clotting or fibroblast proliferation. Harker et al.[43] have shown that in the case of larger vessels where smooth muscle cells fill the role of mesenchymal cells, if one can prevent smooth muscle proliferation, atherosclerosis won't develop. Pickrell et al.[77] have had considerable success arresting radiation-induced pulmonary fibrosis under conditions suggesting an inhibition of fibroblast proliferation. Release of CIG into plasma ordinarily carefully controlled may lead to considerable pulmonary injury.

Dividing, developing, and neoplastic cells all have less surface fibronectin. However, the ways in which they arrive at this state reflect not only the performance of this increased cell proliferation, but the ability of the cell to interact with the fibronectin-collagen matrix to perform what the cell views its role to be. Loss of LETS protein during viral transformation may reflect reduced production or increased removal.[18] Adams et al.[1] report that transformation of chick embryo fibroblasts leads to a five-fold reduction of translatable m-RNA for cell surface protein, a 10-fold reduction of m-RNA for two collagen precursors, and an increased m-RNA for two membrane polypeptides. This suggested that the transformed cell line was prepared to proliferate, and would not produce either fibronectin or collagen to impede the progress of its proliferation. The molecular event initiating this has yet to be defined, but these events are in an area which can control protein synthesis without altering DNA of the original cell by controlling transcription rates of specific m-RNAs. This is contrasted by Zetter and Martin[97] with the developing mouse embryo where fibronectin was absent from the proliferating outer cells but present in the inner cell mass. Moreover, its quantity increased with time of growth, and it was associated with the embryonic ectoderm, both in mouse embryo and in a line with many of the same properties, teratocarcinoma cells. In the normal developing mouse embryo, fibronectin seems to be associated with differentiation. However, in embryonal carcinoma lines this correlation cannot be made.[97] Stenman et al.[86] reported that interphase cells had roughly equivalent concentration of intracellular and cell surface fibronectin. This was not changed when cells were making DNA. Mitotic cells had reduced amounts of cell surface but not intracellular fibronectin. Fibronectin first appeared on the surface of flattening telophase cells. Moreover, fibronectin was present in the extracellular matrix surrounding the cells. Rather than being involved in growth control, fibronectin plays a structural role in interaction of the cells with the environment.[86] In both the dividing and neoplastic cell, fibronectin on the surface is reduced. However, in the neoplastic cell the translating machinery for both fibronectin and collagen is shut down. This is to be contrasted with the more temporary arrangement in dividing (mitotic) cells, where only the surface fibronectin is reduced so that the cell can obtain enough room to divide. Finally, in developing mouse embryo, fibronectin is associated with differentiation. Three different methods of cell interaction with the associated matrix reaffirm the ability of the cell to act in a certain way and to shape the matrix so that this can occur.

V. SUMMARY

Bornstein et al.[12] have proposed a model in which many protein producing cells rest in a meshwork of cell surface associated protein. This meshwork is composed at least in part of collagen and fibronectin (a protease-sensitive protein). In support of this they cite the work of Bornstein and Ash,[11] indicating that collagen and fibronectin have approximately the same extracellular distribution. Fibronectin binds to collagen through the α_1(I)-CB7 portion.[54] However, digestion of pericellular collagen or procollagen did not affect the fibrillar distribution of fibronectin, suggesting collagen to be unnecessary to maintain the extracellular matrix.[89] Binding of fibronectin to collagen, procollagen, or fibrin may be inhibited by anions, especially proteoglycans.[54] Fibronectin, and thus the external meshwork, binds to the internal cytoskeleton, presumably eliciting a contact-inhibition signal of some sort,[46] and stabilizing these proteins on the cell surface.[2] The fact that cytocholasin B releases cell-associated fibronectin and causes intracellular microfilaments to disperse[61] lends support to this hypothesis.

The interaction of many protein-producing cells and the extracellular meshwork provides a basis for describing the behavior of fibroblasts, corner cells of Kapanci (both mesenchymal cells), endothelial cells, and perhaps type II epithelial cells in the pulmonary alveolus, as well as platelets. Type I pulmonary epithelial cells with very tight junctions probably do not interact in this fashion, because they do not divide. For instance, endothelial cells release a presumably cleaved form of soluble fibronectin (CIG) into plasma. CIG is recruited by platelets, probably proportionate to their relative concentrations. CIG recruitment in turn leads to attachment and to intravascular coagulation. The balance of endothelial turnover and coagulation seems to be a critical one.

Mesenchymal cells at rest produce connective tissue, probably proportionate to some signal, possibly c-AMP.[5] Dividing cells elaborate less fibronectin (and have less on their surface) but keep a readily available intracellular supply.[86] This is consistent with fibronectin being associated with differentiation in the developing embryo[97] and with less fibronectin and collagen m-RNA being present in transformed cells.[1] The cells seem to control their interaction with the matrix at the secretion level "fine tuning" or at the protein translation level ("coarse adjustment"). The stimulus and events which lead to the cell interacting with its matrix in this manner are far from clear. However, in neither case would it be necessary to alter the basic DNA pattern, especially that of the collagen or fibronectin. Control in the case of neoplasia could be altered at the translation or post-translation level. Further work in this exciting area will be watched eagerly.

The following paragraph contains speculation as to *possible* significance of these findings. Mesenchymal cells in injured lung presumably proliferate to fill an existing void of dead or damaged cells. Interaction of such cells with the extracellular matrix could be initiated by severing the meshwork from the microfilaments. Since microfibrils and microfilaments are involved in protein secretion, the cell could then secrete less as it received the message that cell division was "rational". Mesenchymal cells could then divide to contact inhibition (reattachment to microfibril of fibronectin). At this point they could begin to make collagen; this production rate could be secondarily controlled by a mediator, perhaps c-AMP. If the proliferation stimulus from injury were of just the right type (which is as yet undefined), control could be altered at translation and neoplasia could result. Thus the lung cells could, by specific interaction with their extracellular matrix (and involving fibronectin), progress to a variety of differing lung diseases.

REFERENCES

1. **Adams, S. L., Sobel, M. E., Howard, B. H., Olden, K., Yamada, K. M., de Crombrugshe, B., and Pastan, I.,** Levels of translatable mRNAs for cell surface protein, collagen precursors, and two membrane proteins are altered in Rous sarcoma virus transformed chick embryo fibroblasts, *Proc. Natl. Acad. Sci. U.S.A.*, 74(8), 3399, 1977.
2. **Ash, J. F., Lounard, D., and Singer, S. J.,** Antibody-induced linkages of plasma membrane proteins to intracellular actomyosin-containing filaments in cultured fibroblasts, *Proc. Natl. Acad. Sci. U.S.A.*, 74(12), 5584, 1977.
3. **Balin, A. K., Goodman, D. P. B., Rasmussen, H., and Cristofalo, V. J.,** The effect of oxygen tension on the growth and metabolism of WI-38 cells, *J. Cell. Physiol.*, 89, 235, 1976.
4. **Baum, B. J., McDonald, J. A., and Crystal, R. G.,** Metabolic fate of the major cell surface protein of normal human fibroblasts, *Biochem. Biophys. Res. Commun.*, 79, 8, 1977.
5. **Baum, B. J., Moss, J., Breul, S. D., and Crystal, R. G.,** Association in normal human fibroblasts of elevated levels of adenosine 3′:5′-monophosphate with a selective decrease in collagen production, *J. Biol. Chem.*, 253(10), 3391, 1978.
6. **Bartholomew, J. C., Neff, N. T., and Ross, P. A.,** Stimulation of WI-38 cell cycle transit: effect of serum concentration and cell density, *J. Cell. Physiol.*, 89, 251, 1976.
7. **Bice, D. E., Harris, D. L., and Mauderly, J. L.,** Immunization by lung lavage with antigen suspensions, *Fed. Proc.*, 36, 1275, 1977.
8. **Birdwell, C. R., Gospodarowicz, D., and Nicolson, G. L.,** Identification, localization, and role of fibronectin in cultured bovine endothelial cells, *Proc. Natl. Acad. Sci. U.S.A.*, 75(7), 3273, 1978.
9. **Bolduc, P. and Reid, L.,** Mitotic index of the bronchial and alveolar lining of the normal rat lung, *Am. Rev. Respir. Dis.*, 114, 1121, 1976.
10. **Boone, C. W.,** Malignant hemangioendotheliomas produced by subcutaneous inoculation of BALB/3T3 cells attached to glass beads, *Science*, 188, 68, 1975.
11. **Bornstein, P. and Ash, J. F.,** Cell surface associated structural proteins in connective tissue cells, *Proc. Natl. Acad. Sci. U.S.A.*, 74(6), 2480, 1977.
12. **Bornstein, P., Duksin, D., Balian, G., Davidson, J. M., and Crouch, E.,** Organization of extracellular protein on the connective tissue cell surface: relevance to cell-matrix interaction *in vitro* and *in vivo*, *Ann. N.Y. Acad. Sci.*, 312, 93, 1978.
13. **Bowness, M.,** The similarity between cold-insoluble globulins and connective tissue structural glycoproteins, paper presented at meeting of West Coast Connective Tissue Workers Society, Keystone, Colo., March 31, 1978.
14. **Boyden, E. A.,** The development of the lung in the pig-tail monkey (*Macaca nemestrina*, L.), *Anat. Rec.*, 186, 15, 1976.

15. **Bray, B. A., Hsu, K. C., Wigger, H. J., and Leroy, E. C.,** Association of fibrinogen and microfibrils with trophoblast basement membrane, *Connect. Tissue Res.*, 3, 55, 1975.
16. **Bray, B. A.,** Presence of fibronectin in basement membranes and acidic structural glycoproteins from human placenta and lung, *Ann. N.Y. Acad. Sci.*, 312, 142, 1978.
17. **Breeze, R. G. and Wheeldon, E. B.,** The cells of the pulmonary airways, *Am. Rev. Respir. Dis.*, 116, 705, 1977.
18. **Buchanan, J. M., Chen, L. B., and Zetter, B. R.,** Are high molecular weight glycoproteins regulators of cellular growth?, *Ann. N.Y. Acad. Sci.*, 312, 293, 1978.
19. **Castor, C. W., Smith, S. F., Ritchie, J. C., and Scott, M. E.,** Connective tissue activation: mechanism and significance, in *Biology of Fibroblast*, Academic Press, New York, 1973, 483.
20. **Chen, L. B., Burridge, K., Murray, A., Walsh, M. L., Copple, C. D., Bushnell, A., McDougall, J. K., and Gallimore, P. H.,** Modulation of cell surface glycocalyx: studies on large external, transformation-sensitive protein, *Ann. N.Y. Acad. Sci.*, 312, 366, 1978.
21. **Chung, E., Rhodes, R. K., and Miller, E. J.,** Characterization of basement membrane collagens, *Fed. Proc. Abstr.*, 35, 1520, 1976.
21a. **Chung, E., Rhodes, R. K., and Miller, E. J.,** Isolation of three collagenous components of probable basement membrane origin from several tissues, *Biochem. Biophys. Res. Commun.*, 71(4), 1167, 1976.
22. **Ciechanover, A. and Hershko, A.,** Early effects of serum on phospholipid metabolism in untransformed and oncogenic virus-transformed cultured fibroblasts, *Biochem. Biophys. Res. Commun.*, 73, 85, 1976.
23. **Clements, J. A. and King, R. J.,** Composition of the surface active material, in *The Biochemical Basis of Pulmonary Function*, Crystal, R. G., Ed., Marcel Dekker, New York, 1976, 363.
24. **Davis, G. S., Brody, A. R., and Craighead, J. E.,** Analysis of airspace and interstitial mononuclear cell populations in human diffuse interstitial lung disease, *Am. Rev. Respir. Dis.*, 118, 7, 1978.
25. **Davis, G. S., Brody, A. R., Landis, J. N., Graham, W. B. G., Craighead, J. E., and Green, G. M.,** Quantitation of inflammatory activity in interstitial pneumonitis by bronchofiberscopic pulmonary lavage, *Chest*, 69, 265, 1976.
26. **Davison, P. F.,** Homeostasis in extracellular tissues: insights from studies on collagen, *Crit. Rev. Biochem.*, 1, 201, 1973.
27. **Dulbecco, R. and Elkington, J.,** Induction of growth in resting fibroblastic cell cultures by Ca^{++}, *Proc. Natl. Acad. Sci. U.S.A.*, 72, 1584, 1975.
28. **Ebert, R. V., Kronenberg, R. S., and Terracio, M. J.,** Study of the surface secretion of the bronchiole using radioautography, *Am. Rev. Respir. Dis.*, 114, 567, 1976.
29. **Elsdale, T. and Bard, J.,** Cellular interactions in morphogenesis of epithelial mesenchymal systems, *J. Cell Biol.*, 63, 343, 1974.
30. **Elsdale, T. and Bard, J.,** Collagen substrata for studies on cell behavior, *J. Cell Biol.*, 54, 626, 1972.
31. **Elsdale, T. and Bard, J.,** Cellular interactions in mass cultures of human diploid fibroblasts, *Nature (London)*, 236, 152, 1972.
32. **Elsdale, T. and Foley, R.,** Morphogenetic aspects of multilayering in petri dish cultures of human fetal lung fibroblasts, *J. Cell Biol.*, 41, 298, 1969.
33. **Fishman, A. P. and Pietra, G. G.,** Handling of bioactive materials by the lung (I and II), *N. Engl. J. Med.*, 291, 884, 953, 1974.
34. **Ford, R. J. and Kuhn, C.,** Immunologic competence of alveolar cells. I. The plaque-forming response to particulate and soluble antigens, *Am. Rev. Respir. Dis.*, 107, 763, 1973.
35. **Foster, J. A., Mecham, R. P., and Franzblau, C.,** A high molecular weight species of soluble elastin, *Biochem. Biophys. Res. Commun.*, 72, 1399, 1976.
36. **Fung, Y. C. and Sobin, S. S.,** Theory of sheet flow in lung alveoli, *J. Appl. Physiol.*, 26, 472, 1969.
37. **Gabbiani, G., Le Lous, M., Bailey, A. J., Bazin, S., and Delaunay, A.,** Collagen and myofibroblasts of granulation tissue. A chemical, ultrastructural and immunologic study, *Virchows Arch. B*, 21, 133, 1976.
38. **Gabbiani, G., Majno, G., and Ryan, G. B.,** The fibroblast as a contractile cell: the myo-fibroblast, in *Biology of Fibroblast*, Kulonen, E. and Pikkarainen, J., Eds., Academic Press, New York, 1973, 139.
39. **Goldstein, R. H., Faris, B., Hu, C. L., Snider, G. L., and Franzblau, C.,** The fate of newly synthesized lung collagen after endotracheal administration of ^{14}C-proline to hamsters, *Am. Rev. Respir. Dis.*, 117, 281, 1978.
40. **Gray, P. N., Cullum, M. E., and Griffin, M. J.,** Population density and regulation of cell division in 3T3 cells, *J. Cell. Physiol.*, 89, 225, 1976.
41. **Grazi, E., de Flora, A., and Pontremoli, S.,** The inhibition of phosphoglucose isomerase by D-erythrose 4-phosphate, *Biochem. Biophys. Res. Commun.*, 2, 121, 1960.
41a. **Gross, J.,** Collagen biology: structure, degradation, and disease, *Harvey Lect.*, 68, 351, 1974.

42. **Hance, A. J. and Crystal, R. G.,** The connective tissue of lung, *Am. Rev. Respir. Dis.,* 112, 657, 1975.

43. **Harker, L. A., Ross, R., Slichter, S. J., and Scott, C. R.,** Homocystine-induced arteriosclerosis. The role of endothelial cell injury and platelet response in its genesis, *J. Clin. Invest.,* 58, 731, 1976.

44. **Haynes, R. C. and Larner, J.,** Adrenocorticotropic hormone; adrenocortical steroids and their synthetic analogs; inhibitors of adrenocortical steroid biosynthesis, in *The Pharmacological Basis of Therapeutics,* 5th ed., Goodman, L. S. and Gilman, A., Eds., Macmillan, New York, 1975, 1472.

44a. **Hiti-Harper, J., Wohl, H., and Harper, E.,** Platelet factor 4: an inhibitor of collagenase, *Science,* 199, 991, 1978.

45. **Howard, B. V., Macarak, E. J., and Gunson, D.,** Characterization of the collagen synthesized by endothelial cells in culture, *Fed. Proc. Abstr.,* 35, 1519, 1976.

46. **Hunt, R. C. and Brown, J. C.,** Interaction of an L-cell surface protein with the cytoskeleton, *Ann. N.Y. Acad. Sci.,* 312, 207, 1978.

47. **Hynes, R. O., Ali, I. U., Destree, A. T., Mautner, V., Perkins, M. E., Senger, D. R., Wagner, D. D., and Smith, K. K.,** A large glycoprotein lost from the surface of transformed cells, *Ann. N.Y. Acad. Sci.,* 312, 317, 1978.

48. **Kapanci, Y., Assimacopoulos, A., Irle, C., Zwahlen, A., and Gabbiani, G.,** "Contractile interstitial cells" in pulmonary alveolar septa: a possible regulator of ventilation/perfusion ratio? Ultrastructural, immunofluorescence, and *in vitro* studies, *J. Cell Biol.,* 60, 375, 1974.

49. **Kawamoto, T. and Nagai, Y.,** Developmental changes in glycosaminoglycans, collagen and collagenase activity in embryonic chick skin, *Biochim. Biophys. Acta,* 437, 190, 1976.

50. **Katzenstein, A. L. A., Bloor, C. M., and Leibow, A. A.,** Diffuse alveolar damage — the role of oxygen, shock, and related factors, *Am. J. Pathol.,* 85, 210, 1976.

51. **Kefalides, N. A.,** Structure and biosynthesis of basement membranes, *Int. Rev. Connect. Tissue Res.,* 6, 63, 1973.

52. **Kaski-Oja, J., Mosher, D. F., and Vaheri, A.,** Cross-linking of a major fibroblast surface associated glycoprotein (fibronectin) catalyzed by blood coagulation factor XIII, *Cell,* 9, 29, 1976.

53. **Kirkman, H. N. and Hendrickson, E. M.,** Glucose 6-phosphate dehydrogenase from human erythrocytes, *J. Biol. Chem.,* 237, 2371, 1962.

54. **Kleinman, H. K., McGoodwin, E. B., and Klebe, R. J.,** Localization of the cell attachment region in Types I and II collagens, *Biochem. Biophys. Res. Commun.,* 72, 426, 1976.

54a. **Kleinman, H. K., McGoodwin, E. B., Martin, G. R., and Klebe, R. J.,** Binding of cell attachment protein to collagen: effects of chemical modifications, *Ann. N.Y. Acad. Sci.,* 312, 436, 1978.

55. **Koch, M. A. and Diringer, H.,** A difference in the breakdown of phosphatidylinositol in normal and SV40 transformed mouse fibroblasts, *Biochem. Biophys. Res. Commun.,* 55, 305, 1973.

55a. **Koch, M. A. and Diringer, H.,** Isolation of cyclic inositol-1,2-phosphate from mammalian cells and a probable function of phosphatidylinositol turnover, *Biochem. Biophys. Res. Commun.,* 58, 361, 1974.

56. **Kornfeld, S.,** The effect of 5′-AMP and UDP-D-glucose on UDP-glucose pyrophosphorylase activity in rat liver, *Fed. Proc.,* 24, 536, 1965.

57. **Kravis, T. C., Ahmed, A., Brown, T. E., Fulmer, J. D., and Crystal, R. G.,** Pathogenic mechanisms in pulmonary fibrosis. Collagen-induced migration inhibition factor production and cytotoxicity mediated by lymphocytes, *J. Clin. Invest.,* 58, 1223, 1976.

58. **Kruse, N. J. and Bornstein, P.,** The metabolic requirements for transcellular movement and secretion of collagen, *J. Biol. Chem.,* 250, 4841, 1975.

59. **Kuhn, C.,** The cells of the lung and their organelles, in *The Biochemical Basis of Pulmonary Function,* Crystal, R. G., Ed., Marcel Dekker, New York, 1976, 3.

60. **Kuhns, W. J., Weinbaum, G., Turner, R., and Burger, M. M.,** Sponge aggregation: a model for studies on cell-cell interactions, *Ann. N.Y. Acad. Sci.,* 234, 58, 1974.

61. **Kurkinen, M., Wartiovaara, J., and Vaheri, A.,** Cytochalasin B releases a major surface associated glycoprotein, fibronectin, from cultured fibroblasts, *Exp. Cell Res.,* 111, 127, 1978.

62. **Lehninger, A. L.,** *Biochemistry,* 2nd ed., Worth Publishers, Inc., New York, 1975, 387.

63. **Mason, R. J.,** Lipid metabolism, in *Biochemical Basis of Pulmonary Function,* Crystal, R. G., Ed., Marcel Dekker, New York, 1976, 127.

64. **Massaro, D. and Massaro, G. D.,** Synthesis, intracellular transport, and secretion of macromolecules by the lung, in *Biochemical Basis of Pulmonary Function,* Crystal, R. G., Ed., Marcel Dekker, New York, 1976, 389.

65. **McCullagh, K. A. and Balian, G.,** Collagen characterization and cell transformation in human atherosclerosis, *Nature (London),* 258, 73, 1975.

66. **McGee, J. O'D., O'Hare, R. P., and Patrick, R. S.,** Stimulation of the collagen biosynthetic pathway by factors isolated from experimentally-injured liver, *Nature (London) New Biol.,* 243, 121, 1973.

67. **Miller, R., Engel, M. B., and Catchpole, H. R.,** Collagen and cellular fractions of blood, *Fed. Proc. Abstr.*, 35, 715, 1976.
68. **Mitchell, R. H.,** Inositol phospholipids and cell surface receptor function, *Biochim. Biophys. Acta,* 415, 81, 1975.
69. **Mosher, D. F.,** Labelling of a major fibroblast surface protein (fibronectin) catalyzed by blood coagulation factor XIIIa, *Biochim. Biophys. Acta,* 491, 205, 1977.
70. **Mosher, D. F., Saksela, O., Keski-Oja, J., and Vaheri, A.,** Distribution of a major surface-associated glycoprotein, fibronectin, in cultures of adherent cells, *J. Supramol. Struct.*, 6, 551, 1977.

70a. **Muggenburg, B. A., Felicetti, S., Silbaugh, S., and Elmquist, C.,** Research communication, 1976.

71. **Otten, J., Johnson, G. S., and Pastan, I.,** Regulation of cell growth by cyclic adenosine 3′,5′-monophosphate. Effect of cell density and agents which alter cell growth on cyclic adenosine 3′,5′-monophosphate levels in fibroblasts, *J. Biol. Chem.*, 247, 7082, 1972.

71a. **Munch-Petersen, A., Kalckar, H. M., Cutolo, E., and Smith, E. E. B.,** Uridyl transferases and the formation of uridine triphosphate, *Nature (London),* 172, 1036, 1953.

72. **Parr, C. W.,** Competitive inhibitors of phosphoglucose isomerase, *Biochem. J.*, 65, 34, 1957.
73. **Pasternak, C. A.,** Relief from contact inhibition, *J. Cell Biol.*, 53, 231, 1972.
74. **Peterson, M. and Leblond, C. P.,** Synthesis of complex carbohydrates in the Golgi region, as shown by radioautography after injection of labeled glucose, *J. Cell Biol.*, 21, 143, 1964.
75. **Pfleger, R. C.,** Type II epithelial cells from the lung of Syrian hamsters: isolation and metabolism, *Exp. Mol. Pathol.*, 27, 152, 1977.

75a. **Pickrell, J. A., Bryant, P. L., and Straus, F. C.,** Research communication, 1976.

76. **Pickrell, J. A., Halliwell, W. H., and Jones, R. K.,** Pulmonary injury mechanisms revealed by cytologic analyses of bronchopulmonary lavage, Inhal. Tox. Res. Inst. Annual Report 1975-1976, LF-56, 1976, 360.

76a. **Pickrell, J. A., Harris, D. V., Mauderly, J. L., and Hahn, F. F.,** Altered collagen metabolism in radiation-induced interstitial pulmonary fibrosis, *Chest,* 69, 311, 1976.

77. **Pickrell, J. A., Straus, F. C., Halliwell, W. H., and Jones, R. K.,** The relation of pulmonary collagen metabolism, inflammation and therapy to radiation-induced pulmonary fibrosis, *Fed. Proc. Abstr.*, 36, 607, 1977.
78. **Rosenquist, T. H., Bernick, S., Sobin, S. S., and Fung, Y. C.,** The structure of the pulmonary interalveolar microvascular sheet, *Microvasc. Res.*, 5, 199, 1973.
79. **Rudland, P. S., Seeley, M., and Seifert, W.,** Cyclic GMP and cyclic AMP levels in normal and transformed fibroblasts, *Nature (London),* 251, 417, 1974.

79a. **Seyer, J. M.,** Basement membrane associated collagens of human lung, *Fed. Proc. Abstr.*, 37(6), 1527, 1978.

80. **Ruoslahti, E. and Engvall, E.,** Immunochemical and collagen binding properties of fibronectin, *Ann. N.Y. Acad. Sci.*, 312, 178, 1978.
81. **Ruoslahti, E. and Sjogren, H. O.,** Specific fibroblast cytotoxicity of antibodies to fibroblast surface antigen, *Int. J. Cancer,* 18, 375, 1976.
82. **Slauson, D. O., Hahn, F. F., Benjamin, S. A., Chiffelle, T. L., and Jones, R. K.,** Inflammatory sequences in acute pulmonary radiation injury, *Am. J. Pathol.*, 82, 549, 1976.
83. **Sobin, S. S., Bernick, S., Tremer, H. M., Rosenquist, T. H., Lindal, R., and Fung, Y. C.,** The fibroprotein network of the pulmonary interalveolar wall, *Chest,* 65, 4S, 1974.
84. **Sobin, S. S., Fung, Y. C., Tremer, H. M., and Rosenquist, T. H.,** Elasticity of the pulmonary alveolar microvascular sheet in the cat, *Circ. Res.*, 30, 440, 1972.
85. **Stachurska, J., Roszkowski, W., Kopéc, M., and Ryzewski, J.,** Effects of bradykinin on rat lymphocytes, *Proc. Soc. Exp. Biol. Med.*, 153, 408, 1976.
86. **Stenman, S., Wartiovaara, J., and Vaheri, A.,** Changes in the distribution of a major fibroblast protein, fibronectin, during mitosis and interphase, *J. Cell Biol.*, 74, 453, 1977.
87. **Stuart, J. M., Postlethwaite, A. E., and Kang, A. H.,** Evidence for cell-mediated immunity to collagen in progressive systemic sclerosis, *J. Lab. Clin. Med.*, 88, 601, 1976.
88. **Thurlbeck, W. M.,** Postnatal growth and development of the lung, *Am. Rev. Respir. Dis.*, 111, 803, 1975.
89. **Vaheri, A., Alitalo, K., Hedman, K., Keski-Oja, J., Kurkinen, M., and Wartiovaara, J.,** Fibronectin and the pericellular matrix of normal and transformed adherent cells, *Ann. N.Y. Acad. Sci.*, 312, 343, 1978.
90. **Van Golde, L. M. G.,** Metabolism of phospholipids in the lung, *Am. Rev. Respir. Dis.*, 114, 977, 1976.
91. **Vracko, R.,** Basal lamina scaffold-anatomy and significance for maintenance of orderly tissue structure, *Am. J. Pathol.*, 77, 314, 1974.
92. **Vuento, M.,** Properties of fibronectin isolated from culture medium of human fibroblasts and from human plasma, *Ann. N.Y. Acad. Sci.*, 312, 401, 1978.

93. **West, J. B.,** Respiratory physiology — the essentials, Williams & Wilkins, Baltimore, 1974, 1.
94. **White, A., Handler, P., and Smith, E. L.,** *Principles of Biochemistry,* 5th ed., McGraw-Hill, New York, 1973, 412.
95. **Willingham, M. C. and Pastan, I.,** Cyclic AMP modulates microvillus formation and agglutinability in transformed and normal mouse fibroblasts, *Proc. Natl. Acad. Sci. U.S.A.,* 72, 1263, 1975.
96. **Zetter, B. R., Martin, G. R., Birdwell, C. R., and Gospodarowicz, D.,** Role of the high-molecular weight glycoprotein in cellular morphology, adhesion, and differentiation, *Ann. N.Y. Acad. Sci.,* 312, 299, 1978.
97. **Zetter, B. R. and Martin, G. R.,** Expression of a high molecular weight cell surface glycoprotein (LETS protein) by preimplantation mouse embryos and teratocarcinoma stem cells, *Proc. Natl. Acad. Sci. U.S.A.,* 75(5), 2324, 1978.

Chapter 10

INTERACTION OF MESENCHYMAL CELLS WITH THE EXTRACELLULAR MATRIX — A SPECULATIVE MODEL

J. A. Pickrell

TABLE OF CONTENTS

It is appropriate at this point (just prior to our discussion about pulmonary disease) to speculate as to what the evidence cited in Chapters 2 through 9 might mean. In fact, we must consider how lung cells interact with the extracellular matrix so that the internal protein-producing machinery of the cell is aware of the level of collagen which is required. Although there may seem to be a good deal of conflicting evidence, the speculative interpretations of this data in earlier chapters enable one to state some hypotheses. A summary of evidence is presented which is suggestive of injury control of (1) the proportion of cell population that is mesenchymal, (2) the nature and rate of collagen DNA transcription, and (3) the efficiency of translation of collagen messenger RNA. Collagen biosynthesis and interaction presumably take precedence over hydroxylation or glycosylation, registration, helix formation, and secretion of procollagen or P_N-collagen. The mesenchymal cell is primarily discussed as the best-known representative of dividing cells of the alveolus.

I. PROPORTION OF CELL POPULATION THAT IS MESENCHYMAL

The extracellular matrix (Figure 1) surrounds virtually all mesenchymal cells, especially those producing collagen. The cell matrix interaction limits the proliferation of fibroblasts. The matrix is determined in shape by a newly characterized protease-sensitive protein, fibronectin,[8] which forms an extracellular network. Initially, this network binds with collagen[2] and presumably subsequently with dermatan sulfate. This complex binds to the cell and microfilaments[17] inside the cell. This binding probably constrains the cell to the point where cell division ceases and collagen synthesis begins. Elastin is somehow placed in the matrix so that it can sit upon the microfibrillar elastin scaffolding where it was cross-linked (see Chapter 6 for details) and so that if it is broken down, considerable quantities of intact collagen chains are solubilized from the matrix.[6] Collagen and possibly elastin have degradative enzymes, collagenase, and elastase bound to their fibers.[14] Since this matrix has a slow turnover, one may assume that these bound enzymes are either inactivated by a reversibly bound antiproteinase, in the inactive proenzyme form, or both. Should excess proteolysis occur, the consequences would be the same, i.e., apparent activation of both enzymes (by cleavage of proenzyme or competition for inhibitor or both). In the case of the Kuettner et al.[11] low molecular weight collagenase inhibitor, it might be impossible to tell because the inhibitor and the "pro" piece have nearly identical molecular weights. Fibronectin, which is extremely protease sensitive, would be broken down, destroying the extracellular matrix, freeing and degrading connective tissue constituents. We have observed this response in collagen after inhalation of NO_2, 20 ppm for 10 of 14 days. Thus, the consequences of proteolysis on one hand are (1) dissolution of matrix, (2) freeing and degrading connective tissue constituents, and (3) cell proliferation to a level where the mesenchymal cell perceives that it is "confluent". On the other hand, the normal cell builds up a matrix and communicates via the microfibrils that it is "confluent", constraining it to the point where cell division ceases and collagen synthesis begins. This is a somewhat involved mechanism by which the numbers of mesenchymal cells relative to other alveolar cells can be controlled. As such, it probably constitutes the coarse adjustment of the level of connective tissue production.

An examination of a few pros and cons of this portion of the model tends to indicate that it explains the data. The argument that collagenase bound to collagen makes no sense can be dealt with by postulating that an inhibitor or a proform of the enzyme is bound to collagen. Then it becomes not only feasible but useful. For collagenase can be secreted continuously by the fibroblast and the amount may be determined by available collagenase: collagen affinity. The argument that this setup (with respect to collagenase-collagen and protease sensitive fibronectin) resembles a time bomb waiting to go off may be countered with the observation that during injury with accompanying cell death there may be a rapid need for mesenchymal cells to proliferate to fill an existing void. It may be necessary to remove portions of the matrix to effect this. Vracko[20] has indicated that the lung is extremely poor in regenerating basement membrane. Considering the "spread out" nature of the alveolus and the need for proteolysis to accompany proliferation, this may merely be reflecting the rather long odds against the successful repair. The odds may be better than one thinks, because Collins et al.[4] and Pickrell et al.[15] have observed resolution after moderate to severe, but different, lung injury. This model seems to be one which will explain most of the data.

II. NATURE AND RATE OF COLLAGEN DNA TRANSCRIPTION

Once the number of cells in an injury has been regulated and established, the rate and type of collagen production may be controlled (Figure 1). Logically, transcription would be a reasonable place for this control to reside. Procollagen binding to the cell membrane accelerates production of membrane-bound ribosomes and collagens.[8a] As procollagen is secreted from the cell it can bind to either fibronectin or heparin on the cell surface.[7,10] Speculatively, competition should exist between them such that the relative proportion of cell surface proteoglycan (heparin) vs. fibronectin might well determine transcription rate of collagen m-RNA. This would be accomplished by attachment of procollagen to the membrane via heparin. One could see as cells were just beginning to secrete procollagen and there was little fibronectin, the equilibrium would be toward binding to the cell and collagen transcription would be increasing. If fibronectin also increased, the equilibrium would gradually shift. More procollagen (probably P_c-collagen) would be bound to fibronectin and cleaved and cross-linked so that synthetic rates would level and actually decline. This presents a much more attractive concept than collagen synthesis proceeding at a fixed rate until it becomes diffusion limited with respect to nutrients. Moreover, transcription of collagen m-RNA would seem to be inversely proportional to quantity of the extracellular matrix. This time, the extracellular matrix is indirectly communicating with the intracellular transcription apparatus and influencing rate of collagen m-RNA transcription.

One may well ask, what does such a system do to determine relative proportions of collagen types? Trypsin cleaves type III but not type I collagen or procollagen;[13] turnover of prelabelled types I and III collagen in proteolysis-type-injury was identical.[9] Let us speculate that the bulk of the type III collagen is in the matrix and that proteolysis cleaves primarily type III procollagen. Moreover, the cell doesn't bind and recognize cleavage products of either collagen. Then, during the early proteolysis of pulmonary injury, cell proliferation would occur, would slow, and types I and III procollagen would be secreted, but type III would be cleaved. Thus, by default, type I procollagen would bind to the heparin on the fibroblast surface causing transcription of type I, m-RNA of collagen. This would increase, level off, and then decline much as total collagen m-RNA transcription rates. As proteolysis decreased, the type III procollagen m-RNA transcription rate would gradually increase to normal. Thus, if measured late in the injury it would not correlate with type III content. Seyer et al.[19] report an increased type I collagen in human idiopathic pulmonary fibrosis. Thus, the type of collagen can also be determined by this intriguing binding. These data suggest that the amount and specific genetic type of collagen m-RNA may be controlled by cell-bound procollagen and proteolysis.

Once again, examining the evidence for and against this method of control, one may say that it provides for modulation of proportions of specific collagen types. However,

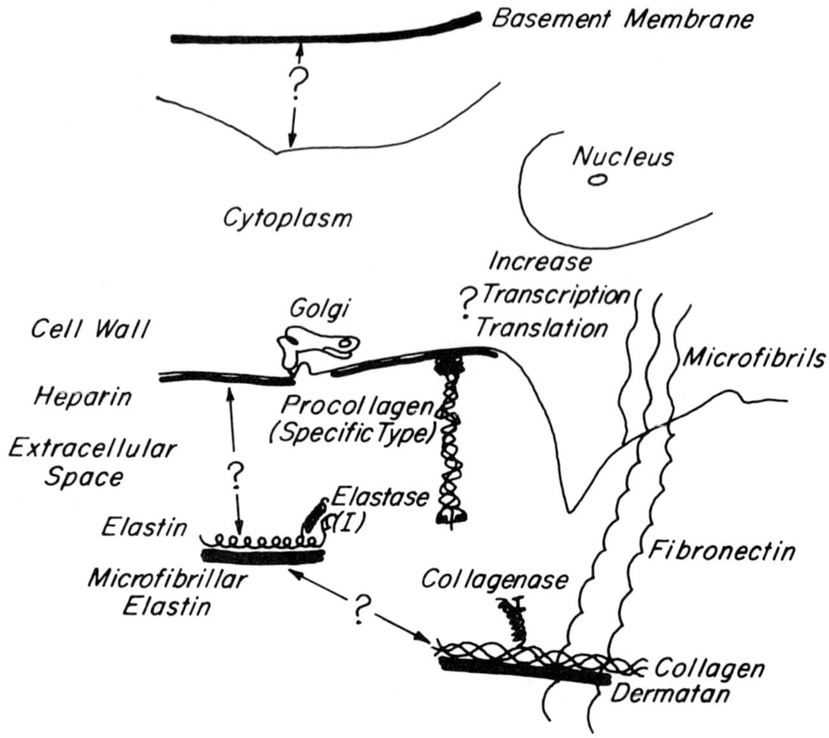

FIGURE 1. A speculative model describing possible interaction of mesenchymal cells producing connective tissue with the extracellar connective tissue matrix is presented. Connective-tissue producing cells are attached or anchored in an undefined manner to basement membrane. These cells are also linked to fibronectin, presumably by their microfibrils, and are coated with heparin. Collagen binds to proteoglycan and fibronectin in such a way that competition would exist for binding of newly secreted procollagen or P-collagen to either cell surface or to extracellular matrix determined by fine structure of fibronectin. This competition probably determines rate of collagen synthesis and blends it to the surrounding matrix. Collagen-bound collagenase provides a rapid way of altering the extracellular matrix. It may be bound to an antiprotease (I) or in a procollagenase form and activated by protelytic enzymes releasing collagen degradation products into the interstitium or even airways. Linkage of elastic fibers of the extracellular matrix to the connective-tissue producing cell is undefined; however, the fiber is composed of an amorphous elastin core and a microfibrillar coating. Elastin bound elastase and its attendant inhibitor (I) seem to be a reasonable but as yet undefined possibility, perhaps acting in a manner similar to collagen-bound collagenase. Elastin is linked to collagen in the extracellular matrix in such a way that elastase action dissolves a large portion of the collagen in the matrix. This linkage is undefined but of great interest in understanding pulmonary molecular anatomy.

one may say that it is difficult to understand why quantity of a collagen precursor varies directly with the rate of transcription. It would be more likely to be the opposite, i.e., procollagen would shut down the reaction. Procollagen is not an "end stage" connective tissue constituent. The cell would need to rapidly produce connective tissue when (1) collagen wasn't being cross-linked or (2) the cells were no longer dividing but there is little extracellular matrix. In both cases, procollagen would be binding to the membrane in increased concentration working to the organism's benefit. Also, against the hypothesis, one might argue that different genes don't have to exist, instead, misreading, mutation, etc., or actually different cells might exist. To counter that, the evidence for type I and III collagen being present in the same cell (cited in Fessler and

Fessler[5]) and on different chromosomes in somatic hybrids,[16] should be cited. Mutations are unlikely because of (1) the uniformity of the response, (2) the large numbers of small differences or point mutations necessary in genes to produce a different collagen type and (3) the glycine triplet structure is conserved reasonably well. Finally, one may say that (1) the nature of the binding to proteoglycans (or glycosaminoglycans), receptors, etc.; (2) the intracellular messenger(s), and (3) the feedback mechanism remain to be demonstrated. Certainly, research in this area should be quite interesting in the future.

III. EFFICIENCY OF TRANSLATION OF COLLAGEN MESSENGER RNA

Even though the cell number and rate and type of collagen are regulated, the response may be modulated still further at the translation level. Fessler and Fessler[5] reviewed evidence indicating that total amount of t-RNA from amino acids reaching collagen cannot be demonstrated to limit translation. However, Carpousis et al.[3] demonstrated a minor isoaccepting species of glycyl t-RNA which is cognate to GGC or GGU and can account for all the increase in glycyl t-RNA in tissues synthesizing collagen. Under the right circumstances, this could influence the efficiency of translating specific m-RNAs.

Finally, cyclic AMP increases will cause transformed fibroblasts to "normalize" their shape, and to produce more collagen. On the other hand, confluent cells whose intracellular cyclic AMP was increased experienced a reduction in collagen production.[1] Thus, levels of cyclic AMP seem to modulate levels of collagen synthesis, although the mechanism is poorly understood. Perhaps an optimum level of cyclic AMP is necessary for optimum collagen production. Cyclic AMP may modulate the differentiated state of normal fibroblasts in collagen production. Cyclic AMP has several mechanisms of action. A recent one is the reversal of phosphorylation of the eIF_2 protein of the ribosomal complex and a concomitant reversal of inhibition of protein synthesis. Collagen synthesis does not vary in the same direction in normal fibroblasts. Perhaps the stimulation is of an inhibitor protein in collagen production. Alternatively, proteins other than collagen may be being produced in greater proportions at the expense of collagen. Finally, Crystal[4a] suggested that this might be a way of rapidly changing collagen synthesis of some lung cells.

In support of their potential control mechanism, Carpousis et al.[3] cite data indicating that a similar increase in glycyl t-RNA but different codons from that of collagen was noted in accelerated fibroin production. Likewise a similar response was noted in $t\text{-}RNA^{gln}$ cognate to CAG and CAA in rabbit hemoglobin synthesis. Finally they cite evidence which showed that under certain circumstances a minor isoaccepting t-RNA species could determine translation rates of different m-RNAs. The minor isoaccepting species could not be replaced with the major one. The cyclic AMP data could be interpreted as indicating conflicting views, i.e., different in transformed and "normal" fibroblasts. Alternatively, it could indicate a modulation of "normal" fibroblasts' collagen synthesis[1] and an activation of cytoskeleton (via energy metabolism) and of collagen production by mechanisms discussed in Chapters 4, 5, and 9. Certainly, all the evidence is not in since Baum et al.[1] were among the first to describe this mechanism. One may also argue that all the mechanisms shown to have biological relevance by Revel and Groner[17] and Lodish[11a] have not been explored for potential control of collagen m-RNA translation. This objection constitutes stimulation to continue this line of investigation. Again, we may point to the possibility that a potential mechanism of the Baum et al.[1] data may be similar to most of those mechanisms reviewed by Revel and Groner.[17] It may be a reversal of the oxidized glutathione inhibition of the translation of some proteins and thus, highly relevant to some lungs especially in light of Rhoades et al.'s[18] observation that lung cyclic AMP decreases in hypoxia. Finally, an isolated mechanism reviewed by Revel and Groner[17] intrigued the author. When cell membrane properties are altered, an influx of Na ions into the cell occurred. This allowed viral m-RNA instead of cellular m-RNA to be translated, since viral m-RNA translation was optimum at this new salt concentration. Could such a mechanism be operating in the on-off type of collagen production in proliferating vs. stationary cells? To my knowledge, no evidence exists either way.

When one examines how the evidence fits together, it seems likely that numbers of mesenchymal cells may be quite important in determining the amount of fibrous connective tissue present in a lesion. As we shall see in Chapters 13 through 17, numbers and location of these mesenchymal cells may influence the course of the disease to the predominant degree. However, some stages of diseases have apparently normal numbers and location of mesenchymal cells. These diseases could have abnormally high or low quantities or specific types of collagen m-RNA translated and reflected in the collagen composition. Negative feedback is an obvious need and its failure has equally obvious consequences, i.e., fibrosis. We shall speculate in Chapters 13 through 17 the possible portions of this mechanism involved in the specific disease state. Alterations of translation efficiency might also be operating, especially in disease states where collagen types do not change. Research on alteration of collagen types has not progressed far enough to imply such evidence indirectly. Thus, a measure of the isoaccepting species of t-RNA cognate to GGC and GGU in the disease state may be necessary to demonstrate this state. To my knowledge, no such measurements have been reported.

We have presented evidence which allows one to speculate on control points at (1) the relative proportion of mesenchymal cells, (2) the efficiency or relative rates of transcription of individual collagen m-RNA, (3) the translation of collagen m-RNAs and hydroxylation of proline in nascent collagen chains (see Chapter 5 for details). Where appropriate, in disease, we will speculate as to the applicability of the model to the data being reviewed. The readers may draw additional conclusions as they choose. Finally, this is a speculative model drawn from data from a variety of disciplines. Time will either validate it or fail to do so. New data in the more speculative areas will be watched with great enthusiasm.

REFERENCES

1. **Baum, B. J., Moss, J., Breul, S. D., and Crystal, R. G.,** Association in normal human fibroblasts of elevated levels of adenosine 3′:5′-monophosphate with a selective decrease in collagen production, *J. Biol. Chem.*, 253(10), 3391, 1978.
2. **Bornstein, P. and Ash, J. F.,** Cell surface associated structural proteins in connective tissue cells, *Proc. Natl. Acad. Sci. U.S.A.*, 74(6), 2480, 1977.
3. **Carpousis, A., Christner, P., and Rosenbloom, J.,** Preferential usage of tRNA isoaccepting species in collagen synthesis, *J. Biol. Chem.*, 252(22), 8023, 1977.
4. **Collins, J. F., Durnin, L. S., and Johanson, W. G., Jr.,** Papain-induced lung injury: alterations in connective tissue metabolism without emphysema, *Exp. Mol. Pathol.*, 29, 29, 1978.

4a. **Crystal, R.,** Posttranslational Control of Collagen Production by Intracellular Degradation, paper presented at the Western Connective Tissue Society Meeting, Seattle, February, 1979.

5. **Fessler, J. H. and Fessler, L. I.,** Biosynthesis of procollagen, *Annu. Rev. Biochem.*, 47, 129, 1978.

6. **Goldstein, R. H., Faris, B., Hu, C. L., Snider, G. L., and Franzblau, C.**, The fate of newly synthesized lung collagen after endotracheal administration of ^{14}C-proline to hamsters, *Am. Rev. Respir. Dis.*, 117, 281, 1978.
7. **Horwitz, A. L., Elson, N. A., and Crystal, R. G.**, Proteoglycans and elastic fibers, in *Biochemical Basis of Pulmonary Function*, Crystal, R. G., Ed., Marcel Dekker, New York, 1976, 273.
8. **Hynes, R. O., Ali, I. U., Destree, A. T., Mautner, V., Perkins, M. E., Senger, D. R., Wagner, D. D., and Smith, K. K.**, A large glycoprotein lost from the surfaces of transformed cells, *Ann. N.Y. Acad. Sci.*, 312, 317, 1978.
8a. **Kao, W. W. Y., Flaks, J. G., and Prockop, D. J.**, Primary and secondary effects of ascorbate on procollagen synthesis and protein synthesis by primary culture of tendon fibroblasts, *Arch. Biochem. Biophys.*, 173, 638, 1976.
9. **Klein, L. and ChandraRajan, J.**, Comparison of collagen turnover (types I versus III) in skin and intestine during rapid growth in rats, *Fed. Proc. Abstr.*, 36, 677, 1977.
10. **Kleinman, H. K., McGoodwin, E. B., Martin, G. R., and Klebe, R. J.**, Binding of cell attachment protein to collagen: effects of chemical modifications, *Ann. N.Y. Acad. Sci.*, 312, 436, 1978.
11. **Kuettner, K. E., Soble, L., Croxen, R., Hiti, J., Harper, E., and Pauli, B.**, Inhibition of tumor collagenases by a cartilage-derived inhibitor, *Fed. Proc. Abstr.*, 36, 677, 1977.
11a. **Lodish, H. F.**, Translational control of protein synthesis, *Annu. Rev. Biochem.*, 45, 39, 1976.
12. **Kurkinen, M., Wartiovaara, J., and Vaheri, A.**, Cytochalasin B releases a major surface associated glycoprotein, fibronectin, from cultured fibroblasts, *Exp. Cell Res.*, 111, 127, 1978.
13. **Miller, E. J., Finch, J. E. Jr., Chung, E., and Butler, W. T.**, Specific cleavage of the native type III collagen molecule with trypsin, *Arch. Biochem. Biophys.*, 173, 631, 1976.
14. **Peréz-Tamayo, R.**, Pathology of collagen degradation — a review, *Am. J. Pathol.*, 92, 509, 1978.
15. **Pickrell, J. A., Diel, J. O., Slauson, D. O., Halliwell, W. H., and Mauderly, J. L.**, Diffuse interstitial fibrosis following radiation-induced lung injury resolves spontaneously if dense scars are not formed, submitted for publication, 1979.
16. **Raj, C. V. S., Church, R. L., Creagan, R. P., and Ruddle, F. H.**, *J. Cell Biol.*, 70, A78, 1976; as cited in **Fessler, J. H. and Fessler, L. I.**, Biosynthesis of procollagen, *Annu. Rev. Biochem.*, 47, 129, 1978.
17. **Revel, M. and Groner, Y.**, Post-transcriptional and translational controls of gene expression in eukaryotes, *Annu. Rev. Biochem.*, 47, 1079, 1978.
18. **Rhoades, R. A., Morrow, R. P., and Eskew, M. L.**, Lung cyclic AMP: selective decrease with hypoxia, *Proc. Soc. Exp. Biol. Med.*, 152, 480, 1976.
19. **Seyer, J. M., Hutcheson, E. T., and Kang, A. H.**, Collagen polymorphism in idiopathic chronic pulmonary fibrosis, *J. Clin. Invest.*, 57, 1498, 1976.
20. **Vracko, R.**, Basal lamina scaffold-anatomy and significance for maintenance of orderly tissue structure, *Am. J. Pathol.*, 77, 314, 1974.

Chapter 11

IMMUNOLOGIC MECHANISMS OF PULMONARY CONNECTIVE TISSUE INJURY

R. Burrell and J. O. Hill

TABLE OF CONTENTS

I. INTRODUCTION

The comparatively recent development of the science of immunopathology has brought the realization that lung connective tissue can be injured by immunologic mechanisms. Owing to its anatomic position and physiologic function, the lung is constantly exposed to an enormous amount of potentially damaging, biologically active material. Likewise, it contains an appreciable amount of lymphoid cells and tissue capable of initiating an immune response.[25]

The expression of immunological defense mechanisms and, in particular, how they may be operating in the lung has been the subject of recent detailed reviews[32b,48a] with complete bibliographies. Therefore, only general introductory statements are appropriate here.

Although the lung's role in ventilation is well understood, the idea of the lung as an immunological organ is now becoming documented. Lymphoid tissue is distributed through the entire lung. Outside the bronchial bifurcations, lymphoid nodules are found and the same sort of arrangement continues as far as the most distant respiratory bronchioles. At this level in the lung they are little more than collections of lymphocytes. The pulmonary lymphatic system is also of great significance.[52a] This mode of lymphatic drainage is very important in clearing the "external" environment of the lung, that is, the pulmonary surfaces along the airways. Beneath the lamina propria of the bronchial tissues, there is an abundance of plasma cells, which are actively involved in the production of immunoglobulin, especially of the IgA class. The alveoli themselves are richly lined with macrophages, cells not only very important in clearance, but also essential in many instances in the initiation and maintenance of the immune response. These cells, along with the other immunocytologic reserves of the lung, e.g., lymphocytes and plasma cells, combine with the cilia, goblet cells, seromucous glands, and alveolar surface fluids to make up the defense mechanisms of this extensive mucous membrane system.

The lung as an immunocompetent organ has been considered as a route of immunization. Immunization via this route, however, is not necessarily reflected in an immune response in the peripheral circulation, nor does systemic immunization necessarily produce a response in the immunological effectors of the lung. These observations have led to the development of the concept of a "compartmentalization" of the immune response, wherein the lung and systemic circulation are viewed as occupying separate but overlapping "compartments".[15]

In order to understand the mechanisms involved in the immune response either locally or systemically, it is necessary to understand the cellular basis of immunity. The effectors of humoral immunity are soluble immunoglobulins while sensitized lymphoid cells are the effectors in the typical cell mediated immune response.

As presently conceived, the capacity to recognize and respond to varied antigenic stimuli resides in at least two physiologically and functionally distinct cell populations. One population, the B- or bone marrow-derived lymphocytes, appears to carry on their surface immunoglobulin that they are capable of synthesizing. The reaction of antigen with this surface bound antibody results in the synthesis of antibody with the appropriate specificity for the inducing antigen. The T- or thymus-derived lymphocyte, on the other hand, represents the other population, and appears to constitute the major portion of a host's entire supply of circulating lymphocytes. This is the cell that mediates the effectors of cell mediated immunity (CMI), again, all the immunological responses in which sensitized lymphoid cells (rather than antibodies) effect antigen recognition. The in vivo manifestations of CMI are defense against viruses and fungi and some species of bacteria as the *Mycobacteria.* Immune surveillance mechanisms and defense against neoplasia, graft rejection, and the autoimmune phenomenon are also illustrative of the roles of the T-cell in cell mediated immunity.

In vitro, many correlates have been described for the measurement of CMI in lymphoic populations. Apparently when a sensitized T-cell contacts its antigen, the cell becomes activated and many physiologically active substances called "lymphokines" are released. Some of these are cytotoxic, having nonspecific toxic activity on living cells, while others will induce nonsensitized lymphocytes to undergo blastogenic transformation. Other soluble mediators emanating from sensitized T-cells are responsible for chemotaxis of other cells, inhibition of viral replication (interferon), and inhibition of macrophage migration.[23a]

The capacity of immunologically committed lymphocytes to function in their ability to control the behavior of mononuclear phagocytes is of great importance, not only in the induction and maintenance of non-specific clearance, but also in another way. Macrophage-lymphocyte interaction in the presence of antigens appears to be a special circumstance, required not just for the activation of T-cells but also for the initiation of antigen-specific antibody synthesis by the B-lymphocyte.

The most numerous cell along the alveolar membranes is the macrophage, a cell whose most obvious role appears to be phagocytosis and clearance. The primary alveolar macrophage system depends on the metabolic and enzymatic activities of the cells and their intracellular factors, which contain, neutralize, and destroy ingested material.[32b] Inhalation studies with bacteria provide excellent models for clearance. These studies have shown how rapidly inhaled organisms disappear from the lung. This process, in the sense of killing and removal, depends upon the integrated function of the alveolar macrophage, other inflammatory cells,[61a,74a] and the mucociliary stream.

The role of the macrophage in immunity is also of importance. In their traditional role, the cells may remove antigenic stimuli. Macrophages, as the targets of soluble mediators as well as participants in immune reactions, have recently been reviewed.[59]

Although the major function of lung-associated immunological tissues is to defend the lung against infectious and noxious agents, these very same immunologic effector mechanisms may lead to lung injury.[9] The lung may either be a direct target or a victim of an "innocent bystander" reaction. Several such immunological mechanisms may be examined for their role in injury to lung connective tissue.

Perhaps the most common form of immune injury is due to antibody of the IgE class, which fixes to receptor sites on most cells and basophiles. Following reaction with antigen, a stress or signal is transmitted to the basophile, causing it to release pharmacologic mediators that are responsible for the signs and symptoms of immediate types of allergy, e.g., certain types of extrinsic asthma.[47] Chronic bronchial asthma can lead to certain types of tissue damage, such as smooth muscle hypertrophy and mucous membrane metaplasia; it is of interest to the present subject that alveolar basement membrane thickening may also occur. The precise mechanism of this thickening is unknown.

Other forms of injury to interstitial connective tissue result when this tissue itself is the direct target of immunologic effectors. As we will see, connective tissue substances such as collagen and reticulin may become antigenic in certain chronic pulmonary diseases, inciting humoral antibodies reactive with these constituents. Such reactions may promote to further injury. Antibodies to both interstitial connective tissue and alveolar basement membrane are known. Following reaction with antigen, the antibody may activate the complement system; many of these complement cleavage components possess innate inflammatory properties. Antibody can also cause injury by occluding vital function, as when membranes are coated with antibody. Finally, under certain situations antitissue antibody may be hyperplastic.

Formerly, the activation of the complement system has been considered to be stimulated mostly by antigen-antibody reactions, but considerably insight has been gained concerning activation of complement by alternative pathways that do not require initiation by specific antibody.[61] It is likely that such mechanisms can affect the alveolar basement membrane and set in motion a series of events[18,60] involving inflammatory mediators that may eventually lead to a fibrotic process and involvement of other immune mechanisms.[6,70]

An often-mentioned mechanism of immune injury to lung tissue is that brought about by immune complexes activating complement within the pulmonary architecture. Although there is no direct evidence in natural disease that immune complex formation as a result of inhaling antigen leads to immune injury, this possibility, as well as that of damage to lung resulting from circulating immune complexes, must be considered.

A final mechanism of connective tissue damage by immunologic means may be due to cell mediated immunity.[21,27,52] Just as lung connective tissue antibodies may incite humoral antibodies, they may also stimulate specifically sensitized lymphocytes capable of reacting with the inciting antigens. Following such reaction, macromolecular mediators of inflammation known as lymphokines are released by the lymphocytes. Cell mediated immunity is well known for producing chronic pulmonary granuloma disease to such extrinsic antigens as tubercle bacilli, and it now seems possible that similar mechanisms may be directed to intrinsic components of lung connective tissue. A close examination of this mechanism, as well as other immunological mechanisms[5] of lung injury, follows.

II. CONNECTIVE TISSUE INJURY BY CYTOTOXIC ANTIBODY

Although the development of the idea of organ specificity by the Germans in the 1920 culminated in development of the Wasserman reaction, Masugi nephritis, and experimental allergic encephalitis, the significance of lung reactive antibodies has remained eluseive. The main target tissue of neural tissue antibodies was the myelin sheath, while that of kidney antibodies proved to be glomerular basement membrane. The question arose as to the nature of specificity (if any) of lung reactive antibodies. Although crude saline extracts of brain and kidney contained appreciable amounts of serologically detectable antigens, such extracts of lung rarely produced reactive material other than globulin and other serum proteins.[1,31,73] More careful antigenic analysis of the lung led to the demonstration of two definitive targets within the lung, alveolar basement membrane and interstitial connective tissue.

From the study of organ specific reactivity of tissue antibodies, it was learned that lung and kidney constituents cross-reacted.[51,66,80] Much of this cross-reaction is due to the antigenic similarity between the alveolar and glomerular basement membranes. Krakower and Greenspon[51] showed that, as measured immunologically, basement membrane antigen was present in the lung at only $^1/_{40}$ of its concentration in the kidney.

Saline extracts of crude lung homogenates proved to be unsuitable for antibody detection in sera of patients with chronic lung disease; attention was turned to antigens in the insoluble portion of the homogenate. Using this material as antigen and the antiglobulin consumption technique (AGCT), antibodies could be detected in the sera of patients with a variety of chronic pulmonary diseases in an incidence ten times that found in sera from humans free of demonstrable disease.[19] Using crude analytical techniques for analyzing the relative components, collagen was shown to be the main antigenic material, with elastin contributing to the reactivity in some sera.[12] The antigen was insoluble in conventional saline, but at least partially extractable by neutral salt of hydroxylamine methods. Such extracts neutralized reactive sera. Antigen reactivity was usually destroyed by collagenase and elastase digestion and the antibody reacted with known lung collagen preparations.[32] In addition to being found in lung homogenates, the antigen is also produced in human fibroblast cell cultures[32] and found in kidney homogenates.[12]

When glomular basement membrane suspensions were used as antigens to detect antibodies in lung-reactive sera, positive results were obtained in the AGCT, but not by immunofluorescence. The fluorescent antibody technique might not be sensitive enough to detect the reaction; however, the ferritin conjugated antibody technique, and electron microscopy revealed the cause of the AGCT reactivity in the basement membrane suspensions to be due to what was probably interstitial collagen fibril contamination.[12] Thus, the lung antibodies demonstrated in chronic pulmonary diseases, such as coalworkers' pneumonocoiosis, tuberculosis, pulmonary fibrosis, etc., were reactive against interstitial connective tissue. All of this work was done before the time of the biochemical elucidation of the four basic types of collagen. A re-examination of these antibodies using biochemically characterized collagen types would provide useful information about the nature of the interstitial antigen and whether type IV basement membrane collagen is involved.

Hennes et al.[39] earlier had shown human antibody reactivity to presumably a connective tissue antigen, possibly reticulin. Using a more refined antigen, i.e., erythrocytes passively sensitized to purified collagen peptides, Michaeli and Fudenberg[57] detected antibodies in the sera of 70% of patients with emphysema, possibly a reflection of destruction of pulmonary connective tissue. The literature on the immunological reactivity of collagen as an antigen is extensive and has been reviewed elsewhere.[2]

After demonstrating the incidence and nature of these antibodies, the question of their significance remained. Were they merely a reflection of tissue destruction or did they participate in lesion development? Actions of the antibodies have been demonstrated by a variety of means. When passively injected intravenously, lung antibodies obtained from a species of animal different from that being challenged produce an immediate lethal pneumotoxic and nephrotoxic response.[33] These complement fixing antibodies localized in the glomeruli and pulmonary alveoli[34] in a anti-basement membrane pattern. This acute system is widely regarded as a model for Goodpasture's syndrome in human. Basement membrane antibodies have been demonstrated in the pulmonary lesions of patients with this disease.[3] However, when the anti-lung serum was prepared in the homologous species as that challenged with an intravenous administration of that serum, quite different results were obtained. Such administration did not result in acute pneumotoxic signs nor did it result in as much glomerular localization. Rather, homologous antibodies localized in scattered focal patterns on the interalveolar cross walls.[3]

Many studies have shown that the antibodies capable of localizing in this manner were injurious. They have been shown to be cytotoxic in fibroblast cell cultures,[32] enhance tuberculous infection,[11,16] cause increased production of LDH_2 and LDH_3 isoenzymes,[13] cause increased localization of bacteria in the lung cleared from the circulation[13] and the airways.[15] These antibodies also induce an increase of interstitial alveolar connective tissue leading to a distention of the terminal airways[13] and, thus, possibly to a decrease in ventilatory capacity,[14] and they stimulate macrophages to produce a collagen stimulating factor.[53] The latter factor was demonstrated in an in vitro model of fibrogenesis, where collagen production is evaluated by increased hydroxyproline production in confluent fibroblast cell cultures.[10,41] The antibodies themselves, although reactive with fibroblasts, were unable to stimulate increased hydroxyproline production. Only after the stimulation of macrophages was this effect observed.[53]

Thus antibodies for lung connective tissue, arising as a result of long standing disease or injury, can further damage the lung by localizing on the interstitial tissue, stimulating fibrogenesis through the agency of macrophages, and possibly by injuring the alveolar capillary membrane. In such cases, the lung tissue itself is the antigen, but theoretical considerations must allow for the possibility that foreign antigen from inhaled sources may affix to lung connective tissue in such a way that subsequent antigen-antibody reaction may injure the tissue. It has been suggested[42,85] that hypersensitivity pneumonitis due to inhaled microorganisms may result from such a mechanism, but the data to support this are scarce and indirect.

III. IMMUNE COMPLEX INJURY

The idea of producing immune injury by means of immune complexes draws precedence from the Arthus reaction, a dermal inflammation due to antigen-antibody complexes forming in the capillary bed, and also from a type of glomerulonephritis, where such complexes localize on and within the glomerular basement membrane. These complexes activate the complement cascade, which mediates several aspects of inflammation brought about by lysosomal enzymes and by platelet activation. Since many (but not all) patients with various forms of hypersensitivity pneumonitis exhibit precipitins to the environmental inhalants inducing this disease, early conjecture[62] postulated an immune complex etiology; however, no experimental studies were able to show such a cause and effect relationship. Although there is not direct evidence that immune complexes resulting from inhaled antigen and local antibody may cause pulmonary injury, the possibility exists that circulating antigen-antibody complexes may localize in alveolar capillaries and initiate injury. This problem has been approached experimentally by injecting pre-formed antigen-antibody complexes intravenously.[75] An acute, hemorrhagic alveolitis was produced that was complement and neutrophile dependent. In similar but longer term studies,[8] a chronic interstitial pneumonitis, characterized by alveolar capillary wall thickening, interstitial fibrosis, and fibrinogen deposition was produced.

If such fibrosis can be induced artificially by intravenous injection of immune complexes, the question arises as to whether similar changes can arise spontaneously in humans as a result of circulating complexes. Turner-Warwick[81,81a] reasons that, since the lungs receive virtually the entire cardiac output and are exposed as a filter would be to the entire complement of circulating immunologic effectors, it is not surprising that lung connective tissues are frequently involved in immune injury. She notes that there are a number of diseases composed of widespread pulmonary inflammation and fibrosis in which there also exists a variety of circulating autoantibodies such as antinuclear antibody, rheumatoid factor (antiglobulin), and various tissue antibodies. The suggestion is made that such antibodies to intrinsic antigens may form immune complexes and localize in the lung preferentially, owing to that organ's anatomic relationship to the heart. It has been postulated[45] that antinuclear antibody may complex with nuclear antigens on dead mesothelial cells and that the uptake of these complexes by phagocytes initiates further inflammation to the surrounding connective tissue. Circulating immune complexes were shown to be elevated in most patients with cellular idiopathic interstitial pneumonia, but not in diffuse fibrosis.[28] Antibody and complement deposition was demonstrated histologically in biopsies of patients with elevated immune complex levels.[28,76] In a series of recent reports, data from two other laboratories implicate immune complex etiologies in lung disease. One group[32a] postulates that immune complexes may have an indirect role via interaction with resident alveolar macrophages, effecting an influx of neutrophiles into the lungs of patients with idiopathic pulmonary fibrosis. Eisenberg et al[30a] found granular deposits of immune complexes in the lungs of a majority of patients with *Pneumocystis carinii* pneumonitis, interstitial pneumonitis, and interstitial diseases associated with autoimmune disorders. Only one of twelve patients with pulmonary fibrosis had any evidence of complexes. Although immune complexes may have no role in the genesis of pulmonary disease, they may contribute to any overall etiology, immune or otherwise.

IV. NON-SPECIFIC ACTIVATION OF COMPLEMENT

The complement system is a complex series of proteins, many with enzyme activity, which may become activated through various, well controlled sequences. The consequences of complement activation are varied and serve to amplify the immune response through inflammation. Although antigen-antibody complexes have long been known to activate what is now known as the classical pathway, there has been much recent interest in those agents which may activate alternative pathways in the absence of specific antibody. Since the lung comes into contact with innumerable organic substances through inhalation, the possibility exists that inhalation of sufficient amounts of complement-activating substances may be injurious to the lung.

Following the demonstration that microorganisms associated with hypersensitivity pneumonitis could non-specifically activate complement in vitro,[29,30,55] an animal model of this disease was developed in which unimmunized rabbits could be monitored for depressions in pumonary function and complement level following aerosol challenge of the test substances.[17,60] Nonspecific complement activation stimulates components to act on platelets, causing them to release mediators like histamine.[18] This can produce a decrease in platelets and arterial oxygen tensions following inhalation of sufficient amounts of activator. The inflammation produced by such complement activation may be sufficient to allow the escape of antigen into the peripheral circulation,[15] where immunization on a systemic basis may take place. Cell mediated immunity may then be more important[6] in bringing about the chronic form of the disease once initiated by the complement activation.

Other inhalants which have been shown to be able to activate complement and, thus, be possible agents of pulmonary injury are bacterial endotoxin,[44,63] cotton dust,[22,23] pigeon dropping extract,[4] dextran,[72] lactobacilli,[46] and various fungi.[36,60] In addition to activating platelets, complement activation can also activate macrophages, causing them to release lysosomal enzymes.[75] Continued release of such enzymes by daily inhalation of high concentrations of activators, as in dusty occupational exposure, could result in chronic inflammation and fibrosis.

Although complement activation has not been shown to stimulate release of macrophage collagenase or elastase, complement components with chemotactic activity may serve to draw macrophage and polymorphonuclear leukocytes to the area where they discharge their tissue damaging enzymes.[49] With the recent demonstration that components of the alternative pathway of complement (APC) activation are present in human respiratory secretions[71] and that complement activation via this pathway can occur in the lung,[60] the possibility that the release of collagenase and elastase, as well as lysosomal enzymes, can be mediated by the complement system should receive further attention in the laboratory.

A review of the immunological aspects of lung connective tissue and related injury must mention the work that has been done on the structural similarities of collagen and the first component of the classical pathway of complement, C1q.[67] C1q initiates this complement protein cascade by binding to antigen-antibody complexes. The fact that the helical portion C1q is also susceptible to collagenase stimulates speculation about potential interaction of the complement system and lung connective tissue. In addition, receptors for C1q are also thought to be present on plateletes. Binding of C1q can inhibit collagen-induced release of vasoactive amines from platelets.[79]

We have considered the immunological aspects of lung connective tissue damage that possibly may be mediated by macrophages and/or complement, but there is a more direct mechanism whereby complement may be involved in lung connective tissue injury. Once lung basement membrane is exposed via the action of enzymes or airborne environmental toxicants, the innate biological activities of naked collagen may become manifest. Collagen itself can induce platelet aggregation,[83] mediated possibly by cold insoluble globulin.[46a] Some forms of collagen can activate Hagemen factor,[86] which through a series of enzymological reactions results in the generation of a variety of inflammatory mediators.[65] Hageman factor activation can effect kinin generation, fibrinolysis, and complement activation. By-products of Hageman factor and complement activation are the generation of vasoactive amines such as histamine, which has been shown to accelrate the early formation of collagen precursors and collagen polymerization.[24] Others have reported an increase in lung histamine content in experimental pulmonary fibrosis.[68] Other results of complement activation are the generation of chemotactic factors for mononuclear and polymorphonuclear cells, the cellular effectors of tissue damage.

The key event, therefore, in lung connective tissue damage, by whatever immunological or toxicological mechanism, may be the initial exposure of lung basement membrane and connective tissue components to the "external" environment and the cellular and soluble effectors of inflammation. The type of progressive injury or disease that results may be couched in terms of the types of effectors that become involved and later patterns of inflammation.

V. CELL MEDIATED IMMUNE INJURY

Common features of lung connective tissue damage in pulmonary fibrosis are derangement of parenchymal collagen and chronic inflammation.[52] Because pertubation of connective tissue architecture is an essential feature, it has been proposed that collagen in a deranged form might be recognized as foreign and, therefore, antigenic. Chronic inflammatory lymphocytes infiltrating the interstitium could then, through their various immunological effectors, maintain the injury level or even stimulate further tissue damage.

Using in vitro correlates of cell mediated immunity (CMI), Kravis et al.[52] found that only 17% (2 out of 12) of patients with non-fibrotic lung disorders had significant collagen-reactive lymphocytes as compared to 94% (17 out of 18) of those from patients with idiopathic pulmonary fibrosis (IPF). None of nine controls had reactive cells. There was no organ or species specificity as far as collagen source was concerned, but more patients' cells recognized human lung α_2 chains than α_1 (I) chains. This was probably due to the fact that α_2 chains have more antigenic determinants.[35,56,58,78]

Seyer et al.[77] have presented data indicating that collagen polymorphism is altered in IPF patients. Specifically they found an increase in type 1 collagen and a decrease in type III. In addition, the degree of lysine hydroxylation in the α_1 chains of both types of collagen was reduced in diseased lungs. How these observations relate to the data of Kravis et al. implicating α_2 chains is not understood.

Kravis et al.[52] point out that if collagen-induced injury mediated by cellular immune mechanisms is important in pathogenesis of IPF, then reactivity must be restricted to a local level in the lung. In light of the cross-reactivity between type I collage in different organs,[37,38] if the immune injury were not "compartmentalized", this disease would be a systemic disorder, with other organs involved. That collagen sensitivity in these individuals is generated only at the local level may possibly be because only the lung interstitium is the site of structural disarray and source of antigenic stimulation. Another possibility is the lack of suppressor cell activity in the lung; however, the local immune effector cells have not been isolated for study from these patients. Such studies would be useful in evaluating etiologies and mechanisms.

The CMI in vitro correlate, the macrophage migration inhibition test, measures the release of an inhibitor of macrophage migration from sensitized lymphocytes.[7] The test seems particularly applicable to the study of lung disease because of the relatively large numbers of macrophages in the lung and because these cells contain a number of enzymes, such as collagenase,[43,84] which could have direct toxicity for lung connective tissue. Macrophages could ingest antigen-antibody complexes,[50] stimulating the release of enzymes, promoting futher tissue injury, especially because of the local nature of the antigenic stimulus. Although cell mediated immune processes may be functioning to regulate connective tissue repair, they may also contribute to the pathogenesis of chronic lung disease.

The presence of collagen-reactive lymphocytes in the blood or bronchopulmonary lavage fluid may be a sensitive early indicator of connective tissue injury and lung damage, an important diagnostic and prognostic tool. The lung can function as a relatively independent immune organ, particularly in disease states such as chronic hypersensitivity pneumonitis (CHP) and idiopathic pulmonary fiboris. Reynolds et al.[69] found elevated IgG levels in the lung lavage fluids of CHP and IPF patients. Although pulmonary lymphocytosis was not a feature of IPF patients, the lungs of the pneumonitis patients contained from 38 to 74% lymphocytes. T-lymphocytes, the effectors of cell mediated immunity, predominated. These data indicate the value lung lavage cytology may have in evaluating the cellular aspects of inflammation. Recent data also indicate that not only can the lung function as a relatively independent organ in responding to local immune stimuli,[40] but pulmonary immunity can be observed on a lobe specific basis.[5] Introduction of antigen into specific lung lobes produces an immune response, to a large extent, only in the immunized lobe, while the rest of the lung reflects the systemic immune state. Therefore, in using bronchopulmonary lavage to assess lung cell population for cells sensitized to lung or other antigens, the possibility of a dilution effect of mixing cells from reactive and non-reactive lobes must be considered.

In experiments similar in design to the IPF studies. Dill et al.[27] surveyed patients with a variety of chronic pulmonary diseases for cellular immunity to lung extract antigens. Using techniques similar to Kravis et al.,[52] these authors found anti-lung reactivity in the majority of tested patients with chronic bronchitis and tuberculosis. Patients with sarcoidosis and bronchial carcinoma and their normal controls had no significant autoreactivity. In contrast to the IPF studies, the reactivity observed by Dill et al.[27] was specific for lung tissue extracts with no organ cross-reactivity. They did not use purified connective tissue components or lung lavage cells in their studies, but their data suggest that cell mediated immunity directed against lung connective tissue antigens may not be an exclusive feature of pulmonary fibrosis.

In spite of recent interest in the cellular immune aspects of lung injury, the fact that lung injury may be affected by immune cells is not a recent observation. Cate and Burrell[21] found that animals could be immunized to soluble lung connective tissue extracts. Associated with induced reactivity to the lung antigens were lung pathologic changes. In addition, they demonstrated autoreactivity to this extract in models of three diseases, tuberculosis, berylliosis, and coalworkers' pneumoconiosis.

The mechanisms by which the cells of the immune system and lung connective tissue interact to effect tissue damage is not known. The generation of cytotoxic T-cells, as suggested by some of the above studies, is just one possibility. Other mechanisms must be considered. Johnson and Ziff[48] found that supernatants from cultures of human peripheral blood mononuclear cells, which had been stimulated with a mitogen, enhanced the accumulation of collagen in lung fibroblasts. They proposed that a soluble lymphocyte factor, a lymphokine, was responsible. These data, along with the other information, suggest that a chronic stimulation of the local immune system may be responsible for tissue injury in the lung. Collagen or other connective tissue components could be acting as an antigen, stimulating sensitized lymphocytes to secrete materials which stimulate further accumulation of the antigen (collagen). Considering this hypothesis, lung connective tissue damage may be the result of a failure of normal immunoregulatory mechanisms. Not only have lymphocytes been shown to produce factors which stimulate the accumulation of collagen, these cells also have been shown to release a factor which induces the production of collagenase by synovial cells from patients with rheumatoid arthritis.[26]

Although the situation presently is very complicated, the central issue, that of a role for cell-mediated immunity in lung connective tissue damage, is being reinforced by new data. Postlewaite et al.[64] reported a lymphocyte-derived factor that was chemotactic for fibroblasts. Interestingly, they also found that macrophages, cells plentiful in the lung, are required for the production of this factor. In light of other studies, their data suggest that lymphocytes may not only stimulate collagen accumulation in fibroblasts, but stimulate the accumulation of fibroblasts themselves. In addition, the results help to explain the role of macrophages in wound repair.[54] In subsequent articles,[63a,63b] these authors found that type I to III human collagens and derived peptides themselves are chemotactic for monocytes and fibroblasts.

As accessory and effector cells, the macrophage has received considerable attention as a participant in immune responses[59] A case for a role for macrophages in connective tissue damage could be made in light of their link to the immune system and their complement of enzymes with potential for tissue damage (reviewed in Unanue[82]). The significance of these enzymes, in terms of the immunological mediation of tissue destruction, may be the fact that immune complement activation and subsequent binding of cleavage products to macrophages stimulate the release of lysosomal enzymes.[75] These enzymes may degrade proteoglycans and other components of the glycocalyx that protects the alveolar epithelium and is interspaced between collagen and elastin. It should be emphasized that demonstration of specific immunological features or antigen reactivity in diseases of cell populations from patients with lung disease does not per se allow the conclusions that such a response is responsible for or contributes to the disease process. Regardless, the evidence reviewed here for a role for immune mechanisms in lung connective damage does support these conclusions. With continued study of the natural disease, as well as the development of appropriate disease models, the immune response in this regard can be dissected and reconstructed relative to its significance in lung damage.

REFERENCES

1. **Balchum, O. J. and VanDyke, J.,** Antibodies to lung in pulmonary disease of man, *Arch. Environ. Health,* 8, 139, 1964.

2. **Beard, H. K., Faulk, W. P., Conochie, L. B., and Glynn, L. E.,** Some immunological aspects of collagen, *Prog. Allergy,* 22, 45, 1977.
3. **Beirne, G. J., Octaviano, G. N., Kopp, W. L., and Burns, R. O.,** Immunohistology of the lung in Goodpasture's syndrome, *Ann. Intern. Med.,* 69, 1207, 1968.
4. **Berrens, L., Guikers, C. L. H., and van Dijk, A.,** The antigens in pigeonbreeder's disease and their interaction with human complement, *Ann. N.Y. Acad. Sci.,* 221, 153, 1974.
5. **Bice, D. E., Harris, D. L., Hill, J. O., and Muggenburg, B. A.** Local and systemic immunity following localized deposition of antigen in the lung, *Chest,* 75S, 246, 1979.
6. **Bice, D. E., Salvaggio, J., and Hoffman, E.,** Passive transfer of experimental hypersensitivity pneumonitis with lymphoid cells in the rabbit, *J. Allergy Clin. Immunol.,* 58, 250, 1976.
7. **Bloom, B. R. and Bennett, B.,** The assay of inhibition of macrophage migration and the production of migration inhibitory factor (MIF) and skin reactive factor (SRF) in the guinea pig, in *In Vitro Methods in Cell-Mediated Immunity,* Bloom, B. R. and Glade, P. R., Eds., Academic Press, New York, 1971, 235.
8. **Brentjens, J. R., O'Connell, D. W., Pawlowski, I. B., Hsu, K. C., and Andres, G. A.,** Experimental immune complex disease of the lung: the pathogenesis of a laboratory model resembling certain human interstitial lung diseases, *J. Exp. Med.,* 140, 105, 1974.
9. **Burrell, R.,** Immunological reactions to inhaled physical and chemical agents, in *Handbook of Physiology — Reactions to Environmental Agents,* Lee, D. H. K., Falk, H. L., and Murphy, S. D., Eds., American Physiological Society, Bethesda, Md., 1977, chap. 18.
10. **Burrell, R. and Anderson, M.,** The induction of fibrogenesis by silica-treated alveolar macrophages, *Environ. Res.,* 6, 389, 1973.
11. **Burrell, R. and Cate, C. C.** The effect of lung reactive antibodies on the pathogenesis of tuberculosis, *Clin. Exp. Immunol.,* 9, 809, 1971.
12. **Burrell, R., Esber, H. J., Hagadorn, J. E., and Andrews, C. E.,** Specificity of lung-reactive antibodies in human serum, *Am. Rev. Respir. Dis.,* 94, 743, 1966.
13. **Burrell, R., Flaherty, D. K., DeNee, P. B., Abraham, J. L., and Gelderman, A. H.,** The effect of lung antibody on normal lung structure and function, *Am. Rev. Respir. Dis.,* 109, 106, 1974.
14. **Burrell, R., Flaherty, D. K., and Schreiber, J. E.,** Immunological studies of experimental coalworkers' pneumoconiosis, in *Inhaled Particles IV,* W. H. Walton, Ed., Pergamon Press, Oxford, 1977, 519.
15. **Burrell, R. and Hill, J. O.,** The effect of respiratory immunization on cell-mediated immune effector cells of the lung, *Clin. Exp. Immunol.,* 24, 116, 1976.
16. **Burrell, R. and Lewis, D. M.,** Further studies on the effect of lung antibodies on the pathogenesis of tuberculosis, *J. Lab. Clin. Med.,* 86, 741, 1975.
17. **Burrell, R. and McCullough, M. J.,** Production of thermophilic actinomycete-hay aerosols for use in experimental hypersensitivity pneumonitis, *Appl. Environ. Microbiol.,* 34, 715, 1977.
18. **Burrell, R. and Pokorney, D.,** Mediators of experimental hypersensitivity pneumonitis, *Int. Arch. Allergy Appl. Immunol.,* 55, 161, 1977.
19. **Burrell, R. G., Wallace, J. P., and Andrews, C. E.,** Lung antibodies in patients with pulmonary disease, *Am. Rev. Respir. Dis.,* 89, 697, 1964.
20. **Callerame, M. L., Condemi, J. J., Bohrod, M. G., and Vaughan, J. H.,** Immunologic reactions to bronchial tissues in asthma, *N. Engl. J. Med.,* 284, 459, 1971.
21. **Cate, C. C. and Burrell, R.,** Lung antigen induced cell-mediated immune injury in chronic resporatory diseases, *Am. Rev. Respir. Dis.,* 109, 114, 1974.
22. **Cavagna, G., Foa, V., and Vigliani, E. C.,** Effects in man and rabbits of inhalation of cotton dust or extracts and purified endotoxins, *Br. J. Ind. Med.,* 26, 314, 1969.
23. **Cinkotai, F. F., Lockwood, M. G., and Rylander, R.,** Airborne micro-organisms and prevalence of byssinotic symptoms in cotton mills, *Am. Ind. Hyg. Assoc. J.,* 38, 554, 1977.

23a. **Cohen, S.,** Cell mediated immunity and the inflammatory system, *Hum. Pathol.,* 7, 249, 1976.

24. **Dabrowski, R. and Maslinski, C.,** The effect of histamine on collagen formation and collagen polymerization in the skin wound healing of guinea pigs, *Life Sci.,* 9, 189, 1970.
25. **Dannenberg, A. M., Jr.,** Influence of environmental factors on the respiratory tract — summary and perspectives, *J. Retic. Soc.,* 22, 273, 1977.
26. **Dayer, J. M., Russell, R. G. G., and Krane, S. M.,** Collagenase production by rheumatoid synovial cells; stimulation by a human lymphocyte factor, *Science,* 195, 181, 1977.
27. **Dill, J., Fox, R., Landrigan, P., Macsween, M., Osborn, D., and Rajarman, R.,** A study of lung-specific, cell-mediated immunity in chronic pulmonary diseases, *Clin. Allergy,* 7, 539, 1977.
28. **Dreisin, R. B., Schwarz, M. I., Theofilopoulos, A. N., and Stanford, R. E.,** Circulating immune complexes in the idiopathic interstitial pneumonias, *N. Engl. J. Med.,* 298, 353, 1978.
29. **Edwards, J. H.,** A quantitaitve study on the activation of the alternative pathway of complement by mouldy hay dust and thermophilic actinomycetes, *Clin. Allergy,* 6, 19, 1976.

30. **Edwards, J. H., Baker, J. T., and Davies, B. H.,** Precipitin test negative farmer's lung — activation of the alternative pathway of complement by mouldy hay dusts, *Clin. Allergy,* 4, 379, 1974.

30a. **Eisenberg, H., Barnett, E., and Simmons, D. H.,** Diffuse pulmonary interstitial disease, an immunohistologic study, *Chest,* 79S, 262, 1979.

31. **Esber, H. J. and Burrell, R.,** An immunologic study of experimental silicosis, *Environ. Res.,* 1, 171, 1967.

32. **Esber, H. J. and Burrell, R.,** Further characterization of the specificity of lung-reactive antibodies in human serum, *Arch. Environ. Health,* 21, 502, 1970.

32a. **Gadek, J., Hunninghake, G., Zimmerman, R., Kelman, J., Fulmer, J., and Crystal, R.,** Pathogenetic studies in idiopathic pulmonary fibrosis; control of neutrophil migration by immune complexes, *Chest,* 79S, 264, 1979.

32b. **Green, G. M., Jakab, G. J., Low, R. B., and Davis, G. S.,** Defense mechanisms of the respiratory membrane, *Am. Rev. Respir. Dis.,* 115, 479, 1977.

33. **Hagadorn, J. E. and Mercola, K. E.,** Immunologic and morhpologic studies of the acute effect of anti-lung serum, *Exp. Mol. Pathol.,* 15, 97, 1971.

34. **Hagadorn, J. E., Vazquez, J. J., and Kinney, T. R.,** Immunopathologic studies of an experimental model resembling Goodpasture's syndrome, *Am. J. Pathol.,* 57, 17, 1969.

35. **Hahn, E. and Timpl, R.,** Involvement of more than a single polypeptide chain in the helical antigenic determinants of collagen, *Eur. J. Immunol.,* 3, 442, 1973.

36. **Halprin, G. M., Buckley, C. E., Zitt, M. J., and McMahon, S. M.,** Changes in arteriovenous complement activity induced by inhalation challenge, *Am. Rev. Respir. Dis.,* 108, 343, 1973.

37. **Hance, A. J. and Crystal, R. G.,** The connective tissue of the lung, *Am. Rev. Respir. Dis.,* 112, 657, 1975.

38. **Hance, A. J. and Crystal, R. G.,** Collagen, in *Biochemical Basis of Pulmonary Function,* Crystal, R. G., Ed., Marcel Dekker, New York, 1976, 215.

39. **Hennes, A. R., Moore, M. Z., Carpenter, R. L., and Hammarsten, J. F.,** Antibodies to human lung in patients with obstructive emphysema and pulmonary tuberculosis, *Am. Rev. Respir. Dis.,* 83, 354, 1961.

40. **Henny, C. S.,** Cell-mediated immune reactions in the lung, in *Immunologic and Infectious Reactions in the Lung,* Kirkpatrick, C. H. and Reynolds, H. Y., Eds., Marcel Dekker, New York, 1976, 59.

41. **Heppleston, A. G., and Styles, J. A.,** Activity of a macrophage factor in collagen formation by silica, *Nature (London),* 214, 521, 1967.

42. **Hollingdale, M. R.,** Antibody responses in patients with farmer's lung disease to antigens from *Micropolyspora faeni, J. Hyg.,* 72, 79, 1974.

43. **Horwitz, A. L. and Crystal, R. G.,** Collagenase from rabbit pulmonary alveolar macrophages, *Biochem. Biophys. Res. Commun.,* 69, 296, 1976.

44. **Hudson, A. R., Kilburn, K. H., Halprin, G. M., and McKenzie, W. N.,** Granulocyte recruitment to airways exposed to endotoxin aerosols, *Am. Rev. Respir. Dis.,* 115, 89, 1977.

45. **Hughes, P. and Rowell, N. R.,** Aggravation of turpentine-induced pleurisy in rats by "Homogeneous" and "Speckled" antinuclear antibodies, *J. Pathol.,* 101, 141, 1970.

46. **Huis In 't Veld, J. H. J. and Berrens, L.,** Inactivation of hemolytic complement in human serum by an acylated polysaccharide from a gram-positive rod: possible significance in pigeon-breeder's disease, *Infect. Immun.,* 13, 1619, 1976.

46a. **Hynes, R. O., Ali, I. U., Destree, A. T., Mautner, V., Perkins, M. E., Senger, D. R., Wagner, D. D., and Smith, K. K.,** A large glycoprotein lost from the surfaces of transformed cells, *Ann. N.Y. Acad. Sci.,* 312, 317, 1978.

47. **Ishizaka, K.,** Human reaginic antibodies, *Annu. Rev. Med.,* 21, 187, 1971.

48. **Johnson, R. L. and Ziff, M.,** Lymphokine stimulation of collagen accumulation, *J. Clin. Invest.,* 58, 240, 1976.

48a. **Kaltreider, H. B.,** Expression of immune mechanisms in the lung, *Am. Rev. Respir. Dis.,* 113, 347, 1976.

49. **Kazmierowski, J. A., Gallin, J. I., and Reynolds, H. Y.,** Mechanism of the inflammatory response in primate lungs. Demonstration and partial characterization of an alveolar macrophage-derived chemotactic factor with preferential activity for polymorphonuclear leukocytes, *J. Clin. Invest.,* 59, 273, 1977.

50. **Knapp, W., Menzel, J., Brunner, H., and Steffen, C.** Phagocytosis of soluble collagen-anticollagen complexes and of particulate collagen by peritoneal macrophages, *Z. Immunitaetsforsch. Exp. Klin. Immunol.,* 146, 283, 1974.

51. **Krakower, C. A. and Greenspon, S. A.,** The localization of the "nephrotoxic" antigen(s) in extraglomerular tissues, *Arch. Pathol.,* 66, 364, 1958.

52. **Kravis, T. C., Ahmed, A., Brown, T. E., Fulmer, J. D., and Crystal, R. G.,** Pathogenic mechanisms in pulmonary fibrosis, *J. Clin. Invest.,* 58, 1223, 1976.

52a. **Lauweryns, J. M. and Baert, J. H.,** Alveolar clearance and the role of the pulmonary lymphatics, *Am. Rev. Respir. Dis.,* 115, 625, 1977.

53. **Lewis, D. M. and Burrell, R.,** Induction of fibrogenesis by lung antibody-treated macrophages, *Br. J. Ind. Med.,* 33, 25, 1976.

54. **Leibovich, S. J. and Ross, R.,** The role of the macrophage in wound repair, *Am. J. Pathol.,* 78, 71, 1975.

55. **Marx, J. J., Jr. and Flaherty, D. K.,** Activation of the complement sequence by extracts of bacteria and fungi associated with hypersensitivity pneumonitis, *J. Allergy Clin. Immunol.,* 57, 328, 1976.

56. **Michaeli, D. and Epstein, E. H., Jr.,** Isolation and identification of the antigenic determinants of human collagen, *Isr. J. Med. Sci.,* 7, 462, 1971.

57. **Michaeli, D.and Fudenberg, H. H.** Antibodies to collagen in patients with emphysema, *Clin. Immunol. Immunopathol.,* 3, 187, 1974.

58. **Michaeli, D., Martin, G. R., Kettman, J., Benjamini, E., Leung, D. Y., and Blatt, B. A.,** Localization of antigenic determinants in the polypeptide chains of collagen, *Science,* 166, 1522, 1969.

59. **Nelson, D. S., Ed.,** Immunobiology of the Macrophage, *Academic Press,* New York, 1976.

60. **Olenchock, S. A. and Burrell, R.,** The role of precipitins and complement activation in the etiology of allergic lung disease, *J. Allergy Clin. Immunol.,* 58, 76, 1976.

61. **Osler, A. G.,** The C3 shunt participation in allergic tissue injury, in *Mechanisms in Allergy, Reagin-Mediated Hypersensitivity,* Goodfriend, L., Sehon, A. H., and Orange, R. P., Eds., Marcel Dekker, New York, 1973, 353.

61a. **Pennington, J. E. and Ehrie, M. G.,** Pathogenesis of *Pseudomonas aeruginosa* pneumonia during immunosuppression, *J. Infect. Dis.,* 137, 764, 1978.

62. **Pepys, J.,** *Hypersensitivity Diseases of the Lungs due to Fungi and Organic Dusts,* S. Karger, Basel, 1969.

63. **Pernis, B., Vigliani, E. C., Cavagna, C., and Finulli, M.,** The role of bacterial endotoxins in occupational diseases caused by inhaling vegetable dusts, *Br. J. Ind. Med.,* 18, 120, 1961.

63a. **Postlethwaite, A. E. and Kang, A. H.,** Collagen- and collagen peptide-induced chemotaxis of human blood monocytes, *J. Exp. Med.,* 143, 1299, 1976.

63b. **Postlethwaite, A. E., Seyer, J. M., and Kang, A. H.,** Chemotactic attraction of human fibroblasts to type I, II, and III collagens and collagen-derived peptides, *Proc. Natl. Acad. Sci. U.S.A.,* 75, 871, 1978.

64. **Postlethwaite, A. E., Snyderman, R., and Kang, A. H.,** The chemotactic attraction of human fibroblasts to a lymphocyte-derived factor, *J. Exp. Med.,* 144, 1188, 1976.

65. **Ratnoff, O. D.,** Mediators of inflammation, *J. Allergy Clin. Immunol.,* 58, 438, 1976.

66. **Read, J.,** The pathological changes produced by anti-lung serum, *J. Pathol. Bacteriol.,* 76, 403, 1958.

67. **Reid, K. B.,** A collagen-like amino acid sequence in a polypeptide chain of human C1q (a subcomponent of the first component of complement), *Biochem. J.,* 141, 189, 1974.

68. **Religa, Z. and Maslinski, C.,** Histamine metabolism in experimental silicosis. II. *In vivo* experiements in guinea pigs, *Life Sci.,* 10, 257, 1971.

69. **Reynolds, H. Y., Fulmer, J. D., Kazmierowski, J. A., Roberts, W. C., Frank, M. M., and Crystal, G. R.,** Analysis of cellular and protein content of broncho-alveolar lavage fluid from patients with idiopathic pulmonary fiborsis and chronic hypersensitivity pneumonitis, *J. Clin. Invest.,* 59, 165, 1977.

70. **Richerson, H. B.,** Varieties of acute immunologic damage to the rabbit lung, *Ann. N.Y. Acad. Sci.,* 221, 340, 1974.

71. **Robertson, J., Caldwell, J. R., Castle, J. R., and Waldman, R. H.,** Evidence for the presence of components of the alternative (properdin) pathway of complement activation in respiratory secretions, *J. Immunol.,* 117, 900, 1976.

72. **Salvaggio, J., Kayman, H., and Leskowitz, S.,** Immunologic responses of atopic and normal individuals to aerosolized dextran, *J. Allergy,* 38, 31, 1966.

73. **Scheel, L. D., Smith, B., VanRiper, J., and Fleischer, E.,** Toxicity of silica. II. Characteristics of protein films adsorbed by quartz, *Arch. Ind. Hyg. Occup., Med.,* 9, 29, 1954.

74. **Scherzer, H. and Ward, P. A.,** Lung and dermal vascular injury produced by preformed immune complexes, *Am. Rev. Respir. Dis.,* 117, 551, 1978.

74a. **Schimpff, S. C., Moody, M., and Young, V. M.,** Relationship of colonization with *Pseudomonas aeruginosa* to development of *Pseudomonas* bacteremia in cancer patients, *Antimicorb. Agents Chemother.,* 10, 240, 1970.

75. **Schorlemmer, H. U., Bitter-Suermann, D., and Allison, A. C.,** Complement activation by the alternative pathway and macrophage enzyme secretion in the pathogenesis of chronic inflammation, *Immunology,* 32, 929, 1977.

76. **Schwarz, M. I., Dreisin, R. B., Pratt, D. S., and Stanford, R. E.,** Immunofluorescent patterns in the idiopathic interstitial pneumonias, *J. Lab. Clin. Med.,* 91, 929, 1978.

77. **Seyer, J. M., Hutcheson, E. T., and Kang, A.H.,** Collagen polymorphism in idiopathic chronic pulmonary fibrosis, *J. Clin. Invest.*, 57, 1498, 1976.
78. **Stuart, J. M., Postlethwaite, A. E., and Kang, A. H.,** Evidence for cell-mediated immunity to collagen in progressive systemic sclerosis, *J. Lab. Clin. Med.*, 88, 601, 1976.
79. **Suba, E. A. and Csako, G.,** C1q (C1) receptor on human plateletes: inhibition of collagen-induced platelet aggregation by C1q (C1) molecules, *J. Immunol.*, 117, 304, 1976.
80. **Tamanoi, I., Yagi, Y., Hiramoto, R., and Pressman, D.,** Lung localizing antibodies in anti-lung and anti-kidney serum, *Proc. Soc. Exp. Biol. Med.*, 106, 661, 1961.
81. **Turner-Warwick, M.,** Immunological aspects of systemic diseases of the lung, *Proc. R. Soc. Med.*, 67, 541, 1974.
81a. **Turner-Warwick, M.,** Immune reactions in pulmonary fiboris, *Schweiz. Med. Wochenschr.*, 107, 171, 1977.
82. **Unanue, E. R.,** Secretory function of mononuclear phagocytes, *Am. J. Pathol.*, 83, 396, 1976.
83. **Vaage, J., Bø., G., and Hognestad, J.,** Pulmonary responses to intravascular platelet aggregation in the cat, *Acta Physiol. Scand.*, 92, 546, 1974.
84. **Wahl, L. M., Wahl, S. M., Mergenhagen, S. E., and Martin, G. R.,** Collagenase production by lymphokine-activated macrophages, *Science*, 187, 261, 1975.
85. **Wenzel, F. J., Emanuel, D. A., and Gray, R. L.,** Immunofluorescent studies in patients with farmer's lung, *J. Allergy Clin. Immunol.*, 48, 224, 1971.
86. **Wilner, G. D., Nossel, H. L., and LeRoy, E. C.,** Activation of Hageman factor by collagen, *J. Clin. Invest.*, 47, 2608; 1968.

Chapter 12

SEQUENCE OF EVENTS IN PULMONARY INJURY

J. A. Pickrell

TABLE OF CONTENTS

I. GENERAL

Changes of lung connective tissue metabolism are observed as a consequence of pulmonary injury. The lung responds similarly to a variety of pulmonary insults. This emphasizes that the ways in which the lung can respond to epithelial or endothelial injury may be limited to inflammation, replacement, regeneration, or a distortion of one or more of these. Since few lung diseases are uncomplicated, the cause may be difficult to ascertain.[12] Harrison and Lapp,[18] Witschi,[55] and Rüttner et al.[42] note the importance of using sophisticated analytical techniques to elucidate etiology of lung disease. Differences of response are often due to differences in target cell or in dose or dose rate to the cell(s). The responses represent a balance between types of cells affected, magnitude of the injury, and reparative mechanisms initiated by the injury. The lung is endowed with a complex and interlocking defense system. Excellent review articles[15,16,32,37] on lung defense against inhaled materials describe some aspects of it. They emphasize the importance of deposition and clearance to the pattern of injury. These mechanisms operate at several levels but predominate at the site indicated. Deposition (influenced by particle size)[31,38,39] is determined by nasopharyngeal impaction, bronchoalveolar sedimentation and alveolar diffusion. Clearance which can be defined as response to, inactivation of, or physical removal of the injurious agent; is determined by local and "local-humoral" immune reactions,[3,21,24,41] immunologic activation,[2,7,20,53] modulation of inflammatory complement formation, and macrophage activation;[6,11,29,40,51,52] by phagocytosis, by natural antiproteolytic agents,[4,9,25,33,44,49,50] and by ciliary clearance of particles and debris on a stratified visco-elastic mucus blanket.

Earlier portions of this book define the connective tissue framework of the lung and emphasize its importance. The framework supports the diverse tissues performing nonrespiratory functions of the lung.[19] Likewise, the metabolism of collagen, elastin, proteoglycans, and mucoproteins (mucus glycoproteins) have been reviewed (Chapters 5 through 8). Although it is beyond the scope of this report to discuss the complex phenomena involved in other aspects of the biochemistry of pulmonary function, excellent articles are available on various aspects of it.[8-10,13,14,23,27,47,48] These by no means constitute a complete list. To provide a more complete understanding of the biochemical changes resulting from pulmonary injury, one must first understand the sequence of anatomic changes which result from pulmonary injury. As one compares these reactions with the natural cellular physiology and biochemistry of the lung, it becomes obvious that many represent results of an overzealous defense. If one could arrest this inappropriate defense, the disease in many cases might not develop.

Several review articles document the sequential changes resulting from pulmonary injury.[1,5,22,26,28,34,35,45,46,56] Ryan and Majno[43] reviewed carefully the complex events of acute inflammation. Capillary endothelial and type I alveolar cell damage frequently occur together or with such rapidity that the sequence is difficult to distinguish. Since type I alveolar epithelial cells form a tight junction and endothelial cells a looser one,[43] the initial appearance of septal edema suggests early enothelial damage while the appearance of intraalveolar edema suggests type I alveolar damage. Capillary damage leads to hemorrhage and the formation of hyaline deposits of fibrin outside the vessel. Type I alveolar cell destruction leads to proliferation of type II cells to fill the denuded epithelial areas and to produce surfactant to lower surface tension. Replacement of endothelial cells is by proliferation. By analogy to the vascular injury described by Harker et al.[17] in atherosclerosis, a proliferation of either alveolar contractile cells of fibroblasts may occur if either endothelial cells or type II cells are unable to fill the existing gap. These regenerations will proceed effectively as long as basement membrane has not been interrupted.[54] If basement membrane is interrupted, exposed interstitial collagen initiates coagulation phenomena which involve platelets. This leads to two processes: attempts to replace, which often lead to layering of basement membrane, and, simultaneously, proliferation of fibroblasts and probably either proliferation of or differentiation into contractile cells into vascular, interstitial, and alveolar spaces. As these cells contact the developing extracellular matrix, they elaborate connective tissue and pulmonary fibrosis develops.

Variations of this sequence of events may be viewed, in a highly speculative vein, as a "turning off" the main pathway at a particular point or stage. The initial event is death of endothelial and type I epithelial cells proportional to the intensity of injury. The injury and death of endothelial and epithelial cells is extensive; endothelial and epithelial proliferation are minimal; and compensatory proliferation of mesenchymal cells (fibroblasts and/or alveolar contracile cells) is unsuccessful. Large amounts of proteinaceous fluid will escape from the blood vessels, especially the venules[43] into the septa and alveoli and hylaine membranes of fibrin form. The "edema" and fibrin phase predominate and the subjects die of pulmonary edema. Alternatively, if the injury dose or dose rate is slightly less, the epithelial and endothelial regeneration rate will still be low. However, the mesenchymal cells will be able to proliferate and elaborate connective tissue, resulting in pulmonary fibrosis. A lesser or different pattern of injury, less protracted dose or dose rate will allow epithelial and endothelial proliferation, but result in a low level or local continued proteolysis which weakens support of the basement membranes, leading to alveolar destruction. In many areas there will be a type II cell hyperplasia and eventual conversion to a type I cell more resistant to proteolytic destruction. In other areas, however, alveoli will be lost, and no or unsuccessful regeneration of alveolar basement membrane[54] will occur, leading to emphysema. Finally, injury level may be just great enough so that a few type I epithelial cells or capillary endothelial cells are destroyed. In this case either the endothelial cell or the type II alveolar cell will readily proliferate to fill the existing void. As in the above cases, continued injury may induce altered cells. However, in this case the injury level is low enough that these cells have an increased probability of division and occasionally may become neoplastic. The last three conditions, pulmonary fibrosis, emphysema, or neoplasia, involve alterations of the pulmonary connective tissue metabolism and will be discussed in greater detail (Chapters 13, 14, and 16). Bronchitis-asthma and manifestations of conducting airway disease represent alterations in proteoglycans or mucoproteins (Chapter 15).

Injury to the lung usually occurs at either an alveolar site or in the upper airways. Since the alveolus constitutes a vast majority of the surface area and most of the pulmonary mass, it will be discussed first.

II. ALVEOLAR INJURY

Figure 1 presents the author's concept of alveolar injury. Damage may occur to either endothelial or epithelial (usually type I) cells. Endothelial cells die and are replaced exposing basement membrane, releasing cold insoluble globulin (CIG) and increasing vascular permeability. The exposed basement membrane when combined with platelet recruitment of CIG causes adhesion of platelets to the vessel wall. Edema, complement activation, coagulation, and fibrinolysis are all consequences of this path. In light of Chapter 10, this reflects a dissolution of the extracellular matrix and leads to further proteolysis and collagenolysis, i.e., a freeing of connective tissue followed by significant degradation of it. Edema, complement activation, coagulation, fibrinolysis, proteolysis, and collagenolysis are all contributed to by neutrophils, macrophage accumulation and their effect, and the effect of collagen on cell mediated

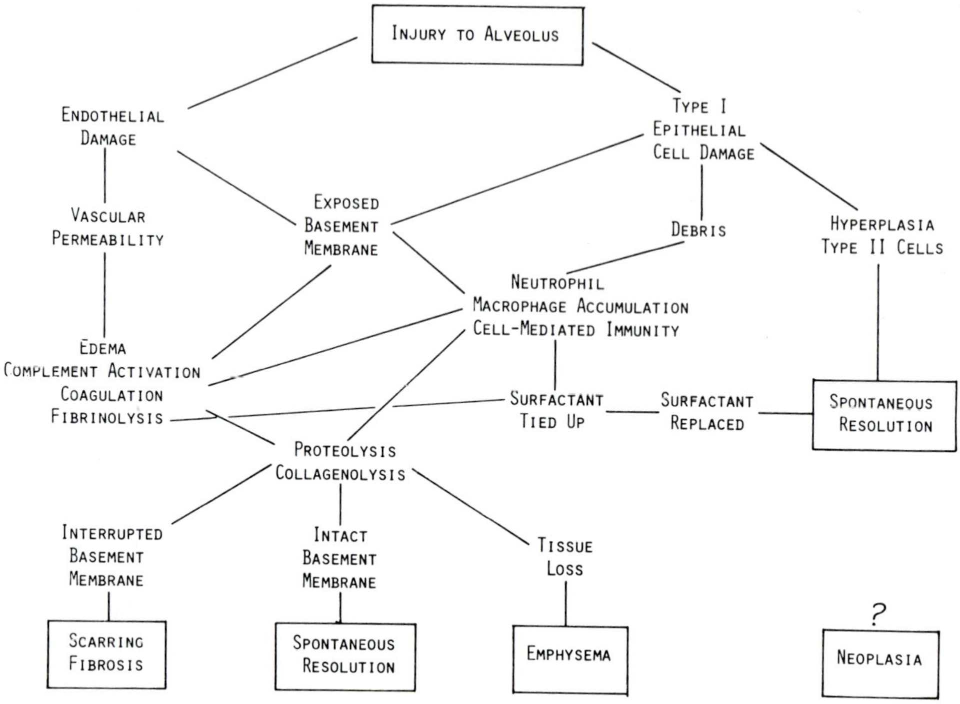

FIGURE 1. Alveolar injury represents damage to endothelium and type I alveolar epithelum. Endothelial damage leads to exposed basement membrane and increased vascular permeability. Edema, complement activation, coagulation and fibrinolysis and an influx of inflammatory cells precede proteolysis and collagenolysis. If basement membrane is severely interrupted, scarring and fibrosis develop. If local interruptions lead to tissue loss, emphysema may result. Finally, intact basement membrane leads to spontaneous resolution. Type I epithelial damage leads to hyperplasia of type II cells or debris. Both may go to spontaneous resolution. However, debris may induce an influx of inflammatory cells and go by an alternate pathway to fibrosis, emphysema, or spontaneous resolution, as described for endothelial damage.

immunity as described in Chapter 11. In fact, in light of Chapter 10, the breakdown of fibronectin, a protease sensitive and matrix determining protein, may be even more critical than fibrinolysis to this process. If basement membrane is interrupted in a significant proportion of places or to a significantly great degree, regeneration of pulmonary architecture will be poor.[54] This leads to the formation of dense fibrous scars, and pulmonary fibrosis of a virtually irreversible nature develops. The author's concept of alveolar injury clearly relates fibrinolysis to irreversible pulmonary fibrosis (to be discussed in Chapter 13). This has been thought by pathologists,[11a,45] to be an essential element in any fibrosis model. If the basement membrane is intact (interstitial injury only) spontaneous resolution may occur even if significant intersititial fibrosis is present as indicated by anatomic, biochemical, and physiological evidence, and considerable injury has occurred.[36] Under certain conditions the proteolysis may be intense and localized, leading to alveolar wall loss, disruption of pulmonary architecture, and emphysema (to be discussed in Chapter 14).

III. INJURY IN UPPER AIRWAYS

Pure epithelial injury is usually repaired by type II cell proliferation, especially if the injury is not sustained. Examples of such injury resulting in disease are rare (Figure 1). Type I epithelial damage leads to hyperplasia of type II cells by an unknown mech-

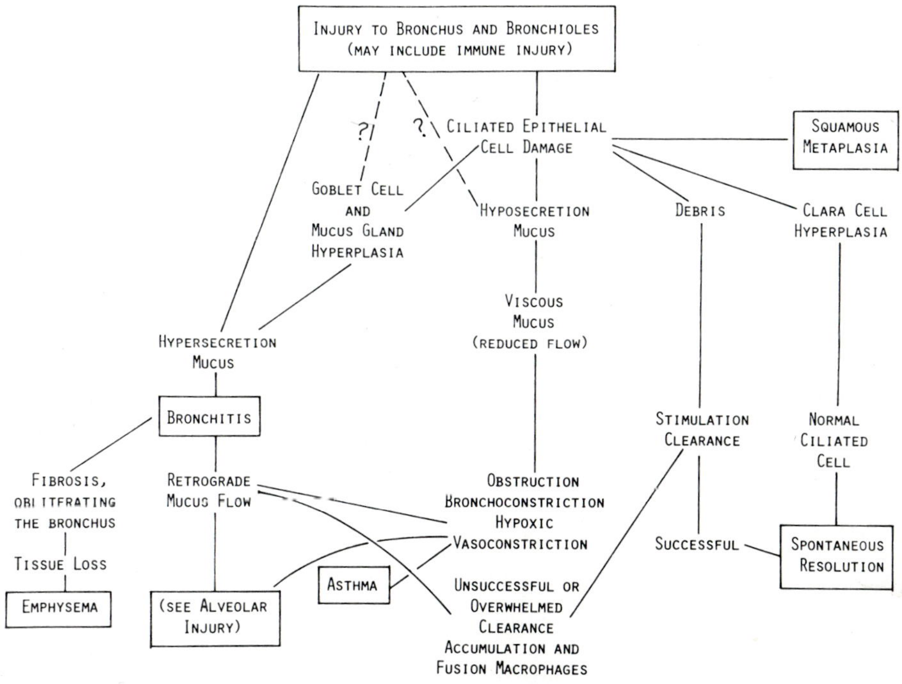

FIGURE 2. Upper airway injury to bronchus or bronchioles may lead to ciliated epithelial cell damage and hypersecretion of mucus either with or without goblet cell and mucus gland hyperplasia. Hypersecretion of mucus may lead to bronchitis, to fibrosis obliterating the bronchus, tissue loss, and emphysema, or to retrograde mucus flow and alveolar injury or fusion of alveolar macrophages. Hyposecretion of mucus may lead to bronchoconstriction, hypoxic vasoconstriction and asthma. Ciliated epithelial damage may lead to squamous metaplasia, or to Clara cell hyperplasia and spontaneous resolution, or to production of debris stimulated and overwhelmed clearance and fusion of pulmonary alveolar macrophages.

anism. The possibility that such cells may be communicating with their extracellular matrix as discussed in Chapter 9 and reviewed for mesenchymal cells in Chapter 10 is an attractive one. However, spontaneous resolution or, at worst, cuboidal (type II cell) hyperplasia, is the most frequent endpoint. Epithelial injury may lead to neutrophil and macrophage accumulations leading to or influencing cell mediated immunity (discussion in Chapter 11). While this leads to surfactant tie-up, the hyperplasia often replaces it and spontaneous resolution occurs. The sensitivity of the two cell populations in most injuries is nearly equivalent as judged by their responses.

Injury to the bronchus and bronchioles (which may include immune injury) is biochemically more complex, especially relating to connective tissue, possibly because it is more poorly understood. Certainly it is more difficult to study because of the small portion of the lung involved. The author's concept of this process is illustrated in Figure 2. Ciliated epithelial cell injury may progress to hyper- or hyposecretion of mucus. Hypersecretion may involve goblet cell hyperplasia accompanying bronchitis (to be discussed in Chapter 15). Retrograde mucus flow leads to the alveolar injury noted in Figure 1, or to an unsuccessful and overwhelmed clearance, inflammation, and fusion of macrophages. Alternatively, ciliated epithelial damage may lead to debris formation, inflammation, and accelerated clearance which may, if unsuccessful (damage is high), lead to accumulation of fused macrophages by the same mechanism or, if successful, lead to spontaneous resolution.

Hyposecretion of mucus reflects a very viscous mucus with an obviously reduced flow. This leads to obstruction, bronchoconstriction, and hypoxic vasoconstriction which in turn leads to alveolar injury (Figure 1). In conditions leading to asthma, there are usually immunologic components.

Squamous metaplasia may result directly from ciliated cell injury. Another consequence of ciliated epithelial cell damage is Clara cell proliferation. A most frequent consequence of this is to produce normal ciliated cells leading to spontaneous resolution. The relation between the two has only been recognized recently and much remains to be done to understand it. However, loss of cilia have been noted as a consequence of inhaling pollutants, so this response may reflect an important determinant of integrity of bronchi and possibly of clearance.

It is to be emphasized that these schemes represent the author's concept of pulmonary injury. They should be useful in following Chapters 13 through 17, since papers usually look at small pieces of these schemes. The author's experience in compiling them has led to validation that if one has two pathologists describing lung injury, a minimum of three opinions may be expected.

REFERENCES

1. **Adamson, I. Y. R., Bowden, D. H., and Wyatt, J. P.,** A pathway to pulmonary fibrosis: an ultrastructural study of mouse and rat following radiation to the whole body and hemithorax, *Am. J. Pathol.,* 58, 481, 1970.
2. **Allison, A. C.,** Immunological surveillance against tumor cells, in *Cancer,* Vol. 4, Becker, F. F., Ed., Plenum Press, New York, 1975, 237.
3. **Austen, K. F.,** Reaction mechanisms in the release of mediators of immediate hypersensitivity from human lung tissue, *Fed. Proc.,* 33, 2256, 1974.
4. **Bell, O. F. and Carrell, R. W.,** Basis of the defect in α-1-antitrypsin deficiency, *Nature (London),* 243, 410, 1973.
5. **Bouhuys, A. and Peters, J. M.,** Control of environmental lung disease, *N. Engl. J. Med.,* 283, 573, 1970.
6. **Bowden, D. H. and Adamson, I. Y. R.,** The alveolar macrophage delivery system. Kinetic studies in cultured explants of murine lung, *Am. J. Pathol.,* 83, 123, 1976.
7. **Burrell, R.,** Immunology of occupational lung diseases, in *Occupational Lung Diseases,* W. K. C., Morgan and A., Seaton, Eds., W. B. Saunders, Philadelphia, 1975, 65.
8. **Clements, J. A. and King, R. J.,** Composition of the surface active material, in *Biochemical Basis of Pulmonary Function,* Crystal, R. G., Ed., Marcel Dekker, New York, 1976, 363.
9. **Cohen, A. B.,** Interrelationships between the human alveolar macrophage and alpha-1-antitrypsin, *J. Clin. Invest.,* 52, 2793, 1973.
10. **Cohen, A. B.,** α-1 Antitrypsin as a systemic determinant of lung structure and function, in *Biochemical Basis of Pulmonary Function,* Crystal, R. G., Ed., Marcel Dekker, New York, 1976, 313.
11. **Colvin, R. B. and Dvorak, H. F.,** Fibrinogen/fibrin on the surface of macrophages: detection, distribution, binding requirements, and possible role in macrophage adherence phenomena, *J. Exp. Med.,* 142, 1377, 1975.

11a. **Dungworth, D.,** Research communication, 1974.

12. **Faulkner, C. S. and Connolly, K. S.,** The ultrastructure of ^{60}Co radiation pneumonitis in rats, *Lab. Invest.,* 28, 545, 1973.
13. **Fisher, A. B.,** Oxygen utilization and energy production, in *Biochemical Basis of Pulmonary Function,* Crystal, R. G., Ed., Marcel Dekker, New York, 1976, 75.
14. **Goerke, J.,** Lung surfactant, *Biochim. Biophys. Acta,* 344, 241, 1974.
15. **Green, G. M.,** In defense of the lung, *Am. Rev. Respir. Dis.,* 102, 691, 1970.
16. **Green, G. M.,** Lung defense mechanisms, *Med. Clin. North Am.,* 57, 547, 1973.
17. **Harker, L. A., Ross, R., Slichter, S. J., and Scott, C. R.,** Homocystine-induced arteriosclerosis. The role of endothelial cell injury and platelet response in its genesis, *J. Clin. Invest.,* 58, 731, 1976.

18. **Harrison, G. and Lapp, N. L.**, Electron microscopic findings in the lungs of miners, *Ann. N.Y. Acad. Sci.*, 200, 73, 1972.
19. **Junod, A. F.**, Metabolism, production and release of hormones and mediators in the lung, *Am. Rev. Respir. Dis.*, 112, 93, 1975.
20. **Kaltreider, H. B.**, Expression of immune mechanisms in the lung, *Am. Rev. Respir. Dis.*, 113, 347, 1976.
21. **Kang, K. Y., Sera, Y., Okochi, T., and Yamamura, Y.**, T-Lymphocytes in asbestosis, *N. Engl. J. Med.*, 291, 735, 1974.
22. **Katzenstein, A. L. A., Bloor, C. M., and Leibow, A. A.**, Diffuse alveolar damage—the role of oxygen, shock, and related factors, *Am. J. Pathol.*, 85, 210, 1976.
23. **King, R. J.**, The surfactant system of the lung, *Fed. Proc.*, 33, 2238, 1974.
24. **Kripke, M. L. and Borsos, T.**, Immune surveillance revisited, *J. Natl. Cancer Inst.*, 52, 1393, 1974.
25. **Kueppers, F. and Black, L. F.**, α_1-Antitrypsin and its deficiency, *Am. Rev. Respir. Dis.*, 110, 176, 1974.
26. **Liebow, A. A.**, Definition and classification of interstitial pneumonias in human pathology. Alveolar Interstitum of the Lung, Int. Symp., Paris, 1974, *Prog. Respir. Res.*, 8, 1, 1975.
27. **Mason, R. J.**, Lipid Metabolism, in *Biochemical Basis of Pulmonary Function,* Crystal, R. G., Ed., Marcel Dekker, New York, 1976, 127.
28. **Masse, R., Nolibe, D., Fritsch, P., Metvier, H., LaFuma, J., and Chrêticn, J.**, Chronic interstitial pneumonitis induced by internal α-irradiation of the lung, *Prog. Respir. Res.*, 8, 74, 1975.
29. **McAdoo, M. H., Dannenberg, A. M., Hayes, C. J., James, S. P., and Sanner, J. H.**, Inhibition of the cathepsin D-type proteinase of macrophages by pepstatin, a specific pepsin inhibitor, and other substances, *Infect. Immun.*, 7, 655, 1973.
30. **Nash, G., Foley, F. D., and Langlinais, P. C.**, Pulmonary interstitial edema and hyaline membranes in adult burn patients, *Hum. Pathol.*, 5, 149, 1974.
31. **Natusch, D. F. S. and Wallace, J. R.**, Urban aerosol toxicity: the influence of particle size, *Science,* 186, 695, 1974.
32. **Newhouse, M., Sanchis, J., and Bienenstock, J.**, Lung defense mechanisms (I,II), *N. Engl. J. Med.*, 295, 990, 1045, 1976.
33. **Ohlsson, K.**, Interaction between endogenous proteases and plasma protease inhibitors *in vitro* and *in vivo, Bayer Symp., V, Proteinase Inhibitors,* Springer-Verlag, Basel, 1974, 96.
34. **Pariente, R.**, Action of oxygen and oxidizers on the lung and bronchioles, *Prog. Respir Res.*, 8, 91, 1975.
35. **Pariente, R., Legrand, M., and Brouet, G.**, Pulmonary ultrastructural aspects of oxygen poisoning under atmospheric pressure in the rat (trans.), *La Presse Med.*, 77, 1073, 1969.
36. **Pickrell, J. A., Diel, J. O., Slauson, D. O., Halliwell, W. H., and Mauderly, J. L.**, Diffuse interstitial fibrosis following radiation-induced lung injury resolves spontaneously if dense scars are not formed, submitted for pub., 1979.
37. **Proctor, D. F.**, The upper airways. I. Nasal physiology and defense of the lungs, *Am. Rev. Respir. Dis.*, 115, 97, 1977.
38. **Raabe, O. G.**, Instruments and methods for characterizing radioactive aerosols, *IEEE Trans. Nucl. Sci.*, NS-19(1), 64, 1972.
39. **Raabe, O. G., Kanapilly, G. M., and Newton, G. J.**, New methods for the generation of aerosols in insoluble particles for use in inhalation studies, in *Inhaled Particles III,* Vol. 1, Walton, W. H., Ed., 1971, 3.
40. **Richmond, V. L.**, *In vitro* hydrolase and phagocytic activities of alveolar macropahges, *J. Lab. Clin. Med.*, 83, 757, 1974.
41. **Rosenbaum, J. T.**, Basophil or IgE-bearing lymphocyte? *N. Engl. J. Med.*, 291, 678, 1974.
42. **Rüttner, J. R., Spycher, M. A., Sticher, H.**, The detection of etiologic agents in interstitial pulmonary fibrosis, *Hum. Pathol.*, 4, 497, 1973.
43. **Ryan, G. B. and Majno, G.**, Acute inflammation — a review, *Am. J. Pathol.*, 86, 183, 1977.
44. **Sandhaus, R. A. and Janoff, A.**, Degradation of human α_1-antitrypsin by hepatocyte acid cathcpsins, *Am. Rev. Respir. Dis.*, 110, 263, 1974.
45. **Slauson, D. O., Hahn, F. F., Benjamin, S. A., Chiffelle, T. L., and Jones, R. K.**, Inflammatory sequences in acute pulmonary radiation injury, *Am. J. Pathol.*, 82, 549, 1976.
46. **Spencer, H.**, Pathogenesis of interstitial fibrosis of the lung, *Prog. Respir. Res.*, 8, 34, 1975.
47. **Tierney, D. F.**, Intermediary metabolism of the lung, *Fed. Proc.*, 33, 2232, 1974.
48. **Tierney, D. F. and Levy, S. E.**, Glucose metabolism, in *Biochemical Basis of Pulmonary Function,* Crystal, R. G., Ed., Marcel Dekker, New York, 1976, 105.
49. **Tuttle, W. C. and Jones, R. K.**, Fluorescent antibody studies of alpha-1-antitrypsin in adult human lung, *Am. J. Clin. Pathol.*, 64, 477, 1975.

50. **Tuttle, W. C. and Westerberg, S. C.,** Alpha-1 globulin trypsin inhibitor in canine surfactant protein, *Proc. Soc. Exp. Biol. Med.,* 146, 232, 1974.
51. **Unanue, E. R.,** Secretory function of mononuclear phagocytes — a review, *Am. J. Pathol.,* 83, 396, 1976.
52. **Unkeless, J. C., Gordon, S., and Reich, E.,** Secretion of plasminogen activator by stimulated macrophages, *J. Exp. Med.,* 139, 834, 1974.
53. **Valentine, F. T.,** Soluble factors produced by lymphocytes, *Ann. N.Y. Acad. Sci.,* 221, 317, 1974.
54. **Vracko, R.,** Basal lamina scaffold-anatomy and significance for maintenance of orderly tissue structure, *Am. J. Pathol.,* 77, 314, 1974.
55. **Witschi, H.,** Exploitable biochemical approaches for the evaluation of toxic lung damage, in *Essays in Toxicology, Vol. 6,* Hayes, W. J., Ed., Academic Press, New York, 1975, 125.
56. **Wolfe, W. G. and DeVries, W. C.,** Oxygen toxicity, *Annu. Rev. Med.,* 26, 203, 1975.

Chapter 13

PULMONARY FIBROSIS

J. A. Pickrell and J. L. Mauderly

TABLE OF CONTENTS

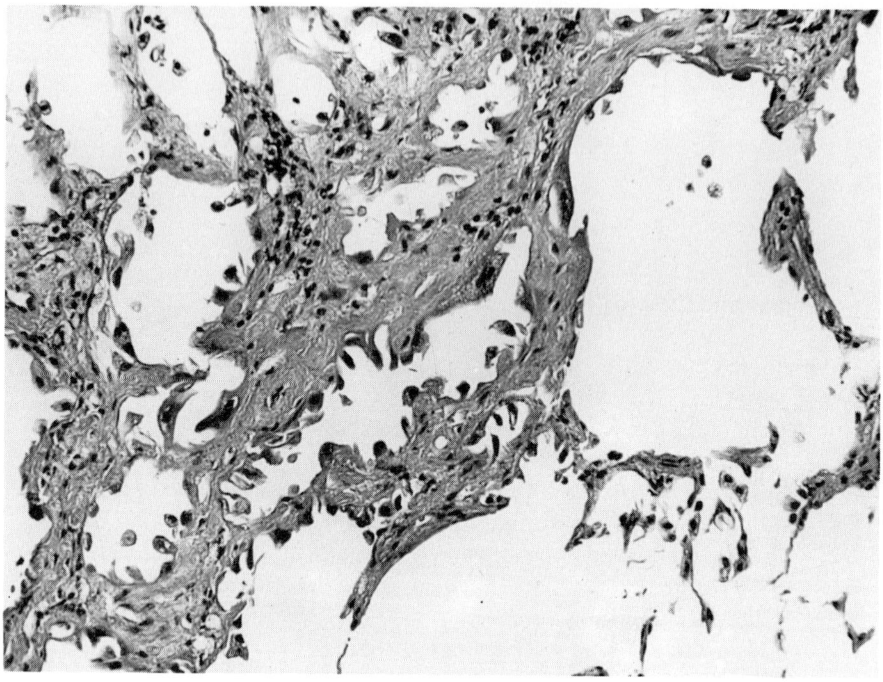

FIGURE 1. Alveolar septal fibrosis with proliferation of alveolar lining cells. (×150, H and E stain.)

I. ETIOLOGIES AND DESCRIPTIONS

Development of pulmonary fibrosis by no means implies a specific etiology, but rather is the end product of a variety of etiologies.[156,175,190] It generally involves each step in the sequence described as leading to pulmonary fibrosis: endothelial and type I cell destruction, type II cell hyperplasia, interruption and layering of basement membrane, mesenchymal cell proliferation, and development of septal and intraalveolar pulmonary fibrosis (Figure 1).

Liebow,[112] in describing the interstitial pneumonitis (IP) conditions, relates fibrosis to factors of chemical, immunologic, ''collagen disease,'' genetic and physical causes, including radiation as usual (U) IP. He also indicates that the superimposition of bronchiolitis obliterans upon basic lung injury as well as the development of desquamative (D)IP, lipid (L)IP, or giant cell (G)IP may lead to the same course. Wolfe and DeVries[205] and Pariente et al.[136] indicate the importance of oxygen toxicity and Katzenstein et al.[96] broaden this to include diffuse alveolar damage of multiple or various origins. Pariente[135] emphasizes the importance of oxidizers in the development of pulmonary fibrosis if the injury is severe and it penetrates to the alveolus.

Pulmonary fibrosis is a common sequelae to radiation exposure. Several investigators[2,49,88,103,117,121,133,166,171,172,180,200] indicate that sufficient quantities of radiation will induce pulmonary fibrosis. Occasionally cardiac fibrosis is noted,[54,121] although whether this is a direct result of radiation damage or secondary to the increased pulmonary vascular resistance is unclear. Slauson et al.[172] emphasize that dissolution of the fibrin deposits (fibrinolysis) is quite important to the continued maintenance of the inflammation and hence to the developing fibrosis. A possible link between inflammation (fibrinolysis) and fibrosis is the activation of T-lymphocytes by bradykinin,[176] bradykinin's link to fibrinolysis, and the link of activated T-lymphocytes to pulmonary fibrosis.[102] Watanabe et al.[200] indicate that mast cells infiltrate alveolar septa and lie close to mesenchymal cells (alveolar interstitial cells), and degranulate so that the associated granules lie between the mast cell and the mesenchymal cell. These granules were not stained with a alcian blue at early stages, suggesting that they contained hyaluronic acid. Later when they did stain with alcian blue they were probably composed of chondroitin sulfate AC and Dermatan sulfate. Lysosomes are activated in response to radiation.[43,143] One often sees vasculitis in early stages of radiation pneumonitis.[143] This may reflect thickening of the vascular basement membrane. Pérez-Tamayo[137] reviewed evidence suggesting that histologic increase in basement membrane material may indicate a local disturbance in collagen degradation and, thus, collagen metabolism.

Ozone has been noted as an inducer of pulmonary fibrosis. Ozone exposures (0.8 ppm for 7 days) induced increased NADH and NADPH diaphorase, LDH, ATPase, and cytochrome oxidase reactivities not only in the central areas which were infiltrated with mononuclear cells but in the adjacent histologically unaffected areas.[20,21] In addition, bronchiolar and ciliary damage have been noted. LDH isoenzyme III increases observed in ozone exposure suggest the source of the LDH increase.[91a]

Mineral dusts frequently lead to the formation of pulmonary fibrosis. Lindy et al.[113] noted an increase in LDH isoenzyme V in silicosis in rats, with no change in LDH(III). Dale[42] noted unilateral fibrosis resulted from unilateral exposure to silica, although mild contralateral effects were present. The fibrogenic effects of various mineral dusts are noted.[12,14] Heppleston et al.[82] reported a lipoproteinosis suggesting that the tissue passes through the inflammatory stage prior to disease formation. Rom and Palmer[159] noted pulmonary effects in asbestosis. Reeves et al.[151] report that asbestos induces considerable pulmonary fibrosis and some neoplasia. Association of fibrosis and neoplasia have been noted.[59]

Drug-induced pulmonary disorders often lead to fibrosis as reviewed by Rosenow[161] and by Martin and Smith,[116] specifically Bleomycin,®[2,9,57] Mecylamine,®[158] Methysergicide,®[66,67,83] Busulfan,®[16,71,131] Diphenylhydantoin,®[114] and Hexamethonium®.[48] Although some of these were reversible, this constitutes a widespread hazard to lung.

The herbicide paraquat causes lung injury which may lead to pulmonary fibrosis. Paraquat produced type I epithelial cell destruction, associated type II cell hyperplasia, and increased surfactant production,[98] leading to pulmonary fibrosis.[173] Thurlbeck and Thurlbeck[184] noted extensive hemorrhage and death following paraquat administration. However, Niden and Khurana[129] gave initially low but progressively increasing doses which were ultimately fibrogenic, passing through each anatomic stage. This is consistent with the lung developing a tolerance to paraquat. It is necessary to just exceed the dosage tolerated and produce continued re-injury to lung. Clearly, initial injury will not sustain itself.

Human pulmonary fibrosis occurs for which one can find no overt cause. It is thus categorized as idiopathic pulmonary fibrosis.[61,167,206] Popovic and Mullane[148] report that biliary obstruction is fibrogenic to rats, progressing through the sequential anatomic changes.

II. PHYSIOLOGIC CHANGES

Several excellent reviews of the effects of interstitial fibrosis on pulmonary function in man have been published.[7,168,202] The increased amount of connective tissue in the parenchymal interstitium results in an abnormally "stiff" lung which requires more effort to expand. The lung pressure-volume curve is shifted markedly to the right, and a major feature is the reduction of both static and dynamic lung compliance. The residual volume may be normal or slightly increased, but both vital capacity and total lung capacity are reduced. The increased effort required to make volume changes in the restricted lung causes the subject to adopt a breathing pattern with progressively higher respiratory frequencies and smaller tidal volumes. As a result, a smaller fraction of each breath reaches the alveoli and thus minute volume must be increased. Alveolar hypoventilation is not usually a feature of the disease, and alveolar oxygen tensions are usually maintained at or above normal levels. There is little if any increase in airway resistance, and forced expiratory flowrates are usually normal. An impairment in alveolar-capillary gas transfer is an early and progressive feature of the disease. Increased thickness of the alveolar-capillary barrier, reduced membrane surface area, and reduced capillary blood volume all contribute to the gas transfer impairment, but a mismatching of ventilation and perfusion is thought to be the major cause. The distribution of inspired gas is abnormally uneven, but not generally to the degree associated with obstructive diseases. As the disease progresses, the oxygen saturation of arterial blood falls, and in severe stages there is carbon dioxide retention and respiratory acidosis.

Similar functional alterations have been reported to occur in experimental interstitial fibrosis induced in dogs by irradiation[118] and in hamsters by endotracheally instilled bleomycin.[174] Arzt[4] reports many of the same changes. Boushy and North[15] note that infiltrative lung disease reduced vital capacity and total lung capacity.

III. CHANGES IN COLLAGEN METABOLISM

A. Idiopathic Pulmonary Fibrosis

Fulmer and Crystal[61] and Crystal et al.[36] have reviewed human idiopathic pulmonary fibrosis and find that hypercellularity is an essential feature. In this disease severe local fibrosis develops, presumably after proceeding through epithelial cell death, attempted replacement, and fibroblast proliferation. The data of Kravis et al.[102] suggest that circulating T-lymphocytes of these patients secrete lymphokines having MIF and cytotoxic activity to collagen coated cells. Reynolds et al.[153] noted increased T-lymphocytes in chronic hypersensitivity pneumonitis but not in idiopathic pulmonary fibrosis. Miller et al.[122] indicated that platelets carry collagen. Thus, platelets or macrophages or both may be involved in this disease. Vital capacity is reduced; however, when it is plotted as a percent of total lung capacity it is only slightly reduced, indicating that considerable volume has been removed from the lung. Severe gas exchange impairment was present occasionally. Morphologically, parenchyma is thickened and intercapillary tissue constitutes over half of the lung tissue ($\simeq$ 16% normal lung)[61] with twofold reductions in airspaces, capillary spaces, and alveolar capillary tissues. DNA/dry weight is increased, indicating the cellularity of the disease. Kawanami et al.[94] observed that anchoring fibrils which attached alveolar epithelial cells to the basal lamina were present in idiopathic fibrosis but not in normal human lungs. Their presence seemed proportional to the severity of disease. He concluded that these were not simply a component of fibrous connective tissue but represented association with cuboidal metaplasia of the alveolar epithelial cells. Whether these develop to attach epithelial cells to the thickened basal lamina and at what phase in the injury they develop awaits further examination. Collagen content is not increased, nor is collagen synthesis increased, even though histologically local collagen deposition is obvious. The mechanism for this remains obscure.[61] Seyer et al.[167] have shown an increase in type I collagen relative to type III collagen and an increased release of collagen by pepsin digestion.

Further work in this area may define more clearly the mechanism involved in the pathogenesis of this type of pulmonary fibrosis.

Are pulmonary collagenous scars properly cross-linked? Less or a different type of organization of pulmonary collagen is present at the tissue level. Correlation of tissue collagen organization and cross-linking has been studied in skin but not in lung. The two tissues may be similar with respect to this correlation. As cutaneous scars become increasingly abnormal, less organization and cross-linking were present. Surprisingly, lysyl oxidase (the cross-linking enzyme) was normal to elevated and α_1/α_2 chain ratios decreased.[100]

B. Silicotic Fibrosis

Although collagen/wet weight is not increased in silicotic guinea pig lungs,[93] silicosis produces an increase in lung weight and total collagen.[99] The source of the silica seems to relate to its fibrogenicity. The semiconductor nature of the silica, which may related to its oxidant potential, is quite important to its fibrogenicity. Likewise, fibrogenic silica reduced the macrophage ability to reduce 2,3,5 triphenyltetrazol chloride. This indicated that the macrophage had contacted an oxidant, and the reduced ATP/ADP is most likely a result of the subsequent interference with oxidative phosphorylation. Bassett and Fisher[6] have shown that chemical interference with oxidative phosphorylation stimulates lung metabolism. Ziskind et al.,[208] reviewing silicosis, noted that silica induces macrophages to discharge protelytic enzymes. Dale[41] induced unilateral fibrosis after unilateral silica exposure. Increasing lung weight and collagen content were noted. Rodkina[157] noted that peptide and protein hydroxyproline content increased in silicosis, indicating increased collagen breakdown and content in silicotic lungs. Since progressive increases in collagen content were noted, synthetic rate presumably increased sufficiently to reflect a positive balance of collagen metabolism. Vasil'yeva and Myagkaya[196] note progressively increased lung weight and collagen content following exposure to silica. Vasil'yeva[195] noted an increase in carbohydrates, uronic acids, and hydroxyproline soluble in sequential extractions of 0.14 or 0.2 *M* NaCl, citrate buffer, and 0.2 *M* NaOH. An activated collagen synthesis or breakdown or both may have been present. However, the high molecular weight hydroxyproline was not separated; determination of which part of collagen metabolism was increased is not possible. Increased proteoglycan metabolism is indicated by the increased uronic acid and carbohydrate. Chvapil et al.[28] summarized their results on silicosis. An increase in hydroxyproline and thus collagen content correlated well with increased ascorbic acid content in exposed lungs. This resembled results seen in a caaragenin-induced granuloma. In the granuloma, citric, lactic, or pyruvic acid remained constant, suggesting that some specificity might be given to the ascorbic acid increase. However, quantity of ascorbate does not influence collagen synthesis of lung or muscle. They found that a single aerosol exposure to silica stimulated the collagen metabolic response maximally. The difference between collagen content, which rose rapidly, and fibrosis, which developed more slowly, were unclear. However, they might represent a conversion of soluble to insoluble collagen or a diffuse interstitial fibrosis going to a more dense fibrosis scarring pattern. Zaidi and Kaw[207] report that malnutrition does not reduce fibrosis in silicotic rats, indicating that pulmonary fibrosis is produced even without adequate nutrition.

Silica produced a reaction in peritoneal macrophages leading to in vitro production of collagen. Heppleston and Styles[81] noted that hydroxyproline was increased when the 50 g supernatant fraction of silicotic peritoneal macrophages was incubated with growing chick embryo fibroblasts. Since the hydroxyproline/DNA increase exceeded that of the hydroxyproline, some killing of the fibroblasts was indicated. How this relates to the suggested interference with macrophage oxidative phosphorylation which exposure to fibrogenic silica induced in macrophages[99] is unclear. However, the interesting observation of Mintz[124] that silica increases mitochondrial NAD/NADH may correlate to an interference with oxidative phosphorylation. Perhaps the observation by Manner et al.[115] that proteolysis of human embryonic lung cells increased the percentage of collagen synthesis due to a reduction of noncollagenous protein synthesis might relate to Heppleston's changes if cell number were increased in his culture. However, DNA content was not increased relative to controls. Heppleston et al.[80,82] further theorized that the known lipoproteinosis of silicosis stimulates macrophage accumulation and that silica causes their death, presumably through an oxidative interference with oxidative phosphorylation. This death leads to elaboration of a fibrogenic stimulus of undefined nature.

Ability to detect this stimulus and reproduce it is far from universal. Our work, and the work of others have indicated that, more often than not, no effect is elicited by the use of activated peritoneal or pulmonary alveolar macrophages. Indeed, if we use macrophages activated in vivo by exposure to aerosols of $^{238}PuO_2$ or $^{239}PuO_2$, we can get a reduction of total hydroxyproline and prolyl hydroxylase, no effect, or a slight increase in collagen synthesis relative to noncollagenous protein.[146a] The reason for difference of response is not clear. This system is extremely complex and very hard to define or control. Aalto et al.[1] report that extract from normal macrophages reduces collagen synthesis and that extract from silicotic macrophages raises it relative to that of normal macrophages, but only to levels when macrophages are not added, not to levels expected in fibrogenesis. Harington et al.[76] report that silicotic macrophages reduce collagen production in fibroblasts maximally stimulated with insulin. In light of insulin's stimulation of glycolysis, important to fibro-proliferation, one wonders if the system was not further complicated. Burrell and Anderson[17] found that silicotic pulmonary alveolar macrophages stimulated the amount of hydroxyproline released in the medium from WI-38 diploid lung fibroblasts. The amount of hydroxyproline was a function of cell concentration. Although 1/10 dilution produced collagen stimulation, a 1/100 dilution had no effect. Lewis and Burrell[111] reported that lung connective tissue antibodies cause macrophages to release a substance which accelerates collagen synthesis in stationary fibroblasts. Media from macrophages cultured with silica more than two years before had the same effect, suggesting that the factor is stable to freezing. Kilroe-Smith et al.[97] also note fibrogenicity of silicotic macrophages which cannot be attributed to unreacted silica. This system shows promise for studying lung disease in vitro but still may require considerable standardization. However, these results are consistent with those of Kravis et al.[102] and Stuart et al,.[181] suggesting an immunologic basis to lung disease, or with those of Liebovich and Ross,[107] indicating that fibroblast proliferation is influenced by a macrophage factor.

C. Oxidation and Macrophages

Parakkal[134] reported that macrophages were involved with collagen resorption. This correlated with Horowitz and Crystal's[86] isolation and partial characterization of pulmonary alveolar macrophage collagenase. Certainly cross-linked fragments of collagenase-digested collagen could be endocytized (taken into the cell) and further degraded by lysosomal proteases at acid pH.[73,77] The relation of collagen resorption to pulmonary injury is most likely a reflection of collagenase's association with rapidly dividing cell systems and possible interruption of basement membrane by digestion of basement membrane collagen. The relation of macrophages to lung injury has been assumed to be that of phagocytosis of cell debris. However, as Unanue[193] has indicated, phagocytosis elaborates protelytic enzymes into the surrounding interstitium.

Fisher et al.[56] suggest that hyperoxia interferes with the oxidative phosphorylation of macrophages, causing increased glucose utilization, lactate production, and decreased CO_2 production. This is similar to the response reported by Klosterkotter and Robock[99] for silicotic macrophage and to that reported by Gray et al.[70] prior to proliferation of 3T3 fibroblasts released from contact inhibition. Plopper et al.[147] notes no effects on macrophage ultrastructure from 3 ppm O_3 for four hr, although O_3 oxidant effects were well known. Macrophage number had doubled with 12 hr and extensive phagocytosis had occurred. The possibility that extensive lysosomal proteases were released concomitant to such phagocytosis must be considered. Karl et al.[92] report that zinc-treated peritoneal macrophages are more resistant to the toxic effects of silica.

Chvapil and Peng[32] reported that both hypoxia and hyperoxia lead to enhanced lipoperoxidation, increased lung lactate, prolyl hydroxylase, inflammation, and increased collagen content, or pulmonary fibrosis. They suggested an interference with oxidative phosphorylation. Välimäki et al.[194] observed anatomic and biochemical changes which support those of Chvapil and Peng.[32] The kinetics of incorporation suggested the possibility of some rapid turnover of collagen. Cunningham et al.[37] noted that hypoxia induced lung growth while elastic recoil remained normal. In newborn rats the number of alveoli increased while in three- and nine-week-old rats the size but not the number of alveoli increased. Thurlbeck[183] reviewed this area and noted both responses, although failing to note the distinction made by Cunningham et al.[37] Chvapil et al.[29] reported that increased collagen relative to noncollagen protein synthesis in hypoxic lung was due to decreased noncollagen protein synthesis. This may reflect a mechanism like that reported by Manner et al.[115] after proteolysis of human embryonic fibroblasts.

Zinc affects inflammation in several organs, including the lung. Zinc deficiency is thought to predispose tissues to lysosomal labilization.[26] Henkin[79] discusses its role in wound healing without arriving at any conclusions, although he feels it to be an important factor in cell division. Fernandez-Madrid et al.[55] report decreased collagen and noncollagenous protein synthesis in wound sponge granuloma in zinc deficiency. So under some conditions, probably lysosomal labilization, zinc does not lead to relative or absolutely accelerated collagen synthesis. However, addition of 10^{-4} to 10^{-8} *M* $ZnSO_4$ to low density fibroblast cultures inhibits fibroblast proliferation from a concentration dependent cytotoxicity. $ZnSO_4$ (10^{-5} to 10^{-7} *M*) added to confluent cultures does not affect cellular proliferation but results in a differentially reduced collagen synthesis.[201] Likewise, Chvapil[26] has noted a reduction in collagen synthesis in CCl_4-induced hepatic injury in rats fed a high zinc diet relative to that of the controls. Thus the role of zinc as a preventor of injury-induced fibrosis requires further clarification. Recent data of Chvapil[26] suggests it may have considerable benefit in reducing the fibrosis of silicosis, although further work will tend to clarify this exciting area.

D. Asbestosis

Asbestos may be deposited in bronchioles and alveoli and initiate inflammation. As indicated by Newhouse et al.,[128] asbestos fibers can be inhaled, because they can be oriented parallel to air flow and reach the deep lung as would particles of much smaller size. They do, however, have much greater probability of impaction. Injection into the thoracic cavity after inhalation may occur because the elongate fibers might work through the parenchyma to the outside, causing pleural granulomas of two types: (1) those discretely walled off, having predominantly giant cells (guinea pigs), and (2) those with no distinct walls containing macrophages and fibroblasts (rats and mice). The species' different response may account for this discrepancy. In rats and mice, macrophages are involved and they cannot phagocytize the large asbestos fibers. The possibility that this may lead to incomplete ("frustrated") phagocytosis should be considered. In this case, protelytic enzymes might be elaborated, leading to fibroblast proliferation. This would seem to suggest that some fibers might be more fibrogenic.[8] However, this concept must be more fully defined. In fact, some asbestos fibers seem to be more toxic,[13] producing some bronchiolar proliferation, alveolar damage, and dense subpleural areas of collagen.

Studies have revealed considerable effect of asbestos on cultured fibroblasts. Richards et al.[155] report that asbestos causes fibroblasts to undergo a rapid "maturation process", reflected by highly dilated endoplasmic cisternae, irregularity of nuclear outline, and membrane microvilli. This is presumed to be evidence of transforming fibroblasts from logarithmic to stationary phase, although alternative explanations relating to toxicity must be considered. Richards et al.[155] reported that chrysotile asbestos, but not bituminous, anthracite, glass, or silica caused increased collagen relative to protein. The other substances, except glass, stimulated cell division, as indicated by increased DNA and hyaluronic acid. Chrysotile had a slightly increased hyaluronic acid and slightly reduced DNA, although neither was prominent. The reason for this apparent discrepancy in proliferation indicators is unclear. Lower levels of asbestos which stimulate DNA do not increase collagen. However, chrysotile seems to delay fibroblast growth at days 7 to 10 and reduces collagen relative to protein; the relation to proteolysis is unclear. Subsequently, DNA returns to normal and collagen increases absolutely and relative to protein. Hyaluronic acid does not agree with DNA in terms of cell proliferation. However, chondroitin does show a return from earlier depressions to normal levels. Persistent long term exposure of lung fibroblasts to chrysotile asbestos over 37 passages in vitro leads to enhancement in cell mat collagen deposition. The mechanism is not clear.[79a]

Asbestos induces increased collagen production, but the mechanism is not defined. Davis and Reeves[44] reported an increase in in vitro hydroxylation of radioactive proline at early times after exposure to asbestos fibers. Later hydroxylation was greatly reduced relative to controls. They reported hydroxyproline/proline ratios of 5 to 50, which are inconsistent with being able to hydroxylate only the 3 position of the gly-pro-pro triplet for 4 hydroxyproline. Thus, a hydroxyproline/proline ratio in excess of one would probably be difficult to achieve. The meaning of their results require further clarification. Flowers[58] reviewed asbestos effect on collagen synthesis. He suggested that the initial effect was one of increased glycolysis, which led to the release of a fibrogenic factor, and increased alpha ketoglutaric acid, which increased proline and hydroxylation of it, causing an increase of collagen and resulting fibrosis. Although not discussed, his data is consistent with the increased glycolysis Gray et al.[70] observed prior to cell division. Further work is needed to unify the intriguing changes noted herein and to relate them to carcinomas induced by asbestos. For instance, "which cell makes the collagen?" Might at least some of the increase be secondary to a type II epithelial cell proliferation? If type II cells which have lost contact inhibition can elaborate surfactant while proliferating perhaps they can also elaborate collagen.

E. Histamine

Histamine may lead to alveolar hypoxia, increased cell proliferation, and increased collagen production. Sandberg[165] noted that 48/80, a histamine releaser, caused granulation tissue in healing wounds to contain 55% more collagen five days after implanting polyvinyl sponges. He indicated that histamine accelerated wound healing. Dabrowski and Maslinski[40] indicated that exogenous or endogenous histamine accelerated "precollagen" formation and collagen polymerization at early times. Later, excessive collagen polymerization was inhibited by histamine. Kahlson and Zederfeldt,[91] cited in Dabrowski and Máslinski,[40] indicated that 48/80 and polymixin B increased breaking strength of wounds, and that semicarbazide (a histidine decarboxylase inhibitor) caused considerable decrease in tensile strength and this impaired healing. Demeszko and Dabrowski[46] report that the amount of collagen is considerably higher in the histamine adapted guinea pigs. They noted increased consumption of oxygen in the presence of glucose and alpha ketoglutarate, raising the possibility that cell division may have occurred preceding the analysis and the development of fibrosis. Religa and Máslinski[152] noted that the histamine content of silicotic lungs and lungs with diffuse fibrosis is increased. Since histamine causes alveolar hypoxia, bronchiolar constriction, and emphysema, these conditions (histamine increase, emphysema, and fibrosis) may be related. A closer examination revealed histamine, histidine decarboxylase (endogenous histamine production), and histamine inactivation to be elevated in silicosis. The presumption is that high endogenous production of histamine might lead to pulmonary fibrosis or at a lower dose level to emphysema.

F. Cigarette Smoke

Cigarette smoke leads to increased lung collagen and to altered macrophage physiology. Rosenkrantz et al.[160] demonstrated a dose-related increase in pulmonary hydroxyproline as a result of mice inhaling cigarette smoke. We take this to indicate increased collagen and the development of pulmonary fibrosis, even though his "extracted collagen" failed to confirm this. Comparison of his Kjeldahl nitrogen values (from "extracted collagen") and hydroxyproline values suggests considerable impurity in his lung collagen and more in his liver collagen. The degree of impurity probably reflected the amount of collagen in the beginning mixture. His hydroxyproline values should reflect the collagen values, although the metabolism of it remains undetermined. Powell and Green[149] indicate that cigarette smoke inhibits glyceraldehyde 3-phosphate dehydrogenase without affecting glucose 6-phosphate dehydrogenase or lactate dehydrogenase. This effect can be reversed by cysteine and suggests a sulfhydryl role in this injury. Holt and Keast[85] indicate that cigarette smoke inhibits protein synthesis in alveolar macrophages. However, when macrophages are exposed to low levels for longer periods of time, both protein and RNA synthesis show marked increases, indicating macrophages' capacity to adapt to a toxic environment. This adaptation probably represents either an induction of glutathione reductase or the methyl glycoxylate shunt which bypasses the GAP-3 dehydrogenase step. The relation of cigarette smoke to cancer again links fibrosis and cancer, presumably at different dose levels and possibly involving different cell types. Considerable further investigation is necessary to define this rather complex area.

G. Connective Tissue Activating Peptide

Castor et al.,[22-25] in a series of papers, outlines the isolation and partial characterization of connective tissue activating peptide in synovial cells. This polypeptide, with a molecular weight of 4,000 to 10,000 daltons, markedly increases glycolysis and the formation of hyaluronic acid, strongly suggesting synovial cell proliferation. Later collagen is presumably increased. Steroids and non-steroid anti-inflammatory agents effectively block this action, suggesting that proliferation or inflammation is involved. McGee et al.[120] isolated from livers of rats treated with CCl_4 one or two proteins or polypeptides with molecular weights less than 5000, which will stimulate both prolyl hydroxylase activity and incorporation of proline into collagen chains. They indicate that these factors are also present in wounds but absent in normal skin, and hypothesize the importance to collagen formative diseases in general. Whether these factors induce fibroblast proliferation or activation, and whether they or similar factors are present in lung remains to be determined.

H. Vascular Factors

Ross et al., in an intriguing series of papers,[75,162,163,178] have investigated the molecular alterations of atherosclerosis, a vascular injury potentially related to the vascular component of pulmonary fibrosis. They note that when endothelial cells are damaged, medial smooth muscle cells migrate to the intima and proliferate. McCullough and Balian[119] reported that these cells become "fibroblast-like" in morphology and switch from making predominantly type III collagen to predominantly type I collagen. Ross' group further demonstrated that platelets had a reduced survival time in atherosclerotic animals and that these platelets contained a factor mitogenic for smooth muscle cells. By using homocysteine, Harker et al.[75] were able to induce endothelial loss, smooth muscle cell migration, and proliferation. In a comparable in vitro smooth muscle cell system[15a] similar proliferation resulted in proportional increases in collagen synthesis with the same amount of collagen synthesized per cell. Fuller et al.[60] noted an increase in aorta active and inactive prolyl hydroxylase, which tends to agree with Ross and Burke's findings of cell proliferation. Concomitant reductions in platelet survival times were noted. Dipyrimadole, which blocks the platelet reaction, blocked the smooth muscle cell proliferation and the atherosclerosis. However, it had no discernible effect on the endothelial cell loss. Thus, the smooth muscle cell proliferation is extremely important to the development of atherosclerosis. The relation of this condition to a similar vasculitis in lung must be considered.

Release of platelet factors may relate to pulmonary injury and to lymphokines in that injury. Steele et al.[177] have noted a reduction in platelet survival time in human chronic airway obstruction. They suggested that platelet suppressant drugs may be of considerable value in reducing the thrombosis of chronic airway obstruction. Johnson et al.[89] note improvement of survival time when oxygen is given to patients with chronic obstructive airway disease. Perhaps platelets are also an important component of vascular injury in pulmonary fibrosis. Certainly Kravis et al.'s[102] work suggests that T-lymphocytes participate in a reaction with collagen which causes them to secrete lymphokines, which will lyse collagen coated cells. When combined with the observation of Miller et al.[122] that platelets carry collagen, it provides some indirect support for this concept. The observation of Kohler and Lipton[101] that platelets are an enriched source of growth promoting activity for 3T3 fibroblasts ($\sim$ 5 times greater than autologous serum) tends to support the plausibility of this hypothesis. Ubatuba et al.[192] observed that antiplatelet serum had no effect upon edema formation. Likewise, Benjamin et al.[11a] noted that thymectomy did not reduce and probably intensified pulmonary fibrin deposition. In neither of these studies was fibrosis allowed to develop. Finally, Benditt[10] presented evidence for atherosclerosis developing from proliferation of a monoclonal cell similar to a smooth muscle cell but having different characteristics. The intriguing question relates to the degree of similarity of atherosclerosis and pulmonary fibrosis. They respond differently to antioxidant therapy, which reduced lipoperoxidation. The therapy was successful in atherosclerosis[127] but not in radiation-induced pulmonary fibrosis.[138]

I. Radiation-Induced Pulmonary Fibrosis

Collagen is the most important altered connective tissue constituent in pulmonary fibrosis[144] in dogs given approximately 20 to 77 Krad total cumulative dose of radiation from ^{144}Ce fused aluminosilicate particles (FAP). Cobalt-60 external thoracic irradiation induces modest increases in lung collagen if given 4 to 6 Krad. Two Krad has little effect. Tsurufugi and Ohuchi[189] report small increases in lung collagen at 1200 rads in mice. Eddy and Casarett[49] present data indicating collagen accumulation in radiation-induced pulmonary fibrosis. Gerber et al.[62] noted increased disappearance of labelled collagen in irradiated animals, suggesting that radiation increases collagen metabolism.

Law et al.[106b] noted considerable time delay in development of ana c fibrosis. Only small amounts of collagen increase were noted. These were most pr bunced near the LD_{50}. Tseveleva[188] indicated that plutonium (isotope not specified) c trate given as an intratracheal injection led to increased collagen synthesis, indicated by increased soluble collagen and incorporation of ^3H proline into collagen. This led to increased collagen accumulation. Rantanen[150] indicated that radiation reduces collagen quantity in wound healing sponges. This amount returns to normal and in some cases exceeds it. These findings showed that the concept of a negative collagen balance in radiation injury must be considered. Collins et al.[32a] reported collagen decreases in lobes which received 1000 R once weekly to achieve 3000 to 4000 R. Irradiation to these lobes was severe enough that weight and DNA were reduced to ≃ one half that of controls. This seemed somewhat more severe than in our hamster study[142] (500 R/exposure repeated two times a week) to achieve 4000 or 6000 R because wet weights of lungs did not decrease. They remained about the same or were increased. Thus, these two papers suggest different species' radiation sensitivity with respect to lung. Such differences are not uncommon with respect to whole body. Collins et al.[32a] may have irradiated at a level exceeding the lethal dose to a portion of the mesenchymal cells. Thus, this work may represent an important upper end point for fibrosis and its definition. The compensatory increase of fibrous connective tissue in the remaining lobes could represent a mechanism similar to that[34,106] reviewed by Hance and Crystal[73,74] following partial pneumectomy, although experimental verification of this conjecture may be complex. In our other experiments[141,143,144] the entire lung was theoretically irradiated. Thus, we have no known experience with the type of experiment performed by Collins et al.[32a] It would not seem that their experimental set-up resembled the case of idiopathic pulmonary fibrosis which develops slowly over long periods of time and seems to be a hypercellularity.[61] An important question, as one considers all of this research, is whether radiation injury induces a progression from negative to positive collagen balance.

Pickrell et al.[141-144] have shown that collagen breakdown is increased initially; then there is increased collagen synthesis, quantity, and a return to a less elevated pattern of collagen metabolism. This sequence of events is in agreement with most of the data concerning pulmonary fibrosis, especially radiation-induced pulmonary fibrosis. Moreover, we have noted that the pattern of collagen metabolic changes is similar for ^{90}Y FAP and $^{238}PuO_2$ although they differ with respect to the time over which injury was delivered. All changes of collagen metabolism were similar, differing only in time and magnitude. Early increases of non-collagenous protein incorporation of ^{14}C-proline (Figure 2) and collagen breakdown (Figure 3) preceded any increase in collagen synthesis. Subsequently, increased collagen synthesis (Figure 4) predominated over increased collagen breakdown and the positive balance of collagen metabolism which led to increased collagen content (Figure 5) and pulmonary fibrosis. This was observed earliest in hamsters exposed to ^{90}Y in fused aluminosilicate particles due to a high dose rate and a rapid accumulation of dose. Increased collagen metabolism was observed somewhat later in animals exposed to 100 nCi of $^{238}PuO_2$ and still later in hamsters exposed to 50 nCi of $^{238}PuO_2$. Later reductions of collagen content in hamsters exposed to 50 nCi of $^{238}PuO_2$ were due to a negative collagen balance, reflected by reduced collagen synthesis relative to breakdown. The reduction of collagen content is less in hamsters exposed to 100 nCi of $^{238}PuO_2$. The consistently elevated collagen synthesis observed in these animals at later times appeared to maintain the elevated collagen content. Animals exposed to $^{238}PuO_2$ illustrate a clear-cut radiation dose-effects relationship for pulmonary fibrosis.

Collagen balance may be approximated by subtracting the relative response of collagen breakdown from the relative responses of collagen synthesis relative to non-col-

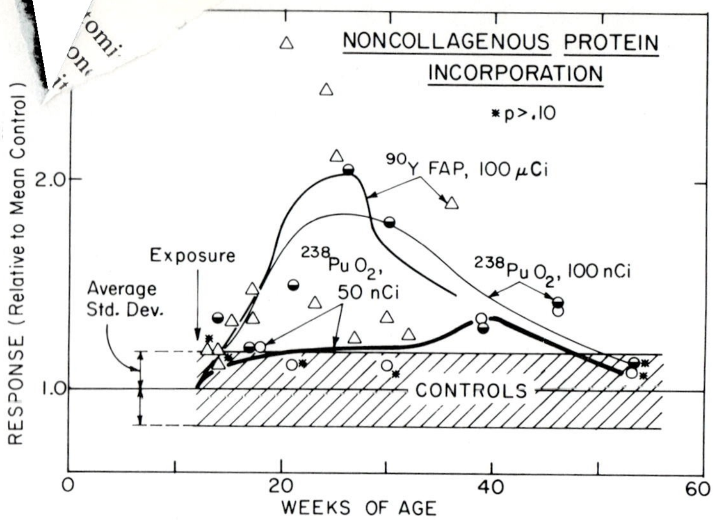

FIGURE 2. Pulmonary noncollagenous protein synthesis is shown as noncollagenous incorporation of proline into pulmonary tissue from exposure at 12 weeks of age to 41 weeks after exposure or 53 weeks of age. ^{90}Y-fused aluminosilicate particles (FAP; Δ) (100 μci) had increased noncollagenous protein synthesis by 3 weeks after exposure. $^{238}PuO_2$ (◒; 100 nCi) also increased, but had returned to normal by 41 weeks after exposure (53 weeks). $^{238}PuO_2$ (O; 50 nCi) increased only at 27 weeks after exposure (39 weeks of age) and was a much more moderate response (* $p > 0.10$).

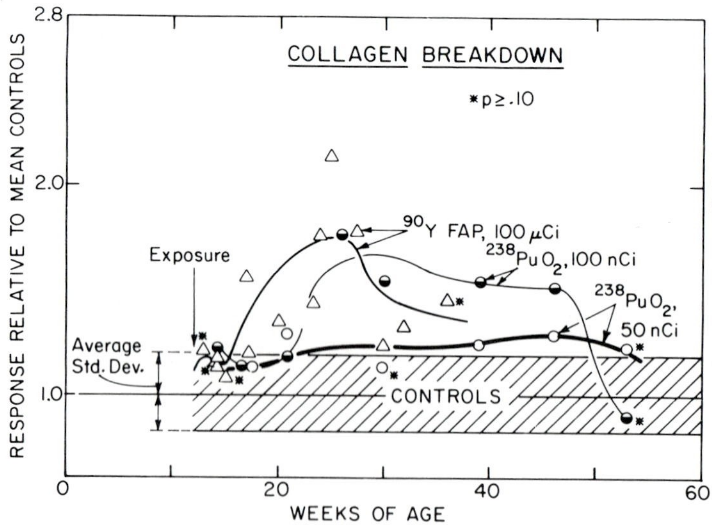

FIGURE 3. Pulmonary collagen breakdown (ultrafilterable hydroxyproline) (legend same as Figure 12) increases for hamsters exposed to ^{90}Y-FAP (Δ) $^{238}PuO_2$; 50 nCi (O) and 100 μCi (◒). By 41 weeks after exposure (53 weeks) it has returned to normal, relative to that of control hamster lungs (* $P > 0.10$).

lagenous protein.[145] The mildly (50 nCi) exposed hamsters have a normal balance which becomes markedly positive. Then it starts to decline and actually becomes negative, indicating clearly why pulmonary fibrosis is less intense and reversible (on a

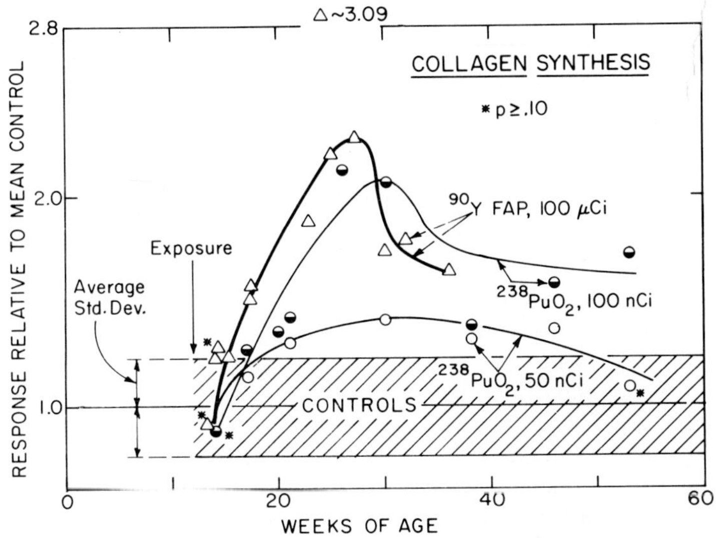

FIGURE 4. Pulmonary collagen synthesis relative to that of non-collagenous protein increases for hamsters exposed to ^{90}Y-FAP (Δ) and $^{238}PuO_2$ (100 nCi, ◒; 50 nCi, ○). In animals exposed to 50 nCi $^{238}PuO_2$ it has returned to normal relative to controls by 41 weeks after exposure (53 weeks of age). However, it remains elevated at that time in lungs of hamsters exposed to 100 μCi of $^{238}PuO_2$ (*$p > 0.10$).

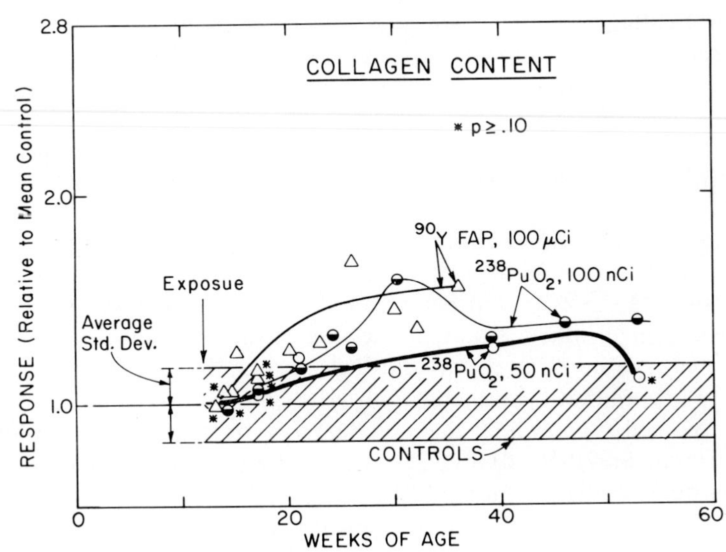

FIGURE 5. Pulmonary collagen content is increased by 8 weeks after exposure to ^{90}Y-FAP (Δ), 14 weeks after exposure to $^{238}PuO_2$ (100 nCi; ◒; 26 weeks of age) and 27 weeks after exposure to $^{238}PuO_2$ (50 nCi; ○; 39 weeks of age). It returns to normal control levels only in animal lungs exposed to 50 nCi of $^{238}PuO_2$ and only at 41 weeks after exposure or 53 weeks of age (*$p > 0.10$).

whole lung basis) in animals sacrificed at later times. When the fibrosis is reversed biochemically, the animals were also normal anatomically and histologically. An important feature of the fibrosis produced at earlier times was that it was almost entirely interstitial fibrosis. Almost no dense fibrous scars were present. To my knowledge, this constituted the first report of anatomic, physiologic, and biochemical fibrosis which was reversible. Counts and Knighten[36a] had produced an acute reversible pulmonary injury subsequent to inhalation of 1% trypsin. Collins et al.[33] induced alterations in connective tissue (collagen and elastin) metabolism after papain inhalation. During the first 2 days, hemorrhage and inflammation were present. The lungs were normal by 2 weeks after exposure. In both studies the lung is clearly able to repair minor injuries. However, in neither case was fibrosis or emphysema produced. Taken together these data clearly indicate that the lung may repair and reverse damage as severe as interstitial fibrosis with reduced compliance and elevated lung collagen.[145] Animals with the higher dose level had dense fibrous scars and the fibrosis was not reversible. Histologic changes and static compliance of the excised lungs support the biochemical analyses. The severly affected animals exposed to 100 nCi of $^{238}PuO_2$ have an early negative phase which rapidly becomes positive, pulling collagen content upward. The balance becomes less positive and negative as content decreases slightly. Finally, the balance approximates zero and collagen content reaches a plateau. ^{90}Y FAP produced a similar but more rapidly occurring pattern. These data illustrate the importance of collagen breakdown and, presumably, tissue injury in developing fibrosis. It is important to note that this modest breakdown increase occurred at a time when total acid phosphatase was normal to decreased and acute inflammation (as indicated by subsequently increased polymorphonuclear leucocytes in lavage fluid) was present. This presumably indicated that the macrophage[17,81,111] was not the determining factor at early times when the negative collagen phase was present. Pérez-Tamayo[137] notes that two stages of hepatic fibrosis are present, an early reversible one in which collagen-bound collagenase is present and a later irreversible one where it is not. The significance relative to the lung and especially to Pickrell et al.'s[145] reversible and irreversible pulmonary fibrosis is unclear. However, in the former case, a negative balance of collagen metabolism (relative breakdown > relative synthesis) was not present. This would be consistent with collagenase being tied up with collagen but not acting. Further work in this area will be necessary before an understanding is reached.

J. Summary

With the notable exception of idiopathic pulmonary fibrosis, collagen metabolism increases prior to the development of pulmonary fibrosis. Whether this increase represents activation of the cells that produce collagen or an increased number of such cells is not clearly determined. Many of the studies measure only collagen content or, at most, collagen synthesis, and thus did little to resolve this controversy. The lung has so many cell types that cytokinetic analyses shed little information upon the problem. Indeed, the cell types which make collagen in normal or injured lungs are not clearly established. For these reasons, only speculative evidence can be offered concerning the pathogenesis of pulmonary fibrosis.

Pickrell et al.[143-145] observed that collagen breakdown increased prior to collagen synthesis, causing an early negative phase of collagen breakdown at a time when lysosomal enzymes were normal and acute inflammation present. This suggested that some injury must precede the accelerated collagen metabolism. The delay of response certainly provided ample time for cell proliferation, which was not unusual in other injured tissues, such as healing wounds (where cytokinetics could be performed). Degradative intracellular enzymes elicit fibroblast proliferation in a variety of tissue culture systems. Finally, steroids block or reduce fibroblast proliferation in tissue culture and arrest radiation-induced pulmonary fibrosis in vivo. Pulmonary collagen synthesis is influenced differently from the synthesis of non-collagenous protein. This line of reasoning supports the concept that proliferation of the cells which produce pulmonary collagen is an integral part of the development of pulmonary fibrosis.

The proliferation of fibroblasts probably relates to proteolysis and to both the mechanisms discussed in Chapter 10 and to the events described in Chapter 12. In the case of injury, excess proteolysis will occur, degrading fibronectin and freeing cells from the extracellular matrix so that they can proliferate. The bound collagenase could be activated, causing solubilization of collagen degradation products so that increased collagen breakdown would be the first change observed. As the cells become what the tissue perceives as confluent and the matrix reforms, the initial procollagen causes the cell to secrete collagen rapidly, and synthesis exceeds breakdown. As the matrix becomes more extensive, most procollagen is matrix rather than cell bound and synthesis levels off. The continual elevation of synthesis in radiation-induced pulmonary fibrosis[143,145] suggests a reoccurrence of this process, i.e., reinjury and/or a reduction in matrix density such that a higher proportion of procollagen is bound to the heparin coated cell membrane. This should maintain elevated synthesis. It is very important in this process to determine whether basement membrane was degraded extensively. If so, then proliferation may be an unsuccessful attempt to repair structure. As such, the architecture is disorganized and the fibrosis seems irreversible. If, however, the initial injury is less and the fibrosis is confined to the interstitium, it seems reversible. This implies that significant remodeling of the collagen in the extracellular matrix can occur at low injury and presumably with no or minimal proliferation. Certainly this is an attractive possibility and the collagen-bound collagenase probably controls it. The mechanism of operation is not speculated on in my or others' model. Further research in this area is expected to be fascinating.

Let us consider the consequences of this proposed mechanism. If this were true it would indicate why pulmonary fibrosis is so difficult to manipulate, and why biological antioxidants and cross-link inhibitors of collagen seemed ineffective, at least at low, non-toxic doses. It would not, however, explain how low degrees of pulmonary fibrosis (largely diffuse interstitial) could resolve spontaneously. To explain this, one must speculatively invoke differential rates of collagen turnover among the specific collagen types or collagen remodeling. A clear-cut understanding of molecular heterogeniety is vital to understanding the pathogenesis of pulmonary fibrosis. Likewise, it is insufficient to describe injury only on a whole lung basis. A clear understanding of the anatomy of this disease and its relation to the physiology and biochemistry are necessary. The importance of interruption of pulmonary basement membranes[198] and its constituent collagen(s) must be further explored. Since local, low grade, pulmonary fibrosis may relate to pulmonary emphysema and to pulmonary neoplasia, this needed understanding may provide considerable enlightenment concerning these two diseases. With the present level of understanding, much work remains to be accomplished. The complexity of the lung's defenses results in only a limited number of possible responses to injury. Most lung injury seems to result from overzealous defense or response to injury.

IV. CHANGES IN PROTEOGLYCAN METABOLISM

Dermatan sulfate, a proteoglycan, may be associated with collagen in the developing fibrosis. Little information exists concerning alterations of proteoglycan metabolism.[73] Vasil'yeva[195] noted increased glycosaminoglycan in silicotic lungs. Lung fibroblasts respond to anthracite dust with increased hyaluronic acid production.[154] Tseveleva,[187] cited in Horwitz et al.,[87] noted that plutonium produced pulmonary fibrosis, together with an increase in total lung glycosaminoglycans, mostly chondroitin and dermatan sulfate. Likewise, Motimiya et al.[125] noted increased dermatan sulfate in a case of pulmonary fibrosis of unspecified origin. Ikenada,[1974] cited in Horwitz et al.,[87] indicated that when bovine lung is treated with collagenase, dermatan sulfate is preferentially released. Finally, Laurent[106a] provides convincing physical arguments demonstrating that collagen binds more effectively to dermatan sulfate or heparin than to chondroitin sulfate. Kawamoto and Nagai[95] have noted that dermatan sulfate increases at the time when collagen is being synthesized most rapidly in chicken embryo skin. This increase is at the expense of hyaluronic acid. Thus, hyaluronic acid may be produced by dividing mesenchymal cells. When these cells make collagen, dermatan sulfate may be necessary to interact with collagen in maintaining lung structure and be produced at the expense of hyaluronic acid. Results in this area are only beginning to be collected and correlated.

V. THERAPEUTIC MANIPULATION OF PULMONARY FIBROSIS

Methods used to manipulate pulmonary fibrosis in general have centered around attempts to influence collagen synthesis without altering the synthesis of noncollagenous proteins. While this has the attractive appearance of specificity, one must realize that somewhere near one half of the body protein is collagen. Thus, if one wishes to exclusively influence lung collagen, this general approach is often nonspecific and toxic if given at effective dose levels.

Attempts to inhibit cross-links have used the lathyrogenic agent, B-aminoproprionitrile, penicillamine, or semicarbizide.[5,110,170] Levene et al.[109] and Chvapil[27] indicated that these agents decrease collagen accumulation in silicotic rats and experimental granuloma. However, proteoglycan synthesis seemed unaffected.[11] Caldwell and Bland[18] showed that penicillamine increases proteoglycan metabolism, suggesting an alternation of collagen. Hoffman et al.[84] indicated that imperfectly cross-linked elastin was probably solubilized. Alternately it indicated a rapid turnover of this fraction of elastin. Grasedyck and Lindner[69] indicated that ^{14}C penicillamine binds rapidly to the newly synthesized collagen. Siegel[170] indicated that penicillamine inhibited the conversion of bifunctional to polyfunctional cross-links. When given at 0.01 to 0.03% in the water, BAPN[140] reduces collagen synthesis (incorporation of ^{14}C proline into collagenous relative to noncollagenous protein; incorporation into collagen breakdown products was usually less than 10% of total incorporation) without altering noncollagen protein synthesis in normal animals. It creates a reproducibly negative collagen balance at three to five weeks after radiation. However, by 12 weeks, when controls still have a negative balance, the BAPN and radiation animals have a positive collagen balance and increased collagen content, suggesting that this regime of BAPN is ineffective in manipulating pulmonary fibrosis.[140]

Colchicine, vinblastine, and vincristine have been used to inhibit the secretion of collagen.[50] Although it seems inherently toxic, Rojkind (cited in Hance and Crystal,[73]) suggested it may have therapeutic benefit to hepatic cirrhosis. Whether it can manipulate pulmonary fibrosis at nontoxic doses remains to be demonstrated. Proline analogs and iron chelators have been used to reduce collagen stability.[27,30,31,68,104] Although both inhibit prolyl hydroxylation, no evidence of in vivo usefulness has been demonstrated to date.[27,30,31] Ooshima et al.[132] reported that reserpine inhibits collagen deposition in vessels of hypertensive rats.

Manipulating fibrinolysis may affect pulmonary fibrosis. Triiodothyronine (T_3) delays by five to nine weeks and minimizes compliance reductions which follow receiving fibrogenic doses of ^{60}Co radiation. T_3 was not toxic at doses given,[191] although it probably raised the metabolic rate. The relation of the therapeutic benefit to increased metabolic rate is unclear, but increased collagen turnover with a temporary negative collagen balance must be considered. Vascular radiation damage is reduced by heparin (anticoagulant), acetyl salacylic acid (ASA, a non-steroid anti-inflammatory drug), prednisone, and by A.M.C.A. (tranexamic acid, cyclic amino caproic acid), an antifibrinolytic agent.[169] These findings suggest that fibrinolysis may be related to platelet degranulation. Since both are associated with dividing cells that produce connective tissue, the suggestion that proliferation is important to the developing fibrosis must be considered. The role of antiproteases[54] which were useful in suppressing tumors is unexplored.

Considerable work on modulation of injury-induced lipoperoxidation has been performed.[47,123,182] Trump and Arstila[186] have elegantly described some of the biological consequences of lipoperoxidation and indicated the desirability of reversing this response. DeLuzio[48] indicated that antioxidants profoundly influenced a variety of chemically-induced hepatic lesions. Wilson et al.[203] indicated the importance of lipoproxidation to vascular damage in choline-deficient rats. This can be reversed by using antioxidants (butylated hydroxyanisole and toluene).[204] Pfleger and Pickrell[138] indicated that these substances would reduce pulmonary lipoperoxidation which resulted from ^{90}Y FAP irradiation. However, no effect was noted upon the connective tissue formation or the resultant death of the animals. These results suggest that to manipulate pulmonary fibrosis one must do more than inhibit lipoperoxidation, although this may prevent the vascular damage of atherosclerosis.

Polyvinyl pyridine-*N*-oxide (PNO, PVNO) reversed the increased collagen production which Heppleston and Styles[81] produced by incubating growing fibroblasts with extract of peritoneal macrophages incubated with silica. Likewise, this compound reversed the increased pulmonary collagen content noted 7.5 months after exposure to silica.[157] These two results indicate that PVNO is of considerable promise in manipulating pulmonary fibrosis, and that activated macrophages are of considerable importance to the developing fibrosis. Rodkina[157] proposes that PVNO changes the surface properties of the silica in some undefined way. This may be correct, since Klosterkötter and Robock[99] have demonstrated the importance of surface interaction of silica with macrophages. Perhaps if one prevents this oxidation of macrophages, damage elicited by silica is inhibited.

Superoxide dismutase may inhibit oxidative-induced collagen accumulation in fibroblasts in vitro (Bhatnagar and Cross, cited in Hance and Crystal[73]). However, Crapo et al.[35] report that it fails to modify the lesions or mortality induced by 100% O_2. Since the aerosolized enzyme can be delivered only to the extracellular space if delivered in small droplets, it could indicate free reaction to be occurring intracellularly[35] or that the enzyme had already been inactivated. Alternatively, since no aerosol size was given, droplets could have been too large to reach the alveolar space. Trnavskä and Trnavsky[185] reported sodium salicilate to be effective in reducing the collagen breakdown present in adjuvant-induced arthritis. Phenylbutazone and chloroquin had less effectiveness. This is consistent with the observation that such drugs have potential but as yet unproven usefulness in such disorders.

Corticosteroids have a broad spectrum of activities including anti-inflammatory and anti-immunologic properties.[78] They induce $\sim$ 0 to 20% weight loss and $\sim$ 80% decrease of thymus weight[59] in Syrian hamsters and reduction of ATP production in rat lymphocytes.[130] Since ATP is important to membrane fluidity, the later change is consistent with lymphocytotoxicity. Fetal rabbit lung takes up glucocorticoids whose binding to cytoplasmic receptors forms a complex which is transferred into the nucleus.[63,64] Although steroids are used in a wide variety of pulmonary conditions, results are quite variable and are often poorly controlled.

Delay of healing induced by corticosteroids may have a negative effect on pulmonary edema but a positive one on fibrosis. Giri et al.[65] reported that steroids did not alter O_3-induced pulmonary edema, although heparin had some protective effect. The correlation between prevention of edema and pulmonary fibrosis is not completely obvious. Langner and Fuller[105] indicated that steroids did not prevent epinepherine-thyroxine-induced arteriosclerosis, although Ehrlich et al.[51] noted that glucocorticoids retarded wound healing. Jeffrey (cited in Gross[72] indicated that dexamethasone (10^{-8} M) or hydrocortisone (10^{-7} M) suppresses collagenase activity without blocking the enzyme directly. Dibutyryl cyclic AMP had the same effect. At somewhat higher doses of Depomedrol® (Upjohn Drug, Kalamazoo, Mich.) we find collagenolysis (ultrafilterable hydroxyproline) to be increased in vivo and in vitro. Eastridge and Hamman[48b]reported that steroids delay healing in pneumothorax. Although this is obviously a hazard in treating pulmonary fibrosis, the inhibition of pleural connective tissue formation suggests that steroids might inhibit pulmonary connective tissue formation. Castellino et al.[19] reported that rapid withdrawal of steroids was followed by the development of radiation injury a few months to six years after radiation. Gradual reduction of steroid dose is usually indicated. However, the steroid therapy while given did seem to delay the fibrosis. Vogel[197] contrasted the effect of penicillamine, which reduced wound breaking strength but had no effect on wound inflammation, with steroids, which inhibited inflammation and size of granuloma formation, but actually increased wound breaking strength at early times.

Let us consider the meaning of these findings. These findings emphasize the anti-inflammatory and anti-proliferative actions of steroids. The reason for the increase in wound breaking strength is unclear. Eisinger[52] reports that the pulmonary disease associated with Goodpasture's syndrome is best controlled by corticosteroids. Juhl et al.[90] reported that prednisone treatment enhanced survival of female patients with compensated non-alcoholic cirrhosis. Picken et al.[139] reported that corticosteroids increase the relative proportion of alveolar type II cells present in lung. This is consistent with Nathan's[126] observation that glucocorticoid treatment enhances lung maturity to the extent that treated lungs held more air than untreated ones. His suggestion that induction of an enzyme (phosphoryl choline glyceride transferase) may provide the basis for its action on lung requires further substantiation. Liebovich and Ross[107] reported that antimacrophage serum and corticosteroids prevented macrophages from coming to the wound, although neither substance had this action when used separately. This is consistent with steroid inhibition of chemotaxis by rising intracellular cyclic AMP in acute inflammation.[164]

Cutroneo[38] indicated that triamcinilone reduced lung prolyl hydroxylase by 40% at 1.5 mg dose in rats. Even at higher doses, this was reversible by approximately nine weeks. Moreover, the assayed reduction of prolyl hydroxylase seemed to be reflected in a similar reduction of inactive prolyl hydroxylase, at least in skin. Although the meaning is not clear, the possibility is that the proportion of cells synthesizing collagen may be less, due to inhibition of proliferation. Alternatively one considers the possibility that prolyl hydroxylase is specifically inhibited. However, this might be expected to require a reduction of active PH with little alteration of inactive PH. In a more recent paper[127] it was reported that glucocorticoids did not cause the accumulation of underhydroxylated collagen, since collagen nascent chain synthesis reduction was the same as hydroxyproline and hydroxylysine formation. Moreover, the polysome makeup did not change greatly. This suggests coordinate regulation of several key steps of collagen biosynthesis at the translational or transcriptional level.[127] This argument is certainly thought-provoking; however, the possibility of the presence of a lower proportion of cells which make collagen at relatively high rates cannot be eliminated without further work. The research in this area continues to show promise for the control of pulmonary disease. Corticosteroids arrest pulmonary fibrosis in vivo and fibroblast proliferation in vitro. When one gives high levels of steroids to manipulate pulmonary fibrosis,[146] collagen balance (relative synthesis — relative breakdown) is initially negative at three and five weeks in both steroid and steroid plus radiation animals. This is due to reduced synthesis and modestly increased breakdown. No effect is noted on acute inflammation as indicated by PMN in lavage fluid. However, the radiation-induced increase of lymphocytes is inhibited. As the steroid is stabilized at a lower dosage, collagen balance gradually returns to normal. Collagen content is not increased, nor is gross evidence of pulmonary fibrosis present. Histologic interpretations indicate a reduction in intensity and a delay of fibrosis of considerable magnitude. These changes indicate that steroids are of considerable use in delaying or inhibiting radiation-induced pulmonary fibrosis. Since synthesis of collagen returned to normal more rapidly than did noncollagenous protein incorporation of proline, we considered the possibility that collagen synthesis was influenced by a different factor than protein synthesis. Similar levels of steroid in culture inhibited proliferation of L-929 and WI-38 fibroblasts, but increased the conversion of synthesized collagen to collagen degradation products. We interpret this to mean that increased collagenolytic capabilities are present, suggesting that the cells are attempting to divide but cannot. Leung and Munck[108] indicate that steroids inhibit the activation of glycolysis which Gray et al.[70] noted prior to cell division in 3T3 cells released from contact inhibition. The reduction in cell number in our cultures is slightly less than the reduction of collagen synthesis we observed in vivo or the reduction of prolyl hydroxylase.[38,39] Further work on steroid manipulation of pulmonary fibrosis will yield therapeutic applications and an understanding of the mechanism of pulmonary fibrosis.

REFERENCES

1. **Aalto, M., Potila, M., and Kulonen, E.,** The effect of silica-treated macrophages on the synthesis of collagen and other proteins *in vitro, Exp. Cell Res.,* 97, 193, 1976.
2. **Adamson, I. Y. R. and Bowden, D. H.,** The type 2 cell as progenitor of alveolar epithelial regeneration, *Lab. Invest.,* 30, 35, 1974.
3. **Adamson, I. Y. R., Bowden, D. H., and Wyatt, J. P.** A pathway to pulmonary fibrosis: an ultrastructural study of mouse and rat following radiation to the whole body and hemithorax, *Am. J. Pathol.,* 58, 481, 1970.
4. **Arzt, G. H.,** Pulmonary function disorders in fibrosis (trans.), *Internist,* 15, 364, 1974.
5. **Barrow, M. V., Simpson, C. F., and Miller, E. J.,** Lathyrism — a review, *Q. Rev. Biol.,* 49, 101, 1974.
6. **Bassett, D. J. P. and Fisher, A. B.,** Metabolic response to carbon monoxide by isolated rat lungs, *Am. J. Physiol.,* 230, 658, 1976.
7. **Bates, D. V. Macklem, P. T., and Christie, R. V.,** Diffuse interstitial fibrosis, in *Respiratory Function in Disease,* 2nd ed., W. B. Saunders, Philadelphia, 1971, 268.
8. **Becklake, M. R.,** Asbestos-related diseases of the lung and other organs: their epidemiology and implications for clinical practice, *Am. Rev. Respir. Dis.,* 114, 187, 1976.
9. **Bedrossian, C. W. M., Luna, M. A., Mackay, B., and Lichtiger, B.,** Ultrastructure of pulmonary bleomycin toxicity, *Cancer,* 32, 44, 1973.
10. **Benditt, E. P.,** The origin of atherosclerosis, *Sci. Am.,* 236, 74, 1977.
11. **Bentley, J. P., Wuthrich, R. C., and Van Bueren, A. M.,** Lathyrism and mucopolysaccharide metabolism in aorta, skin, and cartilage, *Atherosclerosis,* 12, 159, 1970.

11a. **Benjamin, S.,** Research communication, 1976.

12. **Berry, J. P., Henoc, P., Galle, I. P., and Pariente, R.,** Pulmonary mineral dust, *Am. J. Pathol.,* 83, 427, 1976.
13. **Botham, S. K. and Holt, P. F.,** The effects of inhaled crocidolites from transvaal and north-west cape mines on the lungs of rats and guinea-pigs, *Br. J. Exp. Pathol.,* 53, 612, 1972.
14. **Bouhuys, A. and Peters, J. M.** Control of environmental lung disease, *N. Engl. J. Med.,* 283, 573, 1970.

15. **Boushy, S. F. and North, L. B.** Pulmonary function in infiltrative lung disease, *Chest,* 64, 448, 1973.
15a. **Burke, J.,** Research communication, 1976.
16. **Burns, W. A., McFarland, W., and Matthews, M. J.,** Busulfan-induced pulmonary disease, *Am. Rev. Respir. Dis.,* 101, 408, 1970.
17. **Burrell, R. and Anderson, M.,** The induction of fibrogenesis of silica-treated alveolar macrophages, *Environ. Res.,* 6, 389, 1973.
18. **Caldwell, E. J. and Bland, J. H.,** The effect of penicillamine on the rabbit lung, *Am. Rev. Respir. Dis.,* 105, 75, 1972.
19. **Castellino, R. A., Glatstein, E., Turbow, M. M., Rosenberg, S., and Kaplan, H. S.,** Latent radiation injury of lungs and heart activated by steroid withdrawal, *Ann. Intern. Med.,* 80, 593, 1974.
20. **Castleman, W. L., Dungworth, D. L., and Tyler, W. S.,** Cytochemically detected alterations of lung acid phosphatase reactivity following ozone exposure, *Lab. Invest.,* 29, 310, 1973.
21. **Castleman, W. L., Dungworth, D. L., and Tyler, W. S.,** Histochemically detected enzymatic alterations in rat lung exposed to ozone, *Exp. Mol. Pathol.,* 19, 402, 1973.
22. **Castor, C. W.,** Connective tissue activation. IV. Regulatory affects of antirheumatic drugs, *Arthritis Rheum.,* 15, 504, 1972.
23. **Castor, C. W.,** Connective tissue activation. I. The nature, specificity, measurement and distribution of connective tissue activating peptide, *Arthritis Rheum.,* 14, 41, 1971.
24. **Castor, C. W., Prince, R. K., and Dorstewitz, E. L.,** Characteristics of human "fibroblasts" cultivated *in vitro* from different anatomical sites, *Lab. Invest.,* 11, 703, 1962.
25. **Castor, C. W. and Prince, R. K.,** Modulation of the intrinsic viscosity of hyaluronic acid formed by human "fibroblasts" *in vitro*: the effects of hydrocortisone and colchicine, *Biochim. Biophys. Acta,* 83, 165, 1964.
26. **Chvapil, M.,** New aspects in the biological role of zinc: a stabilizer of macromolecules and biological membranes, *Life Sci.,* 13, 1041, 1973.
27. **Chvapil, M.,** Pharmacology of fibrosis and tissue injury, *Environ. Health Perspect.,* 9, 283, 1974.
28. **Chvapil, M., Hurych, J., Cmuchalova, B., Holusa, R., and Ehrlichova, E.,** Conflicting hypotheses on experimental silicotic fibrogenesis: new experimental data, *Environ. Res.,* 1, 89, 1967.
29. **Chvapil, M., Hurych, J., and Mirejovska, E.,** Effect of long-term hypoxia on protein synthesis in granuloma and in some organs in rats, *Proc. Soc. Exp. Biol. Med.,* 135, 613, 1970.
30. **Chvapil, M., Madden, J. W., Carlson, E. C., and Peacock, E. E.,** Effect of *cis*-hydroxyproline on collagen and other proteins in skin wounds, granuloma tissue, and liver of mice and rats, *Exp. Mol. Pathol.,* 20, 363, 1974.
31. **Chvapil, M., Madden, J. W., Peacock, E. E., and Ryan, J. N.,** Effect of 1,10-phenanthroline on acute liver injury induced by dimethylnitrosamine in the rat, *Life Sci.,* 14, 1653, 1974.
32. **Chvapil, M. and Peng, Y. M.,** Oxygen and lung fibrosis, *Arch. Environ. Health,* 30, 528, 1975.
32a. **Collins, J. F., Johanson, W. G., Jr., McCullough, B., Jones, M. A., and Waugh, H. J., Jr.,** Effects of compensatory lung growth in irradiation-induced regional pulmonary fibrosis in the baboon, *Am. Rev. Respir. Dis.,* 117, 1079, 1978.
33. **Collins, J. F., Durnin, L. S., and Johanson, W. G., Jr.,** Papain-induced lung injury: alterations in connective tissue metabolism without emphysema, *Exp. Mol. Pathol.,* 29, 29, 1978.
34. **Cowan, M. J. and Crystal, R. G.,** Lung growth after unilateral pneumonectomy: quantitation of collagen synthesis and content, *Am. Rev. Respir. Dis.,* 111, 267, 1975.
35. **Crapo, J. D., Delong, D. M., Sjostrom, K., Hasler, G. R., and Drew, R. T.,** The failure of aerosolized superoxide dismutase to modify pulmonary oxygen toxicity, *Am. Rev. Respir. Dis.,* 115, 1027, 1977.
36. **Crystal, R. G., Fulmer, J. D., Roberts, W. C., Moss, M. L., Line, B. R., and Reynolds, H. Y.,** Idiopathic pulmonary fibrosis: clinical, histologic, radiographic, physiologic, scintigraphic, cytologic and biochemical aspects, *Ann. Intern. Med.,* 85, 769, 1976.
36a. **Counts, D. F. and Knighten, P.,** Collagen and non-collagen protein synthesis in the lungs of rats exposed to a trypsin aerosol, *Connect. Tissue Res.,* 5, 165, 1977.
37. **Cunningham, E. L., Brody, J. S., and Jain, B. P.,** Lung growth induced by hypoxia, *J. Appl. Physiol.,* 37, 362, 1974.
38. **Cutroneo, K. R.** Anti-inflammatory steroids and collagen metabolism: glucocorticoid mediated decrease of prolyl hydroxylase, *Mol. Pharmacol.,* 11, 44, 1975.
39. **Cutroneo, K. R., Guzman, N. A., and Sharawy, M. M.,** Evidence for a subcellular vesicular site of collagen prolyl hydroxylation, *J. Biol. Chem.,* 249, 5989, 1974.
40. **Dabrowski, R. and Máslinski, C.,** The effect of histamine on collagen formation and collagen polymerization in the skin wound healing of guinea pigs, *Life Sci.,* 9, 189, 1970.
41. **Dale, K.,** A method for inducing unilateral silicosis in rabbits by an injection technique with some observations on lung clearance and quantitative evaluation of experimental silicosis, *Scand. J. Respir. Dis.,* 54, 157, 1973.

42. **Dale, K.**, Lung function studies in experimental silicosis with a radiospirometric technique and some observations on a technique for inducing unilateral silicosis, in *Inhaled Particles III*, Vol. 1, Walton, W. H., Ed. Unwin Bros., Surrey, 1970, 347.
43. **Danpure, C. J. and Taylor, D. M.**, The effect of internally deposited plutonium-239 on the lysosomes of rat liver, *Radiat. Res.*, 59, 679, 1974.
44. **Davis, H. V. and Reeves, A. L.**, Collagen biosynthesis in rat lungs during exposure to asbestos, *Am. Ind. Hyg. Assoc. J.*, 32, 599, 1971.
45. **Davison, P. F.**, Homeostasis in extracellular tissues: insights from studies on collagen, *Crit. Rev. Biochem.*, 1, 201, 1973.
46. **Demeszko, H. and Dabrowski, R.**, Effect of prolonged histamine administration on tissue respiration processes and collagen production in guinea pig lungs, *Bull. Acad. Pol. Sci.*, 17, 717, 1969.
47. **Demopoulos, H. B.**, Control of free radicals in biologic systems, *Fed. Proc.*, 32, 1903, 1973.
48. **DiLuzio, N. R.**, Antioxidants, lipid peroxidation and chemical-induced liver injury, *Fed. Proc.*, 32, 1875, 1973.
48a. **Doniach, I., Morrison, B., and Steiner, R. E.**, Lung changes during hexamethonium therapy for hypertension, *Br. Heart, J.*, 16, 101, 1954.
48b. **Eastridge, C. E. and Hamman, J. L.**, Pneumothorax complicated by chronic steroid treatment, *Am. J. Surg.*, 126, 784, 1973.
49. **Eddy, H. A. and Casarett, G. W.**, Pathology of radiation syndromes in the hamster, *Prog. Exp. Tumor Res.*, 16, 98, 1972.
50. **Ehrlich, H. P. and Bornstein, P.**, Microtubules in transcellular movement of procollagen, *Nature (London) New Biol.*, 238, 257, 1972.
51. **Ehrlich, H. P., Tarver, H., and Hunt, T. K.**, Effects of vitamin A and glucocorticoids upon inflammation and collagen synthesis, *Ann. Surg.*, 177, 222, 1973.
52. **Eisinger, A. J.**, Goodpasture's syndrome: failure of nephrectomy to cure pulmonary hemorrhage, *Am. J. Med.*, 55, 565, 1973.
53. **Eisenstein, R., Schumacher, B., Meineke, C., Matijevitch, B., and Kuettner, K. E.**, Growth regulators in connective tissue. Systemic administration of an aortic extract inhibits tumor growth in mice, *Am. J. Pathol.*, 91(1), 1, 1978.
54. **Fajardo, L. F. and Stewart, J. R.** Pathogenesis of radiation-induced myocardial fibrosis, *Lab. Invest.*, 29, 244, 1973.
55. **Fernandez-Madrid, F., Prasad, A. S., and Oberleas, D.**, Effect of zinc deficiency on nucleic acids, collagen, and noncollagenous protein of the connective tissue, *J. Lab. Clin. Med.*, 82, 951, 1973.
56. **Fisher, A. B., Diamond, S., and Mellen, S.**, Effect of O_2 exposure on metabolism of the rabbit alveolar macrophage, *J. Appl. Physiol.*, 37, 341, 1974.
57. **Fleischman, R. W., Baker, J. R., Thompson, G. R., Schaeppi, U. H., Illievski, V. R., Cooney, D. A., and Davis, R. D.**, Bleomycin-induced intersititial pneumonia in dogs, *Thorax*, 26, 675, 1971.
58. **Flowers, E. S.**, Relationship between exposure to asbestos, collagen formation, ferruginous bodies, and carcinoma, *Am. Ind. Hyg. Assoc. J.*, 35, 724, 1974.
59. **Fraire, A. E. and Greenberg, S. D.**, Carcinoma and diffuse interstitial fibrosis of lung, *Cancer*, 31, 1078, 1973.
60. **Fuller, G. C., Matoney, A. L., Fisher, D. O., Fausto, N., and Cardinale, G. J.**, Increased collagen synthesis and the kinetic characteristics of prolyl hydroxylase in tissues of rabbits with experimental arteriosclerosis, *Atherosclerosis*, 24, 483, 1976.
61. **Fulmer, J. D. and Crystal, R. G.**, The biochemical basis of pulmonary function, in *Biochemical Basis of Pulmonary Function*, Crystal, R. G., Ed., Marcel Dekker, New York, 1976, 419.
62. **Gerber, G. B., Gerber, G., Altman, K. I., and Hempelmann, L. H.**, Studies on the metabolism of tissue proteins. II. Influence of x-irradiation and starvation on the metabolism of collagen, *Int. J. Radiat. Biol.*, 4, 609, 1961.
63. **Giannopoulos, G.**, Glucocorticoid receptors in lung. Mechanism of specific glucocorticoid uptake by fetal rabbit lung nuclei, *J. Biol. Chem.*, 250, 2896, 1975.
64. **Giannopoulos, G.**, Glucocorticoid receptors in lung. Comparison between nonactivated and activated forms of the cytoplasmic glucocorticoid binding protein and their relationship to the nuclear binding protein of fetal rabbit lung, *J. Biol. Chem.*, 250, 2904, 1975.
65. **Giri, S. N., Benson, J., Siegel, D. M., Rice, S. A., and Schiedt, M.**, Effects of pretreatment with anti-inflammatory drugs on ozone-induced lung damage in rats, *Proc. Soc. Exp. Biol. Med.*, 150, 810, 1975.
66. **Graham, J. R.**, Cardiac and pulmonary fibrosis during methysergide therapy for headache, *Am. J. Med. Sci.*, 254, 23, 1967.
67. **Graham, J. R., Suby, H. I., LeCompte, P. R., and Sadowsky, N. L.**, Fibrotic disorders associated with methysergide therapy for headache, *N. Engl. J. Med.*, 274, 359, 1966.
68. **Grant, M. E. and Prockop, D. J.**, The biosynthesis of collagen (I, II and III), *N. Engl. J. Med.*, 286, 194, 242, 291, 1972.

69. **Grasedyck, K. and Lindner, J.**, The behavior of (^{14}C)-D-penicillamine in collagen metabolism, *Connect. Tissue Res.*, 3, 171, 1975.
70. **Gray, P. N., Cullum, M. E., and Griffin, M. J.**, Population density and regulation of cell division in 3T3 cells, *J. Cell. Physiol.*, 89, 225, 1976.
71. **Green, G. I., Levin, R. L., Pierce, L. E., and Witorsch, P.**, Busulfan lung complicated by pneumocystis carinii and cytomegalovirus infection, *Med. Ann. D.C.*, 43, 124, 1974.
72. **Gross, J.**, Aspects of the animal collagenases, in *Biochemistry of Collagen*, Ramachandran, G. N., and Reddi, A. H., Eds., Plenum Press, New York, 1976, 275.
73. **Hance, A. J. and Crystal, R. G.**, The connective tissue of lung, *Am. Rev. Respir. Dis.*, 112, 657, 1975.
74. **Hance, A. J. and Crystal, R. G.**, Collagen, in *Biochemical Basis of Pulmonary Function*, Crystal, R. G., Ed., Marcel Dekker, New York, 1976, 215.
75. **Harker, L. A., Ross, R., Slichter, S. J., and Scott, C. R.**, Homocystine-induced arteriosclerosis. The role of endothelial cell injury and platelet response in its genesis, *J. Clin. Invest.*, 58, 731, 1976.
76. **Harington, J. S., Ritchie, M., King, P. C., and Miller, K.**, The *in-vitro* effects of silica-treated hamster macrophages on collagen production by hamster fibroblasts, *J. Pathol.*, 109, 21, 1973.
77. **Harris, E. D. and Krane, S. M.**, Collagenases (I, II, III), *N. Engl. J. Med.*, 291, 557, 605, 652, 1974.
78. **Haynes, R. C. and Larner, J.**, Adrenocorticotropic hormone; adrenocortical steroids and their synthetic analogs; inhibitors of adrenocortical steroid biosynthesis, in *The Pharmacological Basis of Therapeutics*, 5th ed., Goodman, L. S., and Gilman, A., Eds., Macmillan, New York, 1975, 1472.
79. **Henkin, R. I.**, Zinc in wound healing, *N. Engl. J. Med.*, 291, 675, 1974.

79a. **Hext, P. M., Hunt, J., Dodgson, K. S., and Richards, R. J.**, The effects of long-term exposure of lung fibroblast strains to chrysotile asbestos, *Br. J. Exp. Pathol.*, 58, 160, 1977.

80. **Heppleston, A. G.**, The biological response to silica, in *Biology of Fibroblast*, Kulonen, E., and Pikkarainen, J., Eds., Academic Press, New York, 1973, 529.
81. **Heppleston, A. G. and Styles, J. A.**, Activity of a macrophage factor in collagen formation by silica, *Nature (London)*, 214, 521, 1967.
82. **Heppleston, A. G., Wright, N. A., and Stewart, J. A.**, Experimental alveolar lipoproteinosis following inhalation of silica, *J. Pathol.*, 101, 293, 1969.
83. **Hindle, W., Posner, E., Sweetnam, M. T., and Tan, R. S. H.**, Pleural effusion and fibrosis during treatment with methysergide, *Br. Med. J.*, 1, 605, 1970.
84. **Hoffman, L., Blumenfeld, O. O., Mondshine, R. B., and Park, S. S.**, Effect of DL-penicillamine on fibrous proteins of rat lung, *J. Appl. Physiol.*, 33, 42, 1972.
85. **Holt, P. G. and Keast, D.**, The effect of tobacco smoke on protein synthesis in macrophages, *Proc. Soc. Exp. Biol. Med.*, 142, 1243, 1972.
86. **Horwitz, A. L. and Crystal, R. G.**, Collagenase from rabbit pulmonary alveolar macrophages. *Biochem. Biophys. Res. Commun.*, 69, 296, 1976.
87. **Horwitz, A. L., Elson, N. A., and Crystal, R. G.**, Proteoglycans and elastic fibers, in *Biochemical Basis of Pulmonary Function*, Crystal, R. G., Ed., Marcel Dekker, New York, 1976, 273.
88. **Jennings, F. L. and Arden, A.**, Development of experimental radiation pneumonitis. *Arch. Pathol.*, 71, 437, 1961.
89. **Johnson, T. S., Ellis, J. H., Jr., and Steele, P. P.**, Improvement of platelet survival time with oxygen in patients with chronic obstructive airway disease, *Am. Rev. Respir. Dis.*, 117, 255, 1978.
90. **Juhl, E. Winkel, P., Tygstrup, N.**, Sex, ascites and alcoholism in survival of patients with cirrhosis, *N. Engl. J. Med.*, 291, 271, 1974.
91. **Kahlson, G. and Zederfeldt, B.**, *Acta Chir. Scand.*, 119, 207, 1960; as cited in **Dabrowski, R., and Maslinski, Cz.**, *Life Sci.*, 9(1), 189, 1970.

91a. **Kaneko, J. J.**, Research communication, 1976.

92. **Karl, L., Chvapil, M., and Zukoski, C. F.**, Effect of zinc on the viability and phagocytic capacity of peritoneal macrophages, *Proc. Soc. Exp. Biol. Med.*, 142, 1123, 1973.
93. **Kaw, J. L. and Zaidi, S. H.**, Effect of ascorbic acid on pulmonary silicosis of guinea pigs, *Arch. Environ. Health*, 19, 74, 1969.
94. **Kawanami, O., Ferrans, V. J., Roberts, W. C., Crystal, R. G., and Fulmer, J. D.**, Anchoring fibrils, a new connective tissue structure in fibrotic lung disease, *Am. J. Pathol.*, 92, 389, 1978.
95. **Kawamoto, T. and Nagai, Y.**, Developmental changes in glycosaminoglycans, collagen and collagenase activity in embryonic chick skin, *Biochim. Biophys. Acta*, 437, 190, 1976.
96. **Katzenstein, A. L. A., Bloor, C. M., and Leibow, A. A.**, Diffuse alveolar damage — the role of oxygen, shock, and related factors, *Am. J. Pathol.*, 85, 210, 1976.
97. **Kilroe-Smith, T. A., Webster, I., van Drimmelen, M., and Marasas, L.**, An insoluble fibrogenic factor in macrophages from guinea pigs exposed to silica, *Evniron. Res.*, 6, 298, 1973.
98. **Kimbrough, R. D. and Linder, R. E.**, The ultrastructure of the paraquat lung lesion in the rat, *Environ. Res.*, 6, 265, 1973.

99. **Klosterkotter, W. and Robock, K.**, New aspects on dust and pneumoconiosis research, *Am. Ind. Hyg. Assoc. J.*, 36, 659, 1975.

100. **Knapp, T. R., Daniels, J. R., and Kaplan, E. N.**, Pathologic scar formation. Morphologic and biochemical correlates, *Am. J. Pathol.*, 86, 47, 1977.

101. **Kohler, N. and Lipton, A.**, Platelets as a source of fibroblast growth-promoting activity, *Exp. Cell Res.*, 87, 297, 1974.

102. **Kravis, T. C., Ahmed, A., Brown, T. E., Fulmer, J. D., and Crystal, R. G.**, Pathogenic mechanisms in pulmonary fibrosis. Collagen-induced migration inhibition factor production and cytotoxicity mediated by lymphocytes, *J. Clin. Invest.*, 58, 1223, 1976.

103. **Kurohara, S. S. and Casarett, G. W.**, Effects of single thoracic X-ray exposure in rats, *Radiat. Res.*, 52, 263, 1972.

104. **Lane, J. M., Dehm, P., and Prockop, D. J.**, Effect of the proline analogue axetidine-2-carboxylic acid on collagen synthesis *in vivo*. I. Arrest of collagen accumulation in growing chick embryos, *Biochim. Biophys. Acta*, 236, 517, 1971.

105. **Langner, R. O. and Fuller, G. C.**, Effect of methylprednisolone in epinephrine-thyroxine induced arteriosclerosis, *Proc. Soc. Exp. Biol. Med.*, 141, 999, 1972.

106. **Langston, C., Sachdeva, P., Cowan, M. J., Haines, J., Crystal, R. G., and Thurlbeck, W. M.**, Alevolar multiplication in the contralateral lung after unilateral pneumonectomy in the rabbit, *Am. Rev. Respir. Dis.*, 115, 7, 1977.

106a. **Laurent, T. C.**, Interaction between proteins and glycosaminoglycans, *Fed. Proc.*, 36, 24, 1977.

106b. **Law, M. P., Hornsey, S., and Field, S. B.**, Collagen content of lungs of mice after x-ray irradiation, *Radiat. Res.*, 65, 60, 1976.

107. **Leibovich, S. J. and Ross, R.**, The role of the macrophage in wound repair, *Am. J. Pathol.*, 78, 71, 1975.

108. **Leung, K. and Munck, A.**, Peripheral actions of glucocorticoids, *Annu. Rev. Physiol.*, 37, 245, 1975.

109. **Levene, C. I., Bye, I., and Saffriotti, U.**, The effect of β-aminopropionitrile on silicotic pulmonary fibrosis in the rat, *Br. J. Exp. Pathol.*, 49, 152, 1968.

110. **Levene, C. I.**, Lathyrism, in *Molecular Pathology of Connective Tissues*, Vol. 3, Pérez-Tamayo, R., and Rojkind, M., Eds., Marcel Dekker, New York, 1973, 175.

111. **Lewis, D. M. and Burrell, R.**, Induction of fibrogenesis by lung antibody-treated macrophages, *Br. J. Ind. Med.*, 33, 25, 1976.

112. **Liebow, A. A.**, Definition and classification of interstitial pneumonias in human pathology. Alveolar Interstitium of the Lung, Int. Symp., Paris, 1974, *Prog. Respir. Res.*, 8, 1, 1975.

113. **Lindy, S., Kahanpää, K., Karhunen, P., Halme, J., and Uitto, J.**, Lactate dehydrogenase isoenzymes during the development of experimental fibrosis, *J. Lab. Clin. Med.*, 76, 756, 1970.

114. **Livingston, S., Whitehouse, D., and Pauli, L. L.**, Study of the effects of diphenylhydantoin sodium on the lungs, *N. Engl. J. Med.*, 264, 648, 1961.

115. **Manner, G., Goldring, I, P., and Kuleba, M.**, Effect of proteolytic enzymes on collagen and non-collagen protein synthesis in human lung fibroblasts, *Connect. Tissue Res.*, 2, 283, 1974.

116. **Martin, D. W. and Smith, L. H.**, Drug-induced lung disease: the price of progress, *Calif. Med.*, 119, 48, 1973.

117. **Masse, R., Nolibe, D., Fritsch, P., Metvier, H., LaFuma, J., and Chrétien, J.**, Chronic interstitial pneumonitis induced by internal α-irradiation of the lung, *Prog. Respir. Res.*, 8, 74, 1975.

118. **Mauderly, J. L., Pickrell, J. A., Hobbs, C. H., Benjamin, S. A., Hahn, F. F., Jones, R. K., and Barnes, J. E.**, The effects of inhaled ^{90}Y fused clay aerosol on pulmonary function and related parameters of the Beagle dog., *Radiat. Res.*, 56, 83, 1973.

119. **McCullagh, K. A. and Balian, G.**, Collagen characterization and cell transformation in human atherosclerosis, *Nature (London)*, 258, 73, 1975.

120. **McGee, J. O'D., O'Hare, R. P., and Patrick, R. S.**, Stimulation of the collagen biosynthetic pathway by factors isolated from experimentally-injured liver, *Nature (London) New Biol.*, 243, 121, 1973.

121. **Michaelson, S. M. and Schreiner, B. F.**, Cardiopulmonary effects of upper-body x-irradiation in the dog, *Radiat. Res.*, 47, 168, 1971.

122. **Miller, R., Engel, M. B., and Catchpole, H. R.**, Collagen and cellular fractions of blood, *Fed. Proc. Abstr.*, 35, 715, 1976.

123. **Milvy, P.**, Control of free radical mechanisms in nucleic acid systems: studies in radioprotection and radiosensitization, *Fed. Proc.*, 32, 1895, 1973.

124. **Mintz, S.**, The effects of silica on the free, apparent redox state (NAD + /NADH) of the alveolar macrophage: a possible mitochondrial membrane effect, *Chest*, 69, 298, 1976.

125. **Motomiya, M., Arai, H., Sato, H., Yokosawa, A., Nagai, H., and Konno, K.**, Increase of dermatan sulfate in a case of pulmonary fibrosis, *Tohoku J., Exp. Med.*, 115, 361, 1975.

126. **Nathan, D. M.**, The respiratory distress syndrome and glucocorticoid treatment: the case for enzyme induction, *Mt. Sinai J. Med. N.Y.*, 42, 150, 1975.
127. **Newman, R. A. and Cutroneo, K. R.**, Glucocorticoids selectively decrease the synthesis of hydroxylated collagen peptides, *Mol. Pharacol.*, 14, 185, 1978.
128. **Newhouse, M., Sanchis, J., and Bienenstock, J.**, Lung defense mechanisms (I,II), *N. Engl. J. Med.*, 295, 990, 1045, 1976.
129. **Niden, A. H. and Khurana, M. M. L.**, An animal model for diffuse interstitial pulmonary fibrosis — chronic low dose paraquat ingestion, *Fed. Proc. Abstr.*, 35, 631, 1976.
130. **Nordeen, S. K. and Young, D. A.**, Glucocorticoid action on rat thymic lymphocytes. Experiments utilizing adenosine to support cellular metabolism lead to a reassessment of catabolic hormone actions, *J. Biol. Chem.*, 251, 7295, 1976.
131. **Oliner, H., Schwartz, R., Rubio, F., and Dameshek, W.**, Interstitial pulmonary fibrosis following Busulfun therapy, *Am. J. Med.*, 31, 134, 1961.
132. **Ooshima, A., Fuller, G. C., Cardinale, G. J., Spector, S., and Udenfriend, S.**, Increased collagen synthesis in blood vessels of hypertensive rats and its reversal by antihypertensive agents, *Proc. Natl. Acad. Sci. U.S.A.*, 71, 3019, 1974.
133. **Osborne, G.**, Hyaline membrane following total body radiation, *Lancet*, 1960, 1010, 1960.
134. **Parakkal, P. F.**, Involvement of macrophages in collagen resorption, *J. Cell Biol.*, 41, 345, 1969.
135. **Pariente, R.**, Action of oxygen and oxidizers on the lung and bronchioles, *Prog. Respir. Res.*, 8, 91, 1975.
136. **Pariente, R., Legrand, M., and Brouet, G,.** Pulmonary ultrastructural aspects of oxygen poisoning under atmospheric pressure in the rat (trans.), *La Presse Med.*, 77, 1073, 1969.
137. **Pérez-Tamayo, R.**, Pathology of collagen degradation — a review, *Am. J. Pathol.*, 92, 509, 1978.
138. **Pfleger, R. C. and Pickrell, J. A.**, Effect of injury and antioxidants on pulmonary collagen and lipid metabolism in Syrian hamsters exposed to ^{90}Y fused aluminosilicate particles, in preparation, 1979.
139. **Picken, J., Lurie, M., and Kleinerman, J.**, Mechanical and morphologic effects of long-term corticosteroid administration on the adult rat lung, *Am. Rev. Respir. Dis.*, 110, 746, 1974.
140. **Pickrell, J. A., Halliwell, W. H., Bryant, P. L., and Straus, F. C.**, Pulmonary collagen metabolism in irradiated hamsters and those treated with beta-aminoproprionitrile (BAPN) and others undergoing repeated bronchopulmonary saline lavage, *Inhal. Tox. Res. Inst. Annual Report*, LF-56, p. 356, 1976.
141. **Pickrell, J. A., Harris, D. V., Benjamin, S. A., Cuddihy, R. G., Pfleger, R. C., and Mauderly, J. L.**, Pulmonary collagen metabolism after lung injury from inhaled ^{90}Y in fused clay particles, *Exp. Mol. Pathol.*, 25, 70, 1976.
142. **Pickrell, J. A., Harris, D. V., Hahn, F. F., Belasich, J. J., and Jones, R. K.**, Biological alterations resulting from chronic lung irradiation. III. Effect of partial ^{60}Co thoracic irradiation upon pulmonary collagen metabolism and fractionation in Syrian hamsters, *Radiat. Res.*, 62, 133, 1975.
143. **Pickrell, J. A., Harris, D. V., Mauderly, J. L., and Hahn, F. F.**, Altered collgen metabolism in radiation-induced interstitial pulmonary fibrosis, *Chest*, 69, 311, 1976.
144. **Pickrell, J. A., Harris, D. V., Pfleger, R. C., Benjamin, S. A., Belasich, J. J., Jones, R. K., and McClellan, R. O.**, Biological alterations resulting from chronic lung irradiation. II. Connective tissue alterations following inhalation of ^{144}Ce fused clay aerosol in Beagle dogs, *Radiat. Res.*, 63, 299, 1975.
145. **Pickrell, J. A., Diel, J. O., Slauson, D. O., Halliwell, W. H., and Mauderly, J. L.**, Diffuse interstitial fibrosis following radiation-induced lung injury resolves spontaneously if dense scars are not formed, submitted for publication, 1979.
146. **Pickrell, J. A., Straus, F. C., Halliwell, W. H., and Jones, R. K.**, The relation of pulmonary collagen metabolism, inflammation and therapy to radiation-induced pulmonary fibrosis, *Fed. Proc. Abstr.*, 36, 607, 1977.
146a. **Pickrell, J. A., Wilson, S., Schnizlein, C. T., McCamey, D., and Rodriquez, R.**, Research communication, 1977.
147. **Plopper, C. G., Dungworth, D. L., and Tyler, W. S.**, Pulmonary lesions in rats exposed to ozone. A correlated light and electron microscopic study, *Am. J. Pathol.*, 71, 375, 1973.
148. **Popovic, N. A. and Mullane, J. F.**, Effects of biliary obstruction on pulmonary ultrastructure in the rat, *Am. J. Pathol.*, 68, 97, 1972.
149. **Powell, G. M. and Green, G. M.**, Cigarette smoke — a proposed metabolic lesion in alveolar macrophages, *Biochem. Pharmacol.*, 21, 1785, 1972.
150. **Rantanen, J.**, Radiation injury of connective tissue, a biochemical investigation with experimental granuloma, *Acta Radiol. Suppl.*, 330, 1, 1973.
151. **Reeves, A. L., Puro, H. E., and Smith, R. G.** Inhalation carcinogenesis from various forms of asbestos, *Environ. Res.*, 8, 178, 1974.

152. **Religa, Z. and Måslinski, C.**, Histamine metabolism in experimental silicosis. II. *In vivo* experiments in guinea pigs, *Life Sci.*, 10, 257, 1971.
153. **Reynolds, H. Y., Fulmer, J. D., Kazmierowski, J. A., Roberts, W. C., Frank, M. M., and Crystal, R. G.**, Analysis of cellular and protein content of broncho-alveolar lavage fluid from patients with idiopathic pulmonary fibrosis and chronic hypersensitivity pneumonitis, *J. Clin. Invest.*, 59, 165, 1977.
154. **Richards, R. J. and Wusteman, F. S.**, The effects of silica dust and alveolar macrophages on lung fibroblast grown *in vitro, Life Sci.*, 14, 355, 1974.
155. **Richards, R. J., Wusteman, F. S., and Dodgson, K. S.**, The direct effects of dusts on lung fibroblasts grown *in vitro, Life Sci.* 10, 1149, 1971.
156. **Rigdon, R. H.**, Tissue reaction to foreign materials, *Crit. Rev. Food Sci. Nutr.*, 3, 435, 1975.
157. **Rodkina, B. S.**, Oxyproline content in the composition of peptides of the pulmonary tissue of animals with experimental silicosis, *Ukr. Biokhim. Zh.*, 46, 393, 1974.
158. **Rokseth, R. and Storstein, O.**, Pulmonary complications during mecamylamine therapy, *Acta Med. Scand.*, 167, 23, 1960.
159. **Rom, W. N. and Palmer, P. E. S.**, The spectrum of asbestos-related diseases, *West. J. Med.*, 121, 10, 1974.
160. **Rosenkrantz, H., Esber, H. J., and Sprague, R.**, Lung hydroxyproline levels in mice exposed to cigarette smoke, *Life Sci.*, 8, 571, 1969.
161. **Rosenow, E. C.**, The spectrum of drug-induced pulmonary disease, *Ann. Intern. Med.*, 77, 977, 1972.
162. **Ross, R. and Glomset, J.**, Studies of primate arterial smooth muscle cells in relation to atherosclerosis, *Adv. Exp. Biol. Med.*, 43, 265, 1974.
163. **Ross, R., Glomset, J., Kariya, B., and Harker, L.**, A platelet-dependent serum factor that stimulates the proliferation of artertial smooth muscle cells *in vitro, Proc. Natl. Acad. Sci. U.S.A.*, 71, 1207, 1974.
164. **Ryan, G. B. and Majno, G.**, Acute inflammation — a review, *Am. J. Pathol.*, 86, 183, 1977.
165. **Sandberg, N.**, Accelerated collagen formation and histamine, *Nature (London)*, 194, 183, 1962.
166. **Schreiner, B. F., Michaelson, S. M., and Yuile, C. L.**, The effects of thoracic irradiation upon cardiopulmonary function in the dog, *Am. Rev. Respir. Dis.*, 99, 205, 1968.
167. **Seyer, J. M., Hutcheson, E. T., and Kang, A. H.** Collagen polymorphism in idiopathic chronic pulmonary fibrosis, *J. Clin. Invest.*, 57, 1498, 1976.
168. **Sharp, J. T.**, Fibrosis, diffuse granulomas, and pneumoconiosis, in *Clinical Cardiopulmonary Physiology*, 3rd ed., Gordon, B. L., Carleton, R. A., and Faber, L. P., Eds., Grune & Stratton, New York, 1969, 614.
169. **Sibinga, C. T. S.**, Prevention of vessel wall damage in experimental irradiation, *Bibl. Anat.*, 12, 242, 1973.
170. **Siegel, R. C.**, Collagen cross-linking. Effect of D-penicillamine on cross-linking *in vitro, J. Biol. Chem.*, 252, 254, 1977.
171. **Slauson, D. O. and Dahlstrom, M. A.**, The pulmonary inflammatory response. Cellular events in experimental pulmonary arterial hypersensitivity disease, *Am. J. Pathol.*, 82, 549, 1975.
172. **Slauson, D. O., Hahn, F. F., Benjamin, S. A., Chiffelle, T. L., and Jones, R. K.**, Inflammatory sequences in acute pulmonary radiation injury, *Am. J. Pathol.*, 82, 549, 1976.
173. **Smith, P. and Heath, D.**, Paraquat, *Crit. Rev. Toxicol.*, 4, 411, 1976.
174. **Snider, G. L., Celli, B. R., Goldstein, R. H., O'Brien, J. J., and Lucey, E. C.**, Chronic interstitial pulmonary fibrosis produced in hamsters by endotracheal bleomycin, *Am. Rev. Respir. Dis.*, 117, 289, 1978.
175. **Spencer, H.**, Pathogenesis of interstitial fibrosis of the lung, *Prog. Respir. Res.*, 8, 34, 1975.
176. **Stachurska, J., Roszkowski, W., Kopeć, M., and Ryzewski, J.**, Effects of bradykinin on rat lymphocytes, *Proc. Soc. Exp. Biol. Med.*, 153, 408, 1976.
177. **Steele, P., Ellis, J. H., and Genton, E.**, Platelet survival time in severe chronic airway obstruction, *Chest*, 67, 46S, 1975.
178. **Stemerman, M. B. and Ross, R.**, Experimental arteriosclerosis. I. Fibrous plaque formation in primates, an electron microscope study, *J. Exp. Med.*, 136, 769, 1972.
179. **Stetson, C. G. and Boland, J.**, Experimental radiation pneumonitis. Radiographic and pathologic correlation, *Cancer*, 20, 2170, 1967.
180. **Stone, D. J., Schwartz, M. J., and Green, R. A.**, Fatal pulmonary insufficiency due to radiation effect upon the lung, *Am. J. Med.*, 21, 211, 1956.
181. **Stuart, J. M., Postlethwaite, A. E., and Kang, A. H.**, Evidence for cell-mediated immunity to collagen in progressive systemic sclerosis, *J. Lab. Clin. Med.*, 88, 601, 1976.
182. **Tappel, A. L.**, Lipid peroxidation damage to cell components, *Fed. Proc.*, 32, 1870, 1973.
183. **Thurlbeck, W. M.**, Postnatal growth and development of the lung, *Am. Rev. Respir. Dis.*, 111, 803, 1975.

184. **Thurlbeck, W. M. and Thurlbeck, S. M.,** Pulmonary effects of paraquat poisoning, *Chest,* 69, 276, 1976.
185. **Trnavskâ, Z. and Trnavsky, K.,** Influence of nonsteroidal antirheumatic drugs on collagen metabolism in rats with adjuvant-induced arthritis, *Pharmacology,* 12, 110, 1974.
186. **Trump, B. F. and Arstila, A. U.,** Cellular reaction to injury, in *Principles of Pathobiology,* 2nd ed., LaVia, M. F., and Hill, R. B., Jr., Eds.; Oxford University Press, New York, 1975, 9.
187. **Tseveleva, I. A.,** Collagen biosynthesis in the lungs of rats with radiation injury, *Vopr. Med. Khim.,* 20, 640, 1974.
188. **Tseveleva, I. A.,** Collagen biosynthesis in the lungs of rats with radiation injury, *Vopr. Med. Khim.,* 20, 640, 1974.
189. **Tsurufuji, S. and Ohuchi, K.,** X-irradiation and ageing as reflected in the accumulation and insolubilization of collagen, *Exp. Gerontol.,* 3, 309, 1968.
190. **Turner-Warwick, M.,** A perspective view on widespread pulmonary fibrosis, *Br. Med. J.,* 2, 371, 1974.
191. **Tyree, E. B., Glicksman, A. S., and Nickson, J. J.,** Effect of L-triiodothyronine on radiation-induced pulmonary fibrosis in dogs, *Radiat. Res.,* 28, 30, 1966.
192. **Ubatuba, F. B., Harvey, E. A., and Ferreira, S. H.,** Are platelets important in inflammation? *Agents & Actions,* 5, 31, 1975.
193. **Unanue, E. R.,** Secretory function of mononuclear phagocytes — a review, *Am. J. Pathol.,* 83, 396, 1976.
194. **Välimäki, M., Juva, K., Rantanen, J., Ekfors, T., and Niinikoski, J.,** Collagen metabolism in rat lungs during chronic intermittent exposure to oxygen, *Aviat. Space Environ. Med.,* 46, 684, 1975.
195. **Vasil'yeva, G. N.,** Soluble collagen and protein-carbohydrate component content in the lungs of rats with experimental silicosis (trans.), *Vopr. Med. Khim.,* 17, 277, 1971.
196. **Vasil'yeva, G. N. and Myagkaya, G. L.** Some characteristics of the composition of the insoluble collagen of rat lung under normal conditions and in experimental silicosis (trans.), *Vopr. Med. Khim.,* 16(3), 286, 1970.
197. **Vogel, H. G.,** Effects of D-penicillamine and prednisolone on connective tissue in rats, *Connect. Tissue Res.,* 1, 283, 1972.
198. **Vracko, R.,** Basal lamina scaffold-anatomy and significance for maintenance of orderly tissue structure, *Am. J. Pathol.,* 77, 314, 1974.
199. **Warren, S. and Spencer, J.,** Radiation reaction in the lung, *Am. J. Roentgenol.,* 43, 682, 1940.
200. **Watanabe, S., Watanabe, K., Ohishi, T., Aiba, M., and Kageyama, K.,** Mast cells in the rat alveolar septa undergoing fibrosis after ionizing radiation, *Lab. Invest.,* 31, 555, 1974.
201. **Waters, M. D., Moore, R. D., Amato, J. J., and Houck, J. C.,** Zinc sulfate — failure as an accelerator of collagen biosynthesis and fibroblast proliferation, *Proc. Soc. Exp. Biol. Med.,* 138, 373, 1971.
202. **West, J. B.,** Restrictive diseases, in *Pulmonary Pathophysiology — the Essentials,* Williams & Wilkins, Baltimore, 1977, 92.
203. **Wilson, R. B., Kula, N. S., Newberne, P. M., and Conner, M. W.,** Vascular damage and lipid peroxidation in choline deficient rats, *Exp. Mol. Pathol.,* 18, 357, 1973.
204. **Wilson, R. B., Newberne, P. M., and Kula, N. S.,** Protection by antioxidants against arterial sclerosis of chronic choline-deficiency, *Exp. Mol. Pathol.,* 21, 118, 1974.
205. **Wolfe, W. G. and deVries, W. C.,** Oxygen toxicity, *Annu. Rev. Med.,* 26, 203, 1975.
206. **Yacoub, M. H. and Thompson, V. C.,** Chronic idiopathic pulmonary hilar fibrosis. A clinicopathological entity, *Thorax,* 26, 365, 1971.
207. **Zaidi, S. H. and Kaw, J. L.,** Effect of general dietary deficiency and protein malnutrition on the fibrogenesis caused by silica dust in rats, *Br. J. Ind. Med.,* 27, 250, 1970.
208. **Ziskind, M., Jones, R. N., and Weill, H.,** Silicosis, *Am. Rev. Respir. Dis.,* 113, 643, 1976.

Chapter 14

PULMONARY EMPHYSEMA

J. A. Pickrell and J. L. Mauderly

TABLE OF CONTENTS

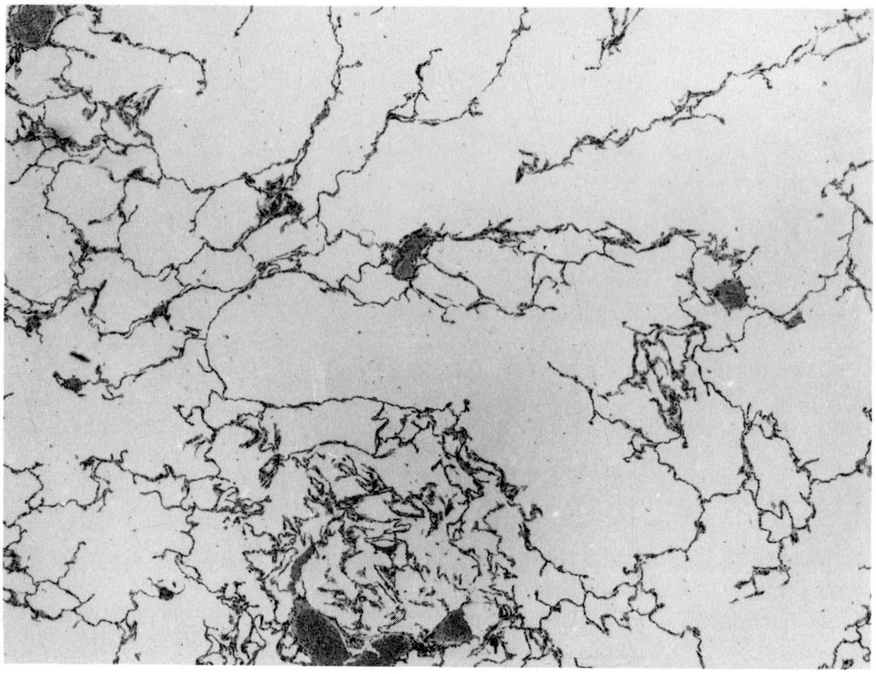

FIGURE 1. Pulmonary emphysema in Syrian hamster induced by intratracheal instillation of elastase. (×35, H and E stain.)

I. ANATOMIC CHANGES

Generally, one may expect injury level to be low enough that epithelial and endothelial proliferation occur, but high enough that proteolysis and inflammation[56] occur. The proteolysis weakens the support of the basement membranes, leading to their destruction. Attempts at repopulation will produce areas of type II epithelial cell hyperplasia with eventual progression to type I cells more resistant to destruction from proteolysis. In other areas, weakening will lead to interruption of basement membrane and alteration of the normal elastic network .[64] Since the membrane is regenerated inadequately and epithelial cells cannot repopulate it,[61a] alveoli will be lost and a varied mesenchymal cell response observed,[55] leading to pulmonary emphysema and a reduction of internal surface area[6] (Figure 1). Causes of emphysema include NO_x, O_3, levels of O_2 near 100%, Cd^{++}, smoking, pollutant gases, and miscellaneous causes. Further causes are reviewed by Bouhuys et al.[4] These produce similar events but will be reviewed to form a cohesive picture.

Exposure to NO_2 leads to emphysema. Evans et al.[17] reported that 17 ppm NO_2 induced an increased labelling index in terminal bronchioles by three days. In peripheral alveoli, type II cells turned over more rapidly. These changes returned to normal by five days. Stephens et al.[67] reported that the same level of exposure for three months induced slight increases in collagen fibrils underlying terminal bronchioles. Young animals developed very large fibrils. A similar resonse was noted for 2 ppm for 2 or more years of exposure. Evans et al.[13] indicated the pulmonary alveolar macrophage to divide in approximately ten hours in response to NO_2 inhalation. Furiosi et al.[20] reported that addition of small amounts of NaCl to the NO_2 aerosol had no effect on its toxicity or upon its ability to induce emphysema. Evans et al.[15] followed kinetics of type II cell proliferation. By 1 hour approximately 90% of the type II cells and approximately 19% of the type I cells are labelled. As label decreases in type II cells (~ 60 to 70%), it increases to approximately 30% in type I cells by 48 hr. This provides evidence for proliferation of type II cells, with subsequent differentiation to type I cells. Evans et al.[14,15] duplicated the previous effort but also provided evidence for an intermediate between type I and II alveolar epithelial cells. In later publications, Evans et al.[16,17] noted that older rats had a higher mortality rate during the first day of exposure from pulmonary edema, that tissue damaged in older rats greatly exceeded that in young rats, that the onset of cell proliferation was slower and the magnitude of type II cell proliferation much greater in old than in young rats. One might speculate that proteolysis which is present in edema seems to be inhibiting cell proliferation rather than stimulating it as would be expected by its degradation of extracellular matrix. Probably the conditions are severe enough to arrest the cell proliferation. When it does occur, in survivors the area damaged and, thus, the response was greater. Finally, Evans[160] indicated that the type I cells newly differentiated from type II cells are more resistant to injury. A critical question concerns the nature of the proliferative stimulus, a need for replacement of type I cells or surfactant or both.

Watanabe et al.[72] described the proximity of the granular pneumocyte to collagen and elastic fibers in developing fibrosis and suggests a relationship to healing. This observation is consistent with Hance and Crystal's[25] observation that type II alveolar epithelial cells make collagen in culture. Whether this produces emphysema or fibrosis is an unresolved question.

Freeman et al.[18] reported the histologic site of injury to be the junction of the terminal and respiratory bronchiole when mixed NO_2 and O_3 exposures were used, indicating their strong resemblance to NO_2 exposures. However, O_3 did tend to produce some fibroblast response, which presumably reflects its greater relative toxicity. These results suggested that smog constituted mostly an O_3 risk while tobacco smoke constituted mostly an NO_2 risk. Both NO_2 and O_3 constitute a risk if one inhales effluents from low temperature coal combustion which has an NO_x and a photochemical hydrocarbon component.

Ozone also produces emphysema after inhalation. Ozone injury extends from the terminal bronchiole to the proximal alveoli, extending slightly more deeply into the lung than does injury from NO_2. Whether this reflects a different type or a different severity of injury remains to be determined. Repair begins in 24 hr, and some adaptation takes place.[66] Ozone initially caused swollen type I epithelial cytoplasm, leading to mitochondrial alterations. This occurred in the presence of normal capillary endothelium.[68] Freeman et al.[18] reported that fibrous elements were rarely deposited at the lowest dose (1 ppm, 8 hrs/day, 18 months) of O_3 but increased proportionately to O_3 dose to 3 ppm, 8 hrs/day for 18 months. Macrophages in lung paralleled this change. Additionally, Stephens et al.[68] notes the loss of ciliary motility induced by O_3. Boatman et al.[3] reported condensed mitochondria with abnormal cristae. Acceleration in type II cell kinetics induced by inhaling ozone resemble those of NO_2. Plopper et al.[51] noted epithelial damage was most prominent in the central area. Some edema occurs, which thickens the blood air exchange membrane.

Oxygen at the 80 to 100% level for up to eight days in squirrel monkeys produces a response very similar to NO_2 and O_3.[23] Specifically, type II cell proliferation is present.[1] Prolonged exposures may be fibrogenic, as reflected by increased collagen metabolism.[47]

Cadmium produces a lung injury similar to that reported for NO_2 or O_3. It interferes with oxidative phosphorylation, suggesting that it is a biological oxidizer.[44] Accidental exposures often produce emphysema approximately 20 years post exposure.[5] Since

Cd^{++} may react with sulfhydryls, this suggests that cadmium may cause damage by its oxidant action. Cadmium damages type I alveolar epithelium and induces type II cell hyperplasia.[70] The cell proliferation peaks at ∼ 4 days after exposure,[49] at the same time as LDH and glucose-6-phosphate dehydrogenase.[27] The changes may be nonspecific response to pulmonary injury similar to those induced by O_2, O_3, and NO_2. Type II cell proliferation would enhance the glucose-6-phosphate dehydrogenase activity. LDH increase would indicate cell damage and an induction of glycolysis.[27] Suffering multiple re-injury leads to centrilobular emphysema.[61] At higher levels or longer periods of time, Miller et al.[43] reported formation of collagen bundles, indicating the close relation of emphysema and fibrosis. Inhalation of tobacco smoke[33] caused only modest central lesions, suggesting that the smoke did not penetrate to most alveoli.

Inhalation of synthetic smog (NO_2, O_3, and SO_x) caused marked hyperplasia of the bronchial lining layer, thickening of alveolar tissue, and increased macrophages in the lesion. This more closely resembles the O_3 effect.[38] Inhalation of exhaust gas causes reduction in body growth. Changes are similar to but more extensive than those of synthetic smog, as indicated by developed emphysema, inflammation, and atalectasis.[35] Silica[78] may occasionally produce emphysema. Small blood vessels in advanced emphysema are similar to those of normals.[45] However, the chronic cor pulmonale related to emphysema seemed to be a function of obliteration of capillaries and an increase in the mass of muscle in arterioles, which probably involves a pressure increase. Michaeli and Fudenberg[41] reported the presence of anticollagen antibodies in patients with emphysema, suggesting that collagen metabolism may be altered in some phase of emphysema. Kilburn et al.[34] and Hahn and Hobbs[24a] used papain to produce emphysema. Alveolar wall collagen was lost by 4 days. However, total lung collagen and elastin did not change by 2 weeks after exposure. Capillaries appeared morphologically to be coiled back after loss of the interalveolar septa. Fibroblasts and type II cells had increased endoplasmic reticulium, this finding suggesting that regeneration as evidenced by increased protein synthesis had occurred. Endothelial damage led to capillary obliteration by 16 days. These findings suggest that collagen may be involved in emphysema. Schuyler et al.[58] were not able to produce anatomic evidence of emphysema using intravenous elastase. They did, however, produce loss of recoil which might have represented submicroscopic lesions, antedating the appearance of morphologic lesions.

II. PHYSIOLOGIC-ANATOMIC CHANGES

Johanson and Pierce[31] reported that treatment of lungs with elastase resulted in increased compliance measured by continuous flow curves obtained from excised lung. They indicated that this change was not due to alteration in surface forces, but rather to a reduction in elastic recoil. Histologic evidence of damaged elastin fibers correlated well with altered recoil. Johnson and Andrews[32] had little success in correlating increasing elastin content and decreasing collagen content with increasing age or with emphysema, although their extraction techniques are known to extract some impurities. Pump[54] postulated that pores of Kohn represented a degenerating emphysematous process which was the first stage in the formation of pulmonary alveolar fenestrae. The area present in 100 fenestrae increased with increasing age, but remained below that of overt emphysema. Atrophy of capillaries and deviation of elastic fibers around the fenestrae were noted. Turino et al.[71] indicated that elastase treatment of trachea increased both collapsibility and distensibility at physiological pressures. However, at higher pressures, no deviation from normal was noted. Snider and Korthy[63] noted decreased internal surface area in hamsters instilled intratracheally with elastase and in which emphysema developed. Air spaces increased to 165% of control (volume) and decreased to less than one half the number of control. About one third of the alveolar volume increase was due to impaired elastic recoil and two thirds to remodeling air-space walls. These changes resembled those of human panlobular emphysema. Senior et al.[59] produced a mild patchy emphysema with little change in pulmonary elastin and considerably more hemorrhage than the pancreatic elastase-induced emphysema. The reasons for differences were poorly understood but might relate to species and substrate specificity of the elastases.

Several excellent reviews of the effects of emphysema on ventilation and gas exchange have been published;[2,8,42,74] therefore, only a summary of the major functional changes will be presented here.

Destruction of alveolar septal tissue results in a loss of elastic recoil, which is reflected by a shift to the left of the entire pressure-volume curve. Static lung compliance is increased, particularly at volumes near total lung capacity. Dynamic lung compliance during quiet breathing may be normal, but compliance becomes frequency-dependent and thus may be reduced if the respiratory frequency is elevated. The loss of elastic recoil tends to increase the resting lung volume (functional residual capacity) and since the total lung capacity may be unaltered or only slightly increased, the vital capacity is usually reduced. A loss of parenchymal support, which normally holds small airways (less than 2 mm) open, results in an early closure of these airways during forced or maximal expiration. Thus, the measured residual volume and closing volume are increased and airflow rates during forced expiration are reduced. There is an abnormally wide range of emptying and filling rates among ventilating units, which contributes to a frequency-dependence of resistance and compliance, uneven intrapulmonary gas distribution, and a mismatching of ventilation and blood perfusion at the alveolar level. Gas exchange efficiency is reduced by a loss of diffusing surface area and mismatching of ventilation and perfusion. As the ventilation and gas exchange abnormalities progress, hypoxemia, carbon dioxide retention, and respiratory acidosis occur.

Functional alterations similar to those observed in human emphysema have been reported for naturally-occurring and experimentally-induced emphysema in horses,[21] dogs,[39] rabbits,[7] rats,[31,50,57] and hamsters.[40,46,62]

Thus elastase, which induces emphysema, seems to reduce the elasticity (recoil) of lung at normal physiological pressures. This is consistent with changes commonly observed in pulmonary emphysema in humans. Increased residual volume/total lung capacity reflects reduced lung recoil. A similar mechanism seems appropriate for reduced forced expiratory volume in 1 second, possibly reflecting the lack of recoil of larger airways, and for reduced mid maximal expiratory flow, suggesting a potential lack of recoil of smaller airways. The lack of alveolar units is reflected by a decreased alveolar surface area, which causes impaired gas exchange. Oxygen exchange is affected at a lower level of injury because of the sigmoid nature of its dissociation curve. However, if severe enough anatomic changes are present, carbon dioxide exchange may be impaired and some shunting of blood may occur.[75]

III. BIOCHEMICAL CHANGES

Since elastase or papain will induce emphysema, one must consider the possibility that elastin may be the principal altered constituent. However, elastase is not completely specific. Moreover, the finding of anticollagen antibodies by Michaeli and Fundenburg[41] suggests that collagen may be involved as well. Kilburn et al.'s[34] finding that collagen fibers are dissolved and fibroblasts stimulated supports this premise. Likewise, Evans et al.[17] suggested that terminal bronchiolar collagen was involved. Freeman et al.,[18] in combined exposure of NO_2 and O_3, noted some fibroblast response which they felt was the ozone component. All this evidence is indirect, because NO_2 or O_3 may be fibrogenic at higher levels; thus, these investigators may be looking at subtly higher levels and observing the collagen component, intermediate between fibrosis and emphysema. Even if so, this suggests a relation of fibrosis to emphysema and an involvement of collagen in the disease process.

Lung collagen changes in emphysema, possibly due to changes in population of cells producing it. Hacker and Flowers[23] noted that 5 ppm NO_2 stimulated collagen synthesis 12 to 24 hours after exposure, suggesting that collagen changes induce a quick response. Collins et al.[10] noted collagen synthetic increases at subemphysematogenic levels of papain where early inflammation was clearly reversed at later times. This indicated that elevated collagen synthesis will not necessarily progress to chronic pulmonary disease. Yu and Keller[77] report a similar increase in collagen synthesis during the development of elastase-treated hamsters. There is no indication of reversibility of this change. Likewise no documentation of anatomic emphysema was provided. Counts[11] and Counts and Knighten[12] noted that collagen content was reduced in 1 day in lungs treated with emphysematogenic levels of trypsin. The increased level of collagen synthesis [23] is understandable, and tends to support the involvement of collagen in emphysema. In contrast, collagen synthesis relative to noncollagen protein remains constant and protein synthesis is decreased after trypsin inhalation.[11,12] Speculatively, the reduction of collagen might lead the fibroblast or contractile cell to proliferate. The level of injury would influence the degree of proliferation (less from the higher level of trypsin). If proliferation was successful, sufficient collagen synthesis would bring the lung to a normal collagen density. Thus, collagen content measured later would appear normal, as observed by Kilburn et al.[34] and numerous other observers, as reviewed by Hance and Crystal.[25] Niinikoski et al.[47] and Chrêtien[8a] observed increased hydroxyproline in lavage fluid, supporting a rapid early breakdown of collagen and linking it to Pickrell et al.'s[50a] observation of a similarly increased breakdown of pulmonary collagen after $^{238}PuO_2$ exposure. Yu and Keller[77] report that collagen, in addition to elastin, is rapidly degraded during development of elastase-induced emphysema. This concept will have to be proven by further experimentation. However, the possibility that lung cell population changes play a role in the pathogenesis of emphysema must be considered.

Snider et al.[60] presented data which support the concept that elastin fibers are the connective tissue element attacked in enzyme-induced experimental emphysema. In a later paper, Stone et al.[69] of the same laboratory presented data to support the concept of long-term binding of elastase to lung tissue as did the data of Janoff et al.[29] This binding may explain, in part, the progressive nature of elastase-induced emphysema. Snider et al.[60] also suggest that digestion of naturally occurring elastin is a more effective predictor of in vivo enzyme-inducing capacities than is benzoyl arginine ethyl ester or artificial pancreatic elastase substrate. Goldstein et al.[22] indicate that digestion of pulmonary parenchyma frees considerable pulmonary collagen, leaving much of it intact. Pickrell, Sass, and Straus[50d] have recovered hydroxyproline-containing material in endobronchial washings of rat and hamster lungs. About three fourths of the hydroxyproline is high molecular weight (membrane cone cut off $\simeq$ 50,000 daltons) in rats. The quantity of hydroxyproline increases in hamsters with 4.4 μg Cd deposited in their lungs and in rats exposed to 20 ppm NO_2 for 120 hrs/week for 2 weeks. In the latter case, only 25% of the hydroxyproline peptides were high molecular weight. This suggests that pulmonary injury destroys cells, frees underlying connective tissue, and degrades some of it. This work supports and is supported by the work of Goldstein et al.,[22] since elastase produced not only an in vitro release of collagen but a protein with an amino acid composition similar to microfibrillar protein. This protein was part of the extracellular matrix and would logically be released if elastin were destroyed. The extent to which other enzymes such as cathepsin operate in this manner remains to be determined. Johansen and Pierce[31] observed changes of the amorphous component of elastin without affecting the microfibrils. As reviewed by Hance and Crystal,[25] proteolysis would certainly accelerate the breakdown of incompletely cross-linked elastin. Whether this would affect the integrity of cross-linked elastin remains to be determined. However, O'Dell et al.[48] were able to induce emphysema (increased mean linear intercept) with copper deficiency and resultant inhibition of lysyl oxidase. Elastin content of lungs was modestly reduced. Similar results were obtained by Harris[26] by inducing copper deficiency.

The efficiency of connective tissue synthesis may determine the severity of emphysema. Chrzanowski et al.[9] reported that elastin content was reduced in alpha$_1$ antitrypsin deficient emphysema from 25 to 35% of the crude connective tissue to 6 to 21%. Since desmosine content was unaffected (1.7 to 2.3 vs 1.4 to 1.8 residues/1000), such analysis would reflect the elastin loss equally well.[28,50b] Elastin content was lowest in bullae and most visibly destroyed parenchyma. Kuhn et al. cited in Kuhn and Starcher[36] indicated that pancreatic elastase actuely destroys elastin, which is resynthesized during subsequent weeks. Kuhn and Starcher[36] indicated elastin resynthesis to be inhibited by use of beta aminoproprionitrile, a lathyrogen which inhibits cross-linking in forming connective tissue fibers. The ability to re-synthesize normal elastin tends to limit resulting structural damage. Starcher et al.[65] indicate that both pulmonary collagen and elastin were increased after intratracheal injection of bleomycin. In an earlier paper, Evans et al.[15] noted that three neonatal pulmonary diseases (respiratory distress syndrome, atalectasis, and hemorrhage) had significantly reduced neutral to charged amino acids in elastin. This may be predisposing factor in lung disease or an immaturity of tissue.

Little definitive work has been done on proteoglycan alterations in emphysema.[25,28] However, the amount of galactoseamine containing proteoglycan was significantly lower in emphysematous relative to normal lungs. Since galactoseamine is also present in other glycoproteins, this index may not reflect the true proteoglycan-elastin changes. The finding that emphysema induces release of proteoglycans suggests, non-specifically, that such are involved. Which proteoglycan is involve remains to be defined. Last et al.[37] provide the initial report of a direct effect of ozone on airway metabolism. Explants demonstrated an initial 1-week decrease followed by a 12-week increase in rate of glycoprotein synthesis during daily exposure to 0.8 ppm (1.9 mg/m^3) for 8 hr/day. They suggest that the changes may be functional (and possibly reversible) rather than structural.

IV. SUMMARY

We have speculated that in emphysema the cell which synthesizes most pulmonary alveolar elastin may not proliferate adequately or it may have no basement membrane to proliferate on. Thus, after initial losses of collagen and elastin, normal collagen density but reduced elastin will be retained. Alternatively, elastin is largely relocated by displacing around fenestrae and a normal elastin content is present. The sequence of molecular events leading to emphysema must be more completely defined by further experimentation. Cells at an intermediate level of proteolysis with an inadequate basement membrane could proliferate briefly and form small pockets of extracellular matrix. The cycle of cell proliferation and connective tissue production could become limited early in the disease process. Lungs would then have abnormal morphology, but a normal overall level of connective tissue, i.e., a normal amount in an abnormal location. The diffuseness of the lesion would be proportionate to the severity of developing emphysema. This is what seems to be seen in a number of these emphysema models, i.e., alveolar loss, reduced internal surface area but apparently normal connective tissue. It would result in collapse of small airways because the connective tissue was poorly distributed. The lower the injury, the more likely the connective tissue is to remain at apparently normal levels, i.e., production and proliferation stimulated only to a low degree. This injury would have to be small enough that it would not stimulate further injury, but merely result in wall loss. Thus re-injury would not occur but merely injury of neighboring normal tissue. Obviously, if this mechanism were widespread, one would see an initial reduction of connective tissue, most likely proportional to intensity of proteolysis. Likewise morphologic alteration would be proportional to level and persistence of proteolysis. That persistence is important is indicated by the return to more nearly normal morphology at three weeks in animals receiving a single aerosol exposure to deposit $\simeq 4\ \mu g\ CdCl_2$ in their lungs.[27a] To further document this model, one must study local chemical and morphologic changes and relate the two. Future work on emphysema should yield especially thought-provoking data.

V. ATTEMPTS AT THERAPEUTIC MANIPULATION

Since elastase can induce emphysema, inhibitors of this enzyme may have therapeutic benefit. Powers et al.[53] have partially characterized inhibitors of elastase and other proteolytic enzymes. It is felt that these may have value in treating $alpha_1$ antitrypsin deficiency. Powers[52] has also attempted characterization of additional elastase inhibitors. Human leucocyte elastase is inhibited by chloromethyl ketones (Ac-$(Ala)_4$-CH_2Cl, Ac-$(Ala)_1$-Pro-Ala-CH_2Cl). However, Ac-$(Ala)_2$-pro-val-CH_2Cl and Ac$(Ala)_2$-pro-Ile CH_2Cl are peptide carbozates which will acylate elastase rapidly, but the binding is irreversible. Thus, they are not effective in vivo. This seems an area of research with exciting possibilities. Watanabe et al.[73] reported little therapeutic benefit from prednisone treatment at a level effective in treating asthma.

Emphysema can be enhanced by inhibition of cross-linking using BAPN.[36] Presumably this also means that other cross-linked inhibitors (penicillamine and semicarbizide) would intensify, not alleviate, pulmonary emphysema. The same is true of copper deficiency or possibly of hypoxia since lysyl oxidase requires a P_{O_2} of approximately 50 mmHg for maximum effectiveness in vitro.[9a] Although this information adds little to the understanding of the pathogenesis of emphysema, it does point out the pitfalls of using inhibitors of connective tissue synthesis to manipulate pulmonary emphysema. Likewise, the information indicates that early inflammatory events may be important determinants of lung injury progressing to emphysema.

REFERENCES

1. **Adamson, I. Y. R. and Bowden, D. H.,** The type 2 cell as progenitor of alveolar epithelial regeneration, *Lab. Invest.*, 30, 35, 1974.
2. **Bates, D. V., Macklem, P. T., and Christie, R. V.,** Pulmonary emphysema, in *Respiratory Function in Disease*, 2nd ed., W. B. Saunders, Philadelphia, 1971, 156.
3. **Boatman, E. S., Sato, S., and Frank, R.,** Acute effects of ozone on cat lungs, *Am. Rev. Respir. Dis.*, 110, 157, 1974.
4. **Bouhuys, A. and Peters, J. M.,** Control of environmental lung disease, *N. Engl. J. Med.*, 283, 573, 1970.

5. **Buell, G.**, Some biochemical aspects of cadmium toxicology, *J. Occup. Med.*, 17, 189, 1975.
6. **Butler, C.**, Lung surface area in various morphologic forms of human emphysema, *Am. Rev. Respir. Dis.*, 114, 347, 1976.
7. **Caldwell, E. J.**, Physiologic and anatomic effects of papain on the rabbit lung, *J. Appl. Physiol.*, 31, 458, 1971.
8. **Cherniack, R. M., Cherniack, L., and Naimark, A.**, Airway Obstruction, in *Respiration in Health and Disease*, 2nd ed., W. B. Saunders, Philadelphia, 1972, 303.
8a. **Chrêtien, J.**, Research communication, 1975.
9. **Chrzanowski, P. J., Keller, S., Fierer, J. A., Mandl, I., and Turino, G. M.**, Elastin content in normal and emphysematous lung parenchyma in man, *Am. Rev. Respir. Dis.*, 113(Abstr.), 199, 1976.
9a. **Chvapil, M.**, Research communication, 1973.
10. **Collins, J. F., Durnin, L. S., and Johanson, W. G., Jr.**, Papain-induced lung injury: alterations in connective tissue metabolism without emphysema, *Exp. Mol. Pathol.*, 29, 29, 1978.
11. **Counts, D.**, Collagen and protein biosynthesis in lung tissue after trypsin inhalation, *Fed. Proc.*, 36, 607, 1977.
12. **Counts, D. F. and Knighten, P.**, Collagen and non-collagen protein synthesis in the lungs of rats exposed to a trypsin aerosol, *Connect. Tissue Res.*, 5, 165, 1977.
13. **Evans, M. J., Cabral, L. J., Stephens, R. J., and Freeman, G.**, Cell division of alveolar macrophages in rat lung following exposure to NO_2. *Am. J. Pathol.*, 70, 199, 1973.
14. **Evans, M. J., Cabral, L. J., Stephens, R. J., and Freeman, G.**, Transformation of alveolar type 2 cells to type 1 cells following exposure to NO_2. *Exp. Mol. Pathol.*, 22, 142, 1975.
15. **Evans, M. J., Cabral, L. C., Stephens, R. J., and Freeman, G.**, Acute kinetic response and renewal of the alveolar epithelium following injury by nitrogen dioxide, *Chest*, 65, 62s, 1974.
16. **Cabral-Anderson, L. J., Evans, M. J., and Freeman, G.**, Effects of NO_2 on the lungs of aging rats, I. Morphology, *Exp. Mol. Pathol.*, 27, 353, 1977.
16a. **Evans, M.**, Research communication, 1976.
17. **Evans, M. J., Cabral-Anderson, L. J., Freeman, G.**, Effect of NO_2 on the lungs of aging rats. II. Cell proliferation, *Exp. Mol. Pathol.*, 27, 366, 1977.
17a. **Evans, M. J., Stephens, R. J., Cabral, L. J., and Freeman, G.**, Cell renewal in the lungs of rats exposed to low levels of NO_2, *Arch. Environ. Health*, 24, 180, 1972.
18. **Freeman, G., Juhos, L. T., Furiosi, N. J., Mussenden, R., Stephens, R. J., and Evans, M. J.**, Pathology of pulmonary disease from exposure to interdependent ambient gases (nitrogen dioxide and ozone), *Arch. Environ. Health*, 29, 203, 1974.
19. **Fulmer, J. D. and Crystal, R. G.**, The biochemical basis of pulmonary function, in *Biochemical Basis of Pulmonary Function*, Crystal, R. G., Ed. Marcel Dekker, New York, 1976, 419.
20. **Furiosi, N. J., Crane, S. C., and Freeman, G.**, Mixed sodium chloride aerosol and nitrogen dioxide in air, *Arch. Environ. Health*, 27, 405, 1973.
21. **Gillespie, J. R. and Tyler, W. S.**, Chronic alveolar emphysema in the horse, *Adv. Vet. Sci. Comp. Med.*, 13, 59, 1969.
22. **Goldstein, R. H., Faris, B., Hu, C. L., Snider, G. L., and Franzblau, C.**, The fate of newly synthesized lung collagen after endotracheal administration of ^{14}C-proline to hamsters, *Am. Rev. Respir. Dis.*, 117, 281, 1978.
23. **Hacker, A. D. and Flowers, E. S.**, Effects of nitrogen dioxide on collagen metabolism in rat lung, *Fed. Proc. Abstr.*, 35, 680, 1976.
24. **Hackney, J. D., Evans, M. J., and Christie, B. R.**, Effects of 60 and 80% oxygen on cell division in lung alveoli of squirrel monkeys, *Aviat. Space Environ. Med.*, 46, 791, 1975.
24a. **Hahn, F. F. and Hobbs, C. H.**, The effect of enzyme-induced pulmonary emphysema in Syrian hamsters on the deposition and long-term retention of inhaled particles, *Arch. Environ. Health*, 34(4), 203, 1979.
25. **Hance, A. J. and Crystal, R. G.**, The connective tissue of lung, *Am. Rev. Respir. Dis.*, 112, 657, 1975.
26. **Harris, E. D.**, A new function for copper in aorta, *Fed. Proc. Abstr.*, 35, 255, 1976.
27. **Hayes, J. S., Snider, G. L. and Palmer, K. C.**, The evolution of biochemical damage in the rat lung after acute cadmium exposure, *Am. Rev. Respir. Dis.*, 113, 121, 1976.
27a. **Henderson, R. F., Rebar, A. H., Pickrell, J. A., and Newton, G. J.**, Early damage indicators in the lung. III. Biochemical and cytologic response in the lung to inhaled metal salts, *Tox. Appl. Pharm.*, 50, 123, 1979.
28. **Horwitz, A. L., Elson, N. A., and Crystal, R. G.**, Proteoglycans and elastic fibers, in *Biochemical Basis of Pulmonary Function*, Crystal, R. G., Ed., Marcel Dekker, New York, 1976, 273.
29. **Janoff, A., Sloan, B., Weinbaum, G., Damiano, V., Sandhaus, R. A., Elias, J., and Kimbel, P.**, Experimental emphysema induced with purified human neutrophil elastase: tissue localization of the instilled protease, *Am. Rev. Respir. Dis.*, 115, 461, 1977.

30. **Johanson, W. G. and Pierce, A. K.,** Effects of elastase, collagenase and papain on structure and function of rat lungs *in vitro, J. Clin. Invest.*, 51, 288, 1972.
31. **Johanson, W. G. and Pierce, A. K.,** Lung structure and function with age in normal rats and rats with papain emphysema, *J. Clin. Invest.*, 52, 2921, 1973.
32. **Johnson, J. R. and Andrews, F. A.,** Lung scleroproteins in age and emphysema, *Chest*, 57, 239, 1970.
33. **Kendrick, J., Nettesheim, P., Guerin, M., Caton, J., Dalbey, W., Griesemer, R., Rubin, I., and Maddox, W.,** Tobacco smoke inhalation studies in rats, *Toxicol. Appl. Pharmacol.*, 37, 557, 1976.
34. **Kilburn, K. H., Dowell, A. R., and Pratt, P. C.,** Morphological and biochemical assessment of papain-induced emphysema, *Arch. Intern. Med.*, 127, 884, 1971.
35. **Kosmider, S., Drozdz, M., Luciak, M., Ludyga, K., Misiewicz, A., Szygula, J., and Zajusz, K.,** The mechanisms of the toxic effect of combustion exhaust gases, *Int. Arch. Arbeitsmed.*, 29, 28, 1971.
36. **Kuhn, C. and Starcher, B.,** The significance of connective tissue repair in elastase-induced emphysema, *Am. Rev. Respir. Dis.*, 113(Abstr.), 209, 1976.
37. **Last, J. A., Jennings, M. D., Schwartz, L. W., and Cross, C. E.,** Glycoprotein secretion by tracheal explants cultured from rats exposed to ozone, *Am. Rev. Respir. Dis.*, 116, 695, 1977.
38. **Loosli, C. G., Buckley, R. D., Hertweck, M. S., Hardy, J. D., Ryan, D. P., Stinson, S., and Serebrin, R.,** Pulmonary response of mice exposed to synthetic smog, *Ann. Occup. Hyg.*, 15, 251, 1972.
39. **Marco, V., Meranze, D. R., Yoshida, M., and Kimbel, P.,** Papain-induced experimental emphysema in the dog, *J. Appl. Physiol.*, 33, 293, 1972.
40. **Martorana, P. A.,** The hamster as a model for experimental pulmonary emphysema, *Lab. Anim. Sci.*, 26, 352, 1976.
41. **Michaeli, D. and Fudenberg, H. H.,** Antibodies to collagen in patients with emphysema, *Clin. Immunol. Immunopathol.*, 3, 187, 1974.
42. **Miller, W. F. and Paez, P. N.,** Physiologic alterations in emphysema. in *Clinical Cardiopulmonary Physiology*, 3rd ed., Gordon, B. L., Carleton, R. A., and Faber, L. P., Eds., Grune & Stratton, New York, 1969, 565.
43. **Miller, M. L., Murthy, L., and Sorenson, J. R. J.,** Fine structure of connective tissue after ingestion of cadmium, *Arch. Pathol.*, 98, 386, 1974.
44. **Mustafa, M. G., Cross, C. E., and Tyler, W. S.** Interference of cadmium ion with oxidative metabolism of alveolar macrophages, *Arch. Intern. Med.*, 127, 1050, 1971.
45. **Naeye, R. L., Mahon, J. K., and Dellinger, W. S.,** Effects of smoking on lung structure of Appalachian coal workers, *Arch. Environ. Health*, 22, 190, 1971.
46. **Niewoehner, D. E. and Kleinerman, J.,** Effects of experimental emphysema and bronchiolitis on lung mechanics and morphometry, *J. Appl. Physiol.*, 35, 25, 1973.
47. **Niinikoski, J., Nikkari, T., and Kulonen, E.,** Pulmonary oxygen toxicity: composition of endobronchial saline extracts of rats during exposure to oxygen, *Aerosp. Med.*, 42, 525, 1971.
48. **O'Dell, B. L., Morgan, R. F., McKenzie, W. N., and Kilburn, K. H.,** Copper deficient rat lung as an emphysema model, *Fed. Proc. Abstr.*, 35, 255, 1976.
49. **Palmer, K. C., Snider, G. L., and Hayes, J. A.,** Cellular proliferation induced in the lung by cadmium aerosol, *Am. Rev. Respir. Dis.*, 112, 173, 1975.
50. **Palecek, F., Palecekova, M., and Aviado, D. M.,** Emphysema in immature rats, *Arch. Environ. Health*, 15, 332, 1967.
50a. **Pickrell, J. A., Harris, D. V., Mauderly, J. L., and Hahn, F. F.,** Altered collagen metabolism in radiation-induced interstitial pulmonary fibrosis, *Chest*, 69, 311, 1976.
50b. **Pickrell, J. A. and Shafer, J.,** Lung connective tissue measurements. I. Amino acid analysis procedures for determination of canine lung connective tissue, *Arch. Intern. Med.*, 127, 891, 1971.
50c. **Plopper, C. G., Dungworth, D. L., and Tyler, W. S.,** Pulmonary lesions in rats exposed to ozone. A correlated light and electron microscopic study, *Am. J. Pathol.*, 71, 375, 1973.
50d. **Pickrell, J. A., Sass, K. S., and Straus, F. C.,** Research communication, 1978.
51. **Plopper, C. G., Dungworth, D. L., and Tyler, W. S.,** Ultrastructure of pulmonary alveolar macrophages *in situ* in lungs from rats exposed to ozone, *Am. Rev. Respir. Dis.*, 108, 632, 1973.
52. **Powers, J. C.,** Synthesis of elastase inhibitors, U.S. Department of Commerce, Springfield, Va., PB 248 391 distributed by Natl. Tech. Info. Serv., 1975.
53. **Powers, J. C., Carroll, D. L., and Tuhy, P. M.,** Synthetic active site-directed inhibitors of elastolytic proteases, *Ann. N.Y. Acad. Sci.*, 256, 420, 1975.
54. **Pump, K. K.,** Emphysema and its relation to age, *Am. Rev. Respir. Dis.*, 114, 5, 1976.
55. **Richards, R. J. and Wusteman, F. S.,** The effects of silica dust and alveolar macrophages on lung fibroblast grown *in vitro, Life Sci.*, 14, 355, 1974.
56. **Ryan, G. B. and Majno, G.,** Acute inflammation — a review, *Am. J. Pathol.*, 86, 183, 1977.
57. **Sahebjami, H. and Vassallo, C. L.,** Exercise stress and enzyme-induced emphysema, *J. Appl. Physiol.*, 41, 332, 1976.

58. **Schuyler, M. R., Rynbrandt, D. J., and Kleinerman, J.**, Physiologic and morphologic observations of the effects of intravenous elastase on the lung, *Am. Rev. Respir. Dis.*, 117, 97, 1978.
59. **Senior, R. M., Tegner, H., Kuhn, C., Ohlsson, K., Starcher, B. C., and Pierce, J. A.**, The induction of pulmonary emphysema with human leukocyte elastase, *Am. Rev. Respir. Dis.*, 116, 469, 1977.
60. **Snider, G. L., Hayes, J. A., Franzblau, C., Kagan, H. M., Stone, P. S., and Korthy, A. L.**, Relationship between elastolytic activity and experimental emphysema-inducing properties of papain preparations, *Am. Rev. Respir. Dis.*, 110, 254, 1974.
61. **Snider, G. L., Hayes, J. A., Korthy, A. L., and Lewis, G. P.**, Centrilobular emphysema experimentally induced by cadmium chloride aerosol, *Am. Rev. Respir. Dis.*, 108, 40, 1973.
62. **Snider, G. L., Sherter, C. B., Koo, K. W., Karlinsky, J. B., Hayes, J. A., and Franzblau, C.**, Respiratory mechanics in hamsters following treatment with endotracheal elastase or collagenase, *J. Appl. Physiol.*, 42(2), 206, 1977.
63. **Snider, G. L., and Korthy, A. L.**, Internal surface area and number of respiratory air spaces in elastase-induced emphysema in hamsters, *Am. Rev. Respir. Dis.*, 117, 685, 1978.
64. **Sobin, S. S., Bernick, S., Tremer, H. M., Rosenquist, T. H., Lindal, R., and Fung, Y. C.**, The fibroprotein network of the pulmonary interalveolar wall, *Chest*, 65, 45, 1974.
65. **Starcher, B. C., Kuhn, C., and Overton, J. E.**, Increased elastin and collagen content in the lungs of hamsters receiving an intratracheal injection of bleomycin, *Am. Rev. Respir. Dis.*, 117, 299, 1978.
66. **Stephens, R. J., Evans, M. J., Sloan, M. F., and Freeman, G.**, A comprehensive ultrastructural study of pulmonary injury and repair in the rat resulting from exposures to less than one ppm ozone, *Chest*, 65, 11a, 1974.
67. **Stephens, R. J., Freeman, G., and Evans, M. J.**, Ultrastructural changes in connective tissue in lungs of rats exposed to NO_2, *Arch. Intern. Med.*, 127, 873, 1971.
68. **Stephens, R. J., Sloan, M. F., Evans, M. J., and Freeman, G.**, Alveolar type I cell response to exposure to 0.5 ppm O_3 for short periods, *Exp. Mol. Pathol.*, 20, 11, 1974.
69. **Stone, P. J., Pareira, W., Jr., Biles, D., Snider, G. L., Kagan, H. M., and Franzblau, C.**, Studies on the fate of pancreatic elastase in the hamster lung: ^{14}C-guanidinated elastase, *Am. Rev. Respir. Dis.*, 116, 49, 1977.
70. **Strauss, R. H., Palmer, K. C., and Hayes, J. A.**, Acute lung injury induced by cadmium aerosol, *Am. J. Pathol.*, 84, 561, 1976.
71. **Turino, G. M., Lourenco, R. V., and McCracken, G. H.**, Role of connective tissues in large pulmonary airways, *J. Appl. Physiol.*, 25, 645, 1968.

71a. **Vracko, R.**, Basal lamina scaffold-anatomy and significance for maintenance of orderly tissue structure, *Am. J. Pathol.*, 77, 314, 1974.

72. **Watanabe, F., Mitchell, M. M., and Renzetti, A. D.**, Granular pneumocyte and pulmonary fibrosis, *Chest*, 62, 400, 1972.
73. **Watanabe, S., Renzetti, A. D., and Bigler, A.**, Bronchodilator and corticosteroid effects on regional and total airway resistance in patients with asthma, chronic bronchitis, and chronic pulmonary emphysema, *Am. Rev. Respir. Dis.*, 106, 392, 1972.
74. **West, J. B.**, Obstructive diseases, in *Pulmonary Pathophysiology — the Essentials*, Williams & Wilkins, Baltimore, 1977, 59.
75. **West, J. B.**, *Respiratory Physiology — the Essentials*, Williams & Wilkins, Baltimore, 1974, 1.
76. **Yu, S. Y., Yoshida, A., and Keller, N. R.**, Degradation of lung collagen during development of elastase-emphysema in hamsters, *Fed. Proc. Abstr.*, 36, 1090, 1977.
77. **Yu, S. Y. and Keller, N. R.**, Synthesis of lung collagen in hamsters with elastase-induced emphysema, *Exp. Mol. Pathol.*, 29, 37, 1978.
78. **Ziskind, M., Jones, R. N., and Weill, H.**, Silicosis, *Am. Rev. Respir. Dis.*, 113, 643, 1976.

Chapter 15

CHRONIC BRONCHITIS AND ASTHMA: BIOCHEMISTRY, RHEOLOGY, AND MUCOCILIARY CLEARANCE

R. K. Wolff, J. L. Mauderly, and J. A. Pickrell

TABLE OF CONTENTS

I. CHRONIC BRONCHITIS

The diagnostic criterion for bronchitis is clinical. The usual definition is that a person has chronic bronchitis if they have productive cough or sputum occurring on most days for at least 3 months of a year.[63] This condition is characterized by the presence of chronic excessive mucous secretion in the airways.

One of the basic morphological changes is hypertrophy of the bronchial mucous glands and goblet cell hyperplasia. Reid[73] has shown that in the normal state, the gland's maximum thickness is about one third of the wall, measured between epithelium and cartilage; however, in chronic bronchitis the gland size increases dramatically. Measuring the ratio of gland to wall thickness (Reid index) can give a guideline to the severity of disease.

The prime abnormality in chronic bronchitis is overproduction of secretion and/or its clearance. To more fully understand the disease, a short discussion of the normal mucociliary system and the alterations that result in chronic bronchitis are presented.

A. Mucociliary System

Rhodin[76] and, more recently, Breeze and Sheldon[11] have described the morphology of the airways. A ciliated pseudo-stratified respiratory tract mucosa extends from the trachea down to the terminal bronchioles. The epithelial layer contains goblet cells and submucosal glands of both serous and mucous types. As one moves distally to the periphery of the lung, the percentage of both ciliated and goblet cells decreases. The number of submucosal glands also decreases, so that the number of goblet cells, or submucosal glands, in human airways less than 1 mm in diameter is small.[64] This general picture holds for most mammalian and rodent species (Goco et al.,[34] Korhonen et al.[48]).

Rhodin and Dalhamn[75] have shown that each ciliated cell has about 200 cilia and many microvilli. Dalhamn[22] has shown that ciliary beat frequency is about 22 Hz in the trachea, and Iravani[41] reported similar findings in the trachea and a progressive decrease to about 7 Hz in peripheral airways.

There is general agreement that the mucous blanket consists of two phases. There is a low viscosity periciliary fluid of about 5 μm thickness in the trachea, which bathes the cilia. Above this is a gel phase of higher viscosity material about 5 μm thick. The clawed tips of the cilia touch the upper layer at the top of their stroke.[43] The existence of these two layers is supported by the work of Lucas and Douglas[57] and Bang and Bang.[5] The source of the upper layer is undoubtedly goblet cells and mucous glands; however, the source and control of the periciliary fluid has not been clearly demonstrated.

Whether the upper mucous layer is a continuous blanket or consists of discrete "flakes" or "plaques" is a controversial issue. The work of Iravani and van As[42] and reviewed by van As[94] supports the latter hypothesis. Many other workers have presented data indicating a continuous mucous blanket.[88,59,57] From available data it does appear that the mucous layer thins as the airways become smaller,[59] and there are fewer ciliated cells, as noted earlier. Certainly the velocity of the mucous blanket decreases from the trachea to peripheral airways as shown by Iravani and van As,[42] Asmundsson and Kilburn,[3] and Morrow et al.[65]

Some of the differences in the chronic bronchitis state are as follows. There is goblet cell hypertrophy and hyperplasia and sometimes partial occulusion of the bronchiolar lumen.[62,72] Goblet cells appear frequently in the terminal bronchioles, where, in the normal state, they are quite rare. It is possible, also, that there are abnormalities in periciliary fluid resorption processes. Asmundsson and Kilburn[3] postulated that this might be necessary to prevent airway flooding because of the tremendous decrease in surface area from the periphery to the trachea. As mentioned earlier, Reid[73] showed mucous gland hypertrophy, resulting in a change of the ratio of gland to bronchial wall thickness from the normal 30% to 50% or more.

Since goblet cell numbers increase and mucous gland hypertrophy occurs, it is not surprising that the volume of secretion increases in chronic bronchitis.

1. Biochemistry and Rheology of Bronchial Secretions

The biochemical and rheological changes which contribute to the changes in mucous properties have been thoroughly reviewed recently.[28,52,54] Bronchial mucous is viscoelastic with a gelatinous consistency, having the properties of both a solid and a liquid.

When a force is applied, mucus deforms and, because of its elastic properties, stores energy. However, mucus is not perfectly elastic and some permanent deformation does occur. Its viscous properties are reflected in the fact that it flows when a force is applied and flow rate is proportional to the applied force. Mucus is not a perfect Newtonian fluid since its viscosity falls, and so it thins with increasing shearing force. This means that a measured viscosity is only valid at a given shear rate.

Collected mucoid sputum is 95% water, with 2.3% glycoprotein and 0.1 to 0.5% protein and 0.3 to 0.5% fats dispersed in a sol phase.[61] Biochemical studies of sputum are difficult because of its inhomogeneity and high viscosity, which often necessitates lengthy preparative methods. Analysis may be made of whole sputum or sol or gel, the main problem being solubilization of the gel glycoprotein.

Glycoproteins have a single polypeptide chain to which one or more polysaccharide side chains are attached in a branched fashion with no simple sequence of sugar residues. The peptide core has a large amount of threonine and serine. The side chains are alkali-labile and generally contain neuraminic acid, fucose, galactose, *N*-acetylgalactosamine, and *N*-acetylglucosamine. Neutral and acid glycoproteins exist. The acid radical in bronchial glycoprotein is *N*-acetyl neuraminic acid or sulfate.

The surface epithelium and submucosal glands contain both acid and neutral glycoproteins. These can be identified by histochemical staining. The stains in most common use are the periodic acid-Schiff (PAS) and Alcian blue (AB) techniques. A combined AB/PAS staining shows acid radicals as bright blue and the neutral glycoprotein as pink. There can be different types of glycoprotein in a single cell, and a cell can change the type of glycoprotein it is producing.[44] In man the predominant type of glycoprotein is acid.

Reid in a recent article[74] cited the work of Creeth's group,[20,21] which indicates that there is only one type of bronchial glycoprotein found in sputum. It is of large molecular weight, up to 7×10^6. The data suggests that this molecule is composed of up to ten subunits linked by disulfide bonds. Presumably the subunits consist of the various acid and neutral glycoproteins produced primarily by the goblet cells and submucosal glands.

Bronchial secretions are composed of airway glycoproteins which usually predominate, but also contain serum glycoproteins, which do assume greater importance in diseases, particularly when inflammation and infection are present. Fucose and sulfate are found in purified bronchial glycoprotein but to only a negligible degree in serum glycoproteins. The case for mannose is the reverse and *N*-acetyl neuraminic acid is found in both.

Collection of secretions from the airways is very difficult and so most of the data deal with analysis of sputum, the expectorated fluid which contains bronchial secretions and saliva. Fortunately the saliva contamination does not pose a serious problem related to biochemical analysis.[54]

The fact that sputum is the expectorated fluid makes comparison with the normal state very difficult. In healthy individuals bronchial secretions are moved up the airways to the larynx, then into the oropharynx and are swallowed. The normal volumes of secretions produced in 24 hr have been most reliably estimated as 0.75 mℓ/kg[10] and 0.1 to 0.3 mℓ/kg.[93] In the normal healthy state, no bronchial secretions are expectorated. To provide a comparision, cough and sputum production has been stimulated in normals by the inhalation of the bronchoconstrictor prostaglandin $F_{2\alpha}$.[52]

Despite the difficulties, when careful measurements are made by the same investigators using consistent techniques, meaningful results can be obtained. Lopez-Vidriero et al.[52] and Sturgess et al.[87] have obtained convincing data comparing viscosity changes in disease states with normals who had inhaled prostaglandin $F_{2\alpha}$ to promote expectoration. They found higher viscosities in patients with chronic bronchitis, asthma, and bronchiectasis than the normals.

Lopez-Vidriero et al.[52,53] have summarized some of the changes which take place in chronic bronchitis. The dry macromolecular weight rises from 0.6% in normals, to 1.6% for mucoid sputum and up to 5.1% for purulent sputum. *N*-acetyl neuraminic acid (NANA) levels rise as well, in a parallel fashion, on an μmol/mℓ basis. The rise in NANA levels is attributed to serum transudate since the levels of mannose, a serum glycoprotein also rise, but less dramatically. Lopez-Vidriero[53] and Puchelle et al.[71] have shown viscosity changes directly correlated with NANA and, particularly, fucose. It is felt that fucose is a marker for the bronchial acid glycoprotein which confers most of the rigidity of the fiber-like structure of mucous and so has a predominant influence on viscosity.

The mucin glycoproteins have a fiber-like structure which, along with cross-linking, imparts cohesion and elasticity to the mucus. It appears that much of the rigidity is provided by the acid glycoproteins. The large number of negative ionic charges from NANA and sulfate residues mutually repeal and so stiffen the macromolecules.[44] The fact that fucose, as the marker for mucous glycoprotein, correlates well with viscosity changes[53] supports this view.

Lopez-Vidriero and Reid[53] showed in chronic bronchitis an increase in viscosity from mucoid to mucopurulent to purulent sputum. They found that bronchial glycoprotein, as represented by the fucose marker, showed the strongest correlation with viscosity in their mucoid sputum samples. In the purulent groups the serum exudates appeared to be contributing more to the viscosity. Their paper provides an interesting comparison of the disease states, chronic bronchitis, asthma, cystic fibrosis, and bronchiectasis. All groups showed similar mean viscosity levels but with large deviations in each group.

The cystic fibrosis patients did not have more viscid mucus than the others, and this does not appear to be the controlling feature of the disease. The asthma group showed the greatest variability in viscosity.

There have been relatively few studies of elasticity. Most of the available evidence shows little change in elasticity between non-purulent or purulent sputum or between diseases.[54]

2. Mucociliary Clearance

Most of the available data indicate that clearance of mucus is altered in chronic bronchitis either because of the extra volume which must be cleared or because of alterations in the mucus properties or both. It is also possible that alterations in cilia or percentage of ciliated cells also plays a role.[85] The general features related to mucus changes and clearance are that viscosity rises, elasticity falls, and mucus transport is slowed.[66] More general treatments of mucociliary clearance can be found in the reviews of Newhouse,[66] Wanner,[96] and Proctor.[70]

A variety of studies have shown that, in general, chronic bronchitics have impaired mucociliary clearance. Using Teflon® discs deposited with a fiberoptic bronchoscope, Santa Cruz et al.[83] showed marked slowing of tracheal mucus velocity in 15 patients with chronic obstructive disease. Goodman et al.[35] also observed a severe depression in tracheal mucus velocity in bronchitics.

Noninvasive measurements of bronchial clearance using inhaled aerosols have yielded somewhat variable results. Some groups have reported faster clearance,[58] others normal clearance,[89] while others reported depressed clearance.[82,55,14] The main problem in interpreting these studies is separating purely mucociliary transport effects from changes in clearance patterns resulting from different deposition patterns. Patients with chronic obstructive lung disease tend to have much more proximal aerosol deposition patterns,[82,9] which, in the absence of other factors, will result in faster lung clearance, since most of the aerosol is in larger airways with higher mucus velocities[3,65] and shorter paths to the trachea. This fact is probably responsible for the discrepancy in results obtained by different investigators. Two of the best studies which attempted to obviate the problem of differing deposition pattern are those of Lourenco[55] and Sanchis.[82] Lourenco[55] attempted to control respiratory rate and tidal volume during aerosol depositions and then chose only groups of bronchitics and normals with similar deposition patterns to compare. The bronchitic group did have slower clearance than the normal group. Sanchis[82] used a regional analysis to compare clearance patterns from an inner lung zone representing predominantly large airways. Again, bronchitics showed depressed clearance rates. These studies, coupled with the tracheal studies cited above, present convincing evidence that in chronic bronchitics the clearance of secretions is severely compromised.

3. *Correlations of Clearance with Rheology*

It is quite obvious that mucus transport is a result of the coupling of the cilia with mucus and so the type of mucus can affect transport rates. Absence of mucus has been shown to stop transport in the frog palate preparation. It can then be restored with the application of heterologous or autologous mucus.[79] Other macromolecules, such as guaran, polacrylamide, agarose, and gelatin, when added to the preparation, do show movement, but at slower rates than the native mucus.[46] The work of King et al.[46] indicate that it is the rheologic properties rather than specific biochemical characteristics which are the controlling factors in mucus transport. The thickness of the mucous layer can also be very important. Aharonson et al.[1] have shown that methacholine dramatically increased the volume of secretion flowing up the trachea, but that surface transport of particles was reduced.

King et al.[47] studied the dose-dependent effect of methacholine on viscosity and elasticity of mucus collected from dosed dogs and then its transport on a frog palate preparation. They found an optimal range for mucus transport on the frog palate, but clearance in the dog itself was not measured. These frog palate preparation studies indicate that a combination of high elasticity with low viscosity provide the fastest transport rates. Shih et al[85a] found that mucus clearance rates increased up to a certain elasticity and then decreased. Giordano et al[33a] showed that for normal dogs with elasticities above this critical value, there was, indeed, a slight inverse correlation between clearance and elasticity. Since elasticity does not appear to change much in mucus in the chronic bronchitic state,[54] then viscosity becomes the controlling factor.

Sadoul and Puchelle[80] investigated bronchial clearance, mucus rheology, and in vitro mucociliary transport in bronchitics and normal non-smokers. In a group of 14 bronchitics he found that 8 showed depressed bronchial clearance, which correlated with decreased transport of their mucus in a frog palate preparation. There was an optimum range of viscosity and elasticity values for effective clearance, and either above or below this range clearance was impaired. The worst affected bronchitics had mucus with both very low viscosity and very low recoil.

Sputum from chronic bronchitics is often purulent during disease exacerbations and this in turn affects rheology and clearance. Dulfano et al.[27] found in a group of patients whom he used as their own controls that viscosity rose and elasticity fell when sputum became purulent. In a later study[29] he and Adler investigated clearance. Purulent sputum, with higher viscosity and lower elastic recoil than mucoid sputum, had a slower transport rate on a frog palate preparation. The native frog mucus had the lowest viscocity, highest recoil, and also the fastest transport rate.

B. Therapeutic Measures

A variety of drugs are used in the treatment of chronic bronchitis. Thomson et al.[89-91] have studied the mucolytic agents, bromhexine, quaiphenesin, and S-carboxymethylcysteine and found virtually no effect on mucociliary clearance of inhaled radioaerosols. This fact emerges despite the fact that these agents decrease sputum viscosity in patients (Dulfano et al.[26]). However, at least one mucolytic agent, *N*-acetyl cysteine, has been shown to inhibit ciliary activity.[25] Percussion has been investigated by Pavia et al.[68] and shown to have a slight but not significant effect in improving mucociliary clearance. Chopra et al.[19] have studied postural drainage in beagle dogs and found it to have a beneficial effect on tracheal mucus velocity. Wolff et al[98] found that both exercise and hyperventilation speeded clearance. Although these studies were in normals, it is suggestive that exercise or breathing exercises might be of some help in chronic bronchitis to improve mucociliary clearance.

Bronchodilators are extensively used in the treatment of chronic bronchitis and so their effects on mucus transport, at least as a side effect, are of interest. The β_2 sympathomimetics have been shown to speed mucociliary clearance in normal healthy adults.[100,16,83,32] The effect in chronic bronchitic patients is much diminished (Santa Cruz et al.[83]). Atropine, an anticholinergic agent, has been shown to slow mucociliary clearance in normal subjects[100] and animal studies.[78] However, ipratropium bromide, an anticholinergic agent used therapeutically, appears to have no effect on mucus clearance in bronchitics and possibly even speeds it in normal subjects.[76] Other studies have shown no significant effect.[78]

C. Initiating Factors

Excess mucus production and/or impairment in clearance, particularly in small airways, appear to be prime features in the development of chronic obstructive airways disease.[40] Certainly in advanced states there have been reports of negative correlations between reductions in lung function and gas exchange with sputum viscosity.[18,69,54] Many studies point to the view that small airway obstruction is a first stage in the development of chronic lung disease.[67] It may well be that mucociliary impairment plays an important role in the initiation of the process, as suggested by Hilding.[38]

Cigarette smoking has been clearly linked to the development of chronic bronchitis and so it is interesting to note its effects with respect to mucociliary clearance. Like much of the scientific literature related to cigarette smoking, there have been some conflicting results. In general, most acute in vitro preparations have shown a depression of ciliary activity and mucus transport.[30,7,23] Acute exposures of cigarette smoke to animals and humans have produced either a speeding, no change, or a slowing in mucociliary clearance. Some of these discrepancies may be methodological, but the studies of Yergin et al.[101] and Yeates et al.[100] on tracheal clearance alone support the view that acute smoking can have a variable effect on clearance.

Long term smoking does appear to depress mucociliary clearance. Again, methodological differences and interindividual variability have provided some conflicting data and so only the more definitive studies will be mentioned. By using radioaerosol inhalations and selecting healthy smokers and non-smokers, Lourenco et al.[56] were able to show delayed overall clearance and an accumulation of material in central airways. Sanchis et al[81] found similar results. Both Bohning et al.[8] and Camner and Philipson[13] were able to study smoking-discordant twins and showed depression of clearance in about half of the cases and no change in others. Camner et al.[12] have seen that in the absence of smoking, clearance in twins is strikingly similar. Goodman et al.[36] found dramatic reductions in tracheal mucus velocities in young healthy smokers. Some of the most informative studies are those in which a subject can be used as his own control. Camner et al.[15] found that cessation of smoking resulted in an improvement in mucociliary clearance after three months. Wanner et al.[95] found that chronic exposures of cigarette smoke for 13.5 months to beagles depressed tracheal mucus velocities while lung mechanics did not change. All of the studies cited above involved asymptomatic smokers, but, even so, abnormalities in mucociliary-clearance were present. These findings suggest that either mucociliary clearance defects may contribute to a chronic bronchitic state and/or they provide an early warning of the development of the disease.

The etiology of chronic bronchitis is not well understood, but it appears that chronic irritation from inhaled materials may play a factor. Cigarette smoking has been clearly linked with the development of chronic bronchitis, and its role in impairing clearance has been discussed above. It is possible that inhalation of other particulates and gases might cause the same result. It is quite clear from a number of studies that acute exposures to common atmospheric pollutants do cause alterations in mucociliary clearance. Acute exposures to 5 ppm SO_2 have altered nasal clearance[2, 97] and bronchial clearance in humans. Exposure to sulfuric acid mist at levels as low as 250 $\mu g/m^3$ has depressed mucociliary clearance in donkeys.[84] On chronic exposure to H_2SO_4 Lippmann[50] has shown alterations at levels as low as 100 $\mu g/m^3$. Grose et al.[37] has shown impairment in ciliary activity at concentrations <1 mg/m^3. There has been impairment in tracheal mucus clearance in rats reported for chronic exposures to 5 ppm NO_2.[33]

Both speeding as well as slowing of clearance have been reported, depending on the concentration of pollutant and duration of exposure. High level chronic exposures almost always depress clearance. A speeding of clearance should not be interpreted as beneficial, since it may indicate a hypersecretory state following exposure to the irritant. Iravani and van As[42] have noted faster than normal mucociliary transport in bronchitic rats, even though there were some large eddy areas of very slow or uncoordinated mucus movement. These data indicate that the velocities of some mucus flakes may be higher than normal, but that if particles deposit in the large number of eddy areas they may be cleared very, very slowly. As is the case with many toxic or irritant materials at low doses or concentrations for short periods of time, there is a stimulation of clearance and then at higher concentrations or longer periods of time a depression results. Exactly this type of response was found by Ferin and Leach[31] when measuring SO_2 effects on deep lung clearance. It is possible that, with acute low level exposures, there is an initial increase in secretion which can be coped with and may result in a speeding of clearance from a dilution effect. However, for more chronic exposures or higher levels the degree of secretion may be too high or mucus properties changed such that the mucociliary apparatus is overwhelmed. Inhibition of the cilia is quite possible as well. Then airways obstruction can result and chronic bronchitis or emphysema develop.

This general picture appears to have validity in that many irritant gases have been shown to cause hypersecretion.[44]

It has not been proven that these observed clearance abnormalities proceed to chronic bronchitic states at low level exposures. However, it is highly suggestive that at least in some individuals this would occur. These mucociliary clearance changes, which occur with pollutant exposures, and also abnormalities reported in young smokers by Goodman et al.[36] indicate that mucus clearance abnormalities are a sensitive indicator of airways disease. Often the clearance changes are detected before any pulmonary function defects can be detected.

The underlying biochemical abnormalities which develop in the early stages of disease, causing the clearance changes, have not been well worked out. In one of the few reports available, Last et al.[49] have described glycoprotein abnormalities in animals exposed to 0.5 ppm 0_3. Spicer et al.[86] examined lesions of chronic SO_2 inhalation at a level which produced squamous metaplasia. Mucus goblet cells were sparse in the trachea, but had undergone hypertrophy and hyperplasia in the bronchi and bronchioles. The increased secretion had reduced PAS reaction, suggesting either diminished mucoprotein content or reactivity to PAS. Ciliated cells were diminished or absent in the presence of goblet cell hyperplasia. Sessile polyploid protrusions partially obstructed airways. Mucus occasionally extended distally into alveoli. Secretory cells of the distal respiratory tree were distended and increased in number. Jones and Reid[45] described an increased discharge rate of secretory cells on exposure to cigarette smoke. Also, there was a shift to acid glycoprotein and presumably higher viscosity mucus as discussed earlier. It appears that goblet cells distended with acid glycoprotein are typical of the irritant state.[44] Charles and Menzel[17] noted that ammonium and sulfate ions elicit histamine release from lung fragments. Possibly, if histamine is released in bronchioles, hypersecretion of mucus might occur, leading to a bronchitic state. If bronchioles become blocked, this would induce alveolar hypoxia and diffuse alveolar damage leading to emphysema and fibrosis.[24]

Baskerville[6] used isoprenaline to induce hypertrophy of mucous glands and mimic bronchitis. Isoprenaline induced an increase in size of glandular acini, an increased production of glycoprotein, and a greater proportion of acid glycoprotein, especially sialomucin. A striking globlet cell hyperplasia was seen in the bronchial epithelium. Maeta et al.[60] noted that a sialoglycopeptide was dramatically increased in human pulmonary tuberculosis. Baker et al.[4] reported that two galactosyl transferases, a sial transferase, and an *N*-acetyl galactosaminyl transferase were elevated 1 and 2 months after daily stimulation with methacholine chloride, which should act as a non-specific irritant. Fucosyl transferase was unchanged. These biochemical changes would account for the effects noted by Baskerville[6] and Maeta et al.[60]

Much work remains to be done to determine the initiating events leading to chronic obstructive disease. Biochemical alterations in secretions and clearance abnormalities appear to play a significant role and deserve further examination. Experimental exposures to environmental pollutants show promise of providing models to explore this area.

II. ASTHMA

Asthma is derived from a Greek word which means "to pant". Given such a general term, it is not surprising that there have been a large range of respiratory abnormalities described as asthma. In the last 15 years or so there has been more care taken to define the disease. It is useful to describe asthma as a disease that is characterized by increased responsiveness of the tracheobronchial tree to a multiplicity of stimuli which result in widespread airway constriction that can change in severity either spontaneously or as the result or treatment. Clinical signs are paroxysms of cough, dyspnea, and wheezing.[1a] Severe airway obstruction with resultant hypoxia are characteristic of an asthmatic attack. The airway constriction can be brought on by factors such as exercise or inhaling non-specific irritants. A key feature of the disease is reversibility. Following an acute attack, lung function usually returns to normal. The best understood type of asthma is the immunologically mediated airway response to inhaled antigenic material. This is the "allergic" asthma which one most often thinks of. A review of the clinical features of asthma has recently been given by McFadden and Feldman.[62a] A related disorder not covered in this discussion is hypersensitivity pneumonitis. This disease has been reviewed recently by Roberts and Moore[76a] and involves primarily the distal portions of the lung which have been sensitized after inhalation of a variety of organic dusts.

Several reviews of the effects of asthma on pulmonary function in man have been published.[6a,36a,96a] The principal physiologic feature of an asthmatic attack is a marked increase in airflow resistance caused by bronchoconstriction. All indices of forced expiratory flowrate are reduced and their there is a characteristic improvement following administration of bronchodilators. The vital capacity measured during forced expiration is reduced because of early airway closure at the lower lung volumes, but there may be little or no reduction of vital capacity measured by slow expiration. The lung pressure-volume curve is usually shifted to the right, and static compliance is slightly increased. The total lung capacity and inspiratory capacity are frequently increased, although the mechanism is yet unclear. Pressure-volume curves and inspiratory capacity usually return to normal after bronchodilator treatment. Intrapulmonary gas distribution is abnormally non-uniform, and arterial hypoxemia usually results from a mismatching of ventilation and perfusion. The diffusing capacity for carbon monoxide is usually normal or elevated in uncomplicated asthma. In mild asthma, the arterial carbon dioxide tension is normal, but in severe status asthmaticus, an increasing carbon dioxide tension and accompanying respiratory acidosis signal respiratory failure. Mechanical and gas exchange functions are often normal between attacks in milder cases, but some impairment of ventilatory function is usually present at all times.

There are few if any naturally occurring animal models of the human asthmatic condition, and, therefore, experimental animal studies have been conducted by challenging previously sensitized animals with inhaled antigens.[67b] These "asthma" models produce a transient bronchoconstrictive episode accompanied by functional changes which are similar to those occurring during human asthmatic attacks. Functional changes, marked primarily by an increased airflow resistance, have been produced in guinea pigs using several antigens,[67b] in dogs using extracts of *Ascaris suum*[34a,67b,99a,95a] and dinitrobenzene-ovalbumin,[45b] and in monkey using *Ascaris suum* extract.[67a] Unfortunately, none of these models produces chronic structural and functional alterations which closely resemble human asthma.

Asthma is a very difficult disease to study, given its heterogenity. There is a wide range of types and manifestations of the disease. The immunologic features of the disease are the best studied thus far, and even these are not as yet completely worked out.[68a,76b] Since the disease is poorly defined, biochemical features and aspects of mucociliary clearance are difficult to study and there is limited data available.

On an anatomical level, the features have been summarized by West[96a] as follows. Airways have hypertrophed smooth muscle which contrasts during an attack, causing the observed bronchoconstriction. There can be hypertrophy of mucous glands. During attacks there is edema of the bronchial wall and infiltration by eosinophils. Mucus can be thick, tenacious, and slow-moving. In severe attacks airways can be occuluded by mucus plugs, which may be coughed up in sputum (Curshmann's spirals).

Mucus viscosity has been studied by Lopez-Vidriero and Reid.[53,54] They found a mean increase in viscosity compared to their normals. The increase in viscosity was of the same order as for their chronic bronchitic group. However, the standard deviation of values was much higher than for any other of their disease categories. There was also a tremendous range of values for macromolecular content, fucose, and *N*-acetyl neuraminic acid. Varying degrees of mucous gland hypertrophy may account for these variations. Keal[45a] suggested there were at least two types of response which could lead to the formation of mucus plugs. One was dehydration and the other was a combination of shearing of mucus, changes in glycoprotein linkages, or alterations in bound calcium or other electrolytes. Barton et al.[5a] have suggested that there is an abnormal water-glycoprotein mixture of mucus, which may increase its viscosity and decrease its permeability to water.

Lopez-Vidriero and Reid,[53] in their study, divided asthmatics into subgroups: asthma of late onset (intrinsic) with and without chronic bronchitis, and extrinsic "allergic" asthma with and without chronic bronchitis. Extrinsic asthmatics without chronic bronchitis did not produce sputum between attacks and so probably had little or no gland hypertrophy. During attacks their bronchial glycoprotein profiles appeared normal, but there was a marked increase in serum proteins. Patients with intrinsic asthma with or without chronic bronchitis had glycoprotein profiles similar to chronic bronchitics, strongly suggesting mucus gland hypertrophy, probably as a result of recurrent infection.

There have been very few studies of mucociliary clearance related to asthma. The study of Santa Cruz et al.[83] suggested a slower tracheal mucus velocity for stable asthmatics. Wanner et al.[95a] carried out experiments in mongrel dogs sensitized to *Ascaris suum*. He found a marked depression of mucociliary clearance within 30 min of antigen exposure and continuing to at least 2 hr. These studies suggest a role for impairment of mucociliary clearance in the asthmatic state.

Alterations in mucus biochemistry, rheology, and clearance are a feature of asthma. Since the disease itself is sometimes complicated by chronic bronchitis, many of the same features prevail. However, asthma is a much more variable and capricious disease, which is reflected by the range of data obtained.

III. SUMMARY

Chronic bronchitis is characterized by excess accumulations of secretions in the airways. It seems clear that excessive production of secretion is a prime cause of this condition. Abnormalities in biochemical properties have also been clearly demonstrated, particularly a rise in acid glycoprotein production. Since much of the rigidity is imparted by acid glycoproteins, this rise is a major contribution to the general rise in viscosity in the chronic bronchitic state. Finally, as a consequence of the higher viscosity, mucociliary clearance is inhibited. It is quite clear that this is the case in advanced stages of chronic bronchitis. It also seems quite likely that alterations in mucociliary clearance resulting from cigarette smoking, pollutant exposures, or respiratory infections can play an important initiating role in the disease. At the least, they are sensitive indicators of early stages of chronic bronchitis.

Asthma is a much more capricious disease. When it is complicated by chronic bronchitis, not surprisingly, many of the features of mucus biochemistry, rheology, and clearance are similar. There is a much greater range of values for these parameters in asthma than in chronic bronchitis. However, even in asthmatics without chronic bronchitis, serum glycoproteins are increased during attacks and there is evidence that both mucous rheology and clearance are adversely affected. These could well be contributing factors in prolonging asthmatic attacks. but the degree of their importance in asthma is not well understood at this time.

REFERENCES

1. **Aharonson, E. F., Reasor, M., and Procter, D. F.,** A method for study of normal respiratory mucus, *Fed. Proc.*, 32, 402, 1973.

1a. American Thoracic Society, Definitions and classification of chronic bronchitis, asthma, and pulmonary emphysema, *Am. Rev. Respir. Dis.*, 85, 762, 1962.

2. **Andersen, I., Lundqvist, G. R., Jenson, P. L., and Proctor, D. F.,** Human response to controlled levels of sulfur dioxide, *Arch. Environ. Health*, 28, 31, 1974.

3. **Asmundsson, T. and Kilburn, K. H.,** Mucocilliary clearance rates at various levels in dog lungs, *Am. Rev. Respir. Dis.*, 102, 388, 1970.

4. **Baker, A. P., Chakrin, L. W., and Wardell, J. R.,** Chronic cholinergic stimulation of canine respiratory tissue, *Am. Rev. Respir. Dis.*, 111, 423, 1975.

5. **Bang, B. G. and Bang, F. B.,** Effect of water deprivation on nasal mucous flow, *Proc. Soc. Exp. Biol. Med.*, 106, 516, 1961.

5a. **Barton, A. D., Powers, J. L., and Lopata, M.,** Biochemical characteristics affecting the consistency of bronchial secretions, *Chest*, 63, (Suppl.), 595, 1973.

6. **Baskerville, A.,** The development and persistence of bronchial-gland hypertrophy and goblet-cell hyperplasia in the pig after injection of isoprenaline, *J. Pathol.*, 119, 35, 1976.

6a. **Bates, D. V., Macklem, P. T., and Christie, R. V.,** Spasmodic asthma, in *Respiratory Function in Disease*, 2nd ed., W. B. Saunders, Philadelphia, 1971.

7. **Battista, S. P., DiNunzio, J., and Kensler, C. J.,** Versatile apparatus to study effects of gases, aerosols and drugs on ciliary activity in non-immersed mammalian trachea, *Fed. Proc.*, 21, 701, 1962.

8. **Bohning, D. E., Albert, R. E., Lippmann, M., and Foster, W. M.,** Tracheobronchial particle deposition and clearance, *Arch. Environ. Health*, 30, 457, 1975.

9. **Bohning, D. E., Foster, W. M., and Bergofsky, E. H.,** Flow limiting segments in expiration induced central tracheobronchial particle deposition in COPD, *Fed. Proc.*, 113, 205, 1976.

10. **Boyd, E. M.,** in *Sputum: Fundamentals and Clinical Pathology*, Dulfano, M. J., Ed., Charles C Thomas, Springfield, Ill., 1973, 544.

11. **Breeze, R. G. and Sheldon, E. B.,** The cells of the pulmonary airways, *Am. Rev. Respir. Dis.*, 116, 705, 1977.

12. **Camner, P., Philipson, K., and Friberg, L.,** Tracheobronchial clearance in twins, *Arch. Environ. Health*, 24, 82, 1972.

13. **Camner, P. and Philipson, K.,** Tracheobronchial clearance in smoking: discordant twins, *Arch. Environ. Health*, 25, 60, 1972.

14. **Camner, P., Mossberg, B., and Philipson, K.,** Tracheobronchial clearance and chronic obstructive lung disease, *Scand. J. Respir. Dis.*, 54, 272, 1973.

15. **Camner, P., Philipson, K., and Arvidsson, T.,** Withdrawal of cigarette smoking, *Arch. Environ. Health*, 26, 90, 1973.

16. **Camner, P., Strandberg, K., and Philipson, K.,** Increased mucocilliary transport by adrenergic stimulation, *Arch. Environ. Health*, 29, 79, 1976.

17. **Charles, J. M. and Menzel, D. B.,** Ammonium and sulfate ion release of histamine from lung fragments, *Arch. Environ. Health*, 30, 314, 1975.

18. **Chodosh, S., Medici, T. C., Ishikowa, S., and Enslein, K.,** Relationship of physical sputum characteristics and ventilatory capacity in chronic bronchial disease, *Chest*, 63(Suppl.), 565, 1973.

19. **Chopra, S. K., Taplin, G. V., Simmons, D. H., Robinson, G. O., Jr., Elam, D., and Coulson, A.,** Effects of hydration and physical therapy on tracheal transport velocity, *Am. Rev. Respir. Dis.*, 115, 1009, 1977.

19a. **Cotton, D. J., Bleecker, E. R., Fischer, S. P., Graf, P. D., Gold, W. M., and Nadel, J. A.,** Rapid shallow breathing after *acaus suum*. Antigen inhalation: role of vagus nerves, *J. Appl. Physiol., Respirat. Environ. Exercise Physiol.*, 42, 101, 1977.

20. **Creeth, J. M. and Denborough, M. A.,** The use of equilibrium-density-gradient methods for the preparation and characterization of blood group specific glycoprotein, *Biochem. J.*, 117, 879, 1970.

21. **Creeth, J. M., Bhaskar, K. R., Horton, J., Das, I., Lopez-Vidriero, M. T., and Reid, L.,** The separation and characterization of bronchial glycoproteins by density gradient methods, *Biochem J.*, 167, 557, 1977.

22. **Dalhamn, T.,** Mucous flow and ciliary activity in the trachea of healthy rats and rats exposed to respiratory irritant gases, *Acta Physiol. Scand.*, 36(Suppl. 123), 1, 1956.
23. **Dalhamn, T.,** *In vivo* and *in vitro* ciliotoxin effects of tobacco smoke, *Arch. Environ. Health*, 21, 633, 1970.
24. **Demeszko, H. and Dabrowski, R.,** Effect of prolonged histamine administration on tissue respiration processes and collagen production in guinea pig lungs, *Bull. Acad. Pol. Sci.*, 17, 717, 1969.
25. **Dreisin, R. B. and Mostow, S. R.,** Adverse effect of N-acetyl-L-cysteine on isolated tracheal cilia, *Am. Rev. Respir. Dis.*, 117(Suppl.), 109, 1978.
26. **Dulfano, M. J. and Glass, P.,** An effective mucolytic aerosol in chronic bronchitis, *JAMA*, 207, 1310, 1968.
27. **Dulfano, M. J., Adler, K., and Phillipson, W.,** Sputum viscoelasticity in chronic bronchitis, *Am. Rev. Respir. Dis.*, 104, 88, 1971.
28. **Dulfano, M. J.,** Ed., *Sputum, Fundamanetals and Clinical Pathology*, Charles C. Thomas, Springfield, Ill., 1973.
29. **Dulfano, M. J. and Adler, K. B.,** Physical properties of sputum. VII. Rheologic properties and mucocilliary transport, *Am. Rev. Respir. Dis.*, 112, 341, 1975.
30. **Falk, H. L., Tremer, H. M., and Kotin, P.,** Effect of cigarette smoke and its constituents on ciliated mucus-secreting epithelium, *J. Natl. Cancer Inst.*, 23, 999, 1959.
31. **Ferin, J. and Leach, L. J.,** The effect of SO_2 on lung clearance of TiO_2 particles in rats, *Am. Ind. Hyg. Assoc. J.*, 34, 260, 1973.
32. **Foster, W. M., Bergofsky, E. H., Bohning, D. E., Lippmann, M., and Albert, R. E.,** Effect of adrenergic agents and their mode of action on mucocilliary clearance in man, *J. Appl. Physiol.*, 41, 146, 1976.
33. **Giordano, A. M. and Morrow, P. E.,** Chronic low-level nitrogen dioxide exposure and mucocilliary clearance, *Arch. Environ. Health*, 25, 443, 1972.

33a. **Giordano, A. M., Holsclaw, D., and Litt, M.,** Mucus rheology and mucociliary clearance: normal physiologic state, *Am. Rev. Respir. Dis.*, 118, 245, 1978.

34. **Goco, R. V., Kress, M. B., and Brantigan, O. C.,** Comparison of mucus glands in the tracheobronchial tree of man and animals, *Ann. N.Y. Acad. Sci.*, 106, 555, 1963.

34a. **Gold, W. M., Kessler, G. F., Yu, D. Y. C., and Frick, O. L.,** Pulmonary physiologic abnormalities in experimental asthma in dogs, *J. Appl. Physiol.*, 33, 496, 1972.

35. **Goodman, R. M., Yergin, B. M., Landa, J. F., Golinvaux, M. H., and Sackner, M. A.,** Tracheal mucus velocity in non-smokers, smokers and patients with obstructive lung disease, *Fed. Proc.*, 36, 607, 1977.
36. **Goodman, R. M., Yergin, B. M., Landa, J. F., Golinvaux, M. H., and Sackner, M. A.,** Relationship of smoking history and pulmonary function tests to tracheal mucous velocity in nonsmokers, young smokers, ex-smokers and patients with chronic bronchitis, *Am. Rev. Respir. Dis.*, 117, 205, 1978.

36a. **Gray, F. D.,** Bronchial asthma, in *Clinical Cardiopulmonary Physiology*, 3rd ed., Gordon, B. L., Carleton, R. A., and Faber, L. P., Eds., Grune & Stratton, New York, 1969.

37. **Grose, E. C., Miller, F. J., and Gardner, D. E.,** The effects of ozone and sulfuric acid on ciliary activity of Syrian hamsters, *Am. Rev. Respir. Dis.*, 117(Suppl.), 237, 1978.
38. **Hilding, A. C.,** Mucocilliary insufficiency and its possible relation to chronic bronchitis and emphysema, *Med. Thorac.*, 22, 329, 1965.
39. **Hirsch, J. A., Swenson, E. W., and Wanner, A.,** Tracheal mucous transport in Beagles after long-term exposure to 1 ppm sulfur dioxide, *Arch. Environ. Health*, 30, 249, 1975.
40. **Hogg, J. C., Macklem, P. T., and Thurlbeck, W. M.,** Site and nature of airway obstruction in obstructive lung disease, *N. Engl. J. Med.*, 278, 1355, 1968.
41. **Iravani, J.,** Flimmerbewegung in den intrapulmonalen Luftwegene der Ratte, *Pfluegers Arch.*, 297, 221, 1967.
42. **Iravani, J. and van As, A.,** Mucus transport in the tracheobronchial tree of normal and bronchitic rats, *J. Pathol.*, 106, 81, 1972.
43. **Jefferey, P. K. and Reid, L.,** New features of rat airway epithelium: a quantitative and electron-microscopic study, *J. Anat.*, 120, 295, 1975.
44. **Jeffery, P. K. and Reid, L.,** Respiratory mucous membrane, in *Respiratory Defense Mechanisms*, Brain, J. D., Proctor, D. F., and Reid, L. M., Eds., Marcel Dekker, New York, 1977, 193.
45. **Jones, R. and Reid, L.,** Timing and pattern of secretory cell hyperplasia in airway epithelium, *Am. Rev. Respir. Dis.*, 117(Suppl.), 354, 1978.

45a. **Keal, E. E.,** Biochemistry and rheology of sputum in asthma, *Postgrad. Med. J.*, 47, 171, 1971.

45b. **Kepron, W., James, J. M., Kirk, B., Schon, A., and Tse, K. S.,** A canine model for reaginic hypersensitivity and allergic bronchoconstruction, *J. Allergy Clin. Immunol.*, 59, 64, 1977.

46. **King, M., Gilboa, A., Meyer, F. A., and Silberberg, A.,** On the transport of mucus and its rheologic simulants in ciliated systems, *Am. Rev. Respir. Dis.*, 110, 742, 1974.

47. **King, M. and Viires, N.,** Influence of metacholine chloride on the mechanical properties of canine tracheal mucus, *Fed. Proc.*, 37, 221, 1978.

47a. **King, M., Cohen, C., and Viires, N.,** Influence of vagal tone on rheology and transportability of canine tracheal mucus, *Am. Rev. Resp. Dis.*, 120, 1215, 1979.

48. **Korhonen, L. K., Holopainen, E., and Paavolainen, M.,** Some histochemical characteristics of tracheobronchial tree and pulmonary neoplasms, *Acta Histochem.*, 32, 57, 1969.

49. **Last, J. A., Jennings, M. D., Schwartz, L. W., and Cross, C. E.,** Glycoprotein secretion by tracheal explants cultured from rats exposed to ozone, *Am. Rev. Respir. Dis.*, 116, 695, 1977.

50. **Lippmann M.,** Personal communication, 1978.

51. **Lopez-Vidriero, M. T., Charman, J., Keal, E., de Silver, P. J., and Reid, L.,** Sputum viscosity: correlation with chemical and clinical features in chronic bronchitis, *Thorax*, 28, 401, 1973.

52. **Lopez-Vidriero, M. T., Das, I., and Reid, L. M.,** Airway secretion: source, biochemical and rheological properties, in *Respiratory Defense Mechanism, 1st ed.*, Brain, J. D., Proctor, D. F., and Reid, L. M., Eds., Marcel Dekker, New York, 1977, 289.

53. **Lopez-Vidriero, M. T. and Reid, L.,** Chemical markers from mucous and serum glycoprotein and their relation to viscosity in mucoid and purulent sputum from various hypersectory diseases, *Am. Rev. Respir. Dis.*, 117, 465, 1978.

54. **Lopez-Vidriero, M. T. and Reid, L.,** Bronchial mucus in health and disease, *Br. Med. Bull.*, 34, 63, 1978.

55. **Lourenco, R. V.,** Distribution and clearance of aerosols, *Am. Rev. Respir. Dis.*, 101, 460, 1970.

56. **Lourenco, R. V., Kllmer, M. F., and Borowski, C. J.,** Deposition and clearance of 2μ particles in the tracheobronchial tree of normal subjects: smokers and nonsmokers, *J. Clin. Invest.*, 50, 1411, 1971.

57. **Lucas, A. M. and Douglas, L. C.,** Principles underlying ciliary activity in the respiratory tract. II. A comparison of nasal clearance in man, monkeys and other mammals, *Arch. Oto-Laryngol.*, 20, 518, 1934.

58. **Luchsinger, P. C., Lagarde, B., and Kilfeather, J. E.,** Particle clearance from the human tracheobronchial tree, *Am. Rev. Respir. Dis.*, 97, 1046, 1968.

59. **Luchtel, D. L.,** Ultrastructural observations on the mucous layer in pulmonary airways, *J. Cell Biol.*, 70, 350a, 1976.

60. **Maeta, T., Endo, M., and Yosizawa, Z.,** Glycoproteins and glycosaminoglycans in human pulmonary tuberculosis, *Clin. Chim. Act*, 57, 255, 1974.

61. **Masson, P. L. and Heremans, J. F.,** Sputum proteins, in *Sputum: Fundamentals and Clinical Pathology*, Dulfano, M. J., Ed., Charles C Thomas, Springfield, 1973, 412.

62. **Matsuba, K. and Thurlbeck, W.,** Disease of the small airways in chronic bronchitis, *Am. Rev. Respir. Dis.*, 107, 552, 1973.

62a. **McFadden, Jr., E. R. and Feldman, N. T.,** Asthma: pathophysiology and clinical correlates, *Med. Clin. North Am.*, 61, 1229, 1977.

63. Medical Research Council, Definition and classification of chronic bronchitis for clinical and epidemiological purposes, *Lancet*, 1; 775, 1965.

64. **Miller, W. S.,** The epithelium of the lower respiratory tract, in *Special Cytology*, 2nd ed., Cowdry, E. V., Ed., Hofner, New York, 1932, 133.

65. **Morrow, P. E., Gibb, F. R., and Gazioglu, K. M.,** A study of particulate clearance from the human lungs, *Am. Rev. Respir. Dis.*, 96, 1209, 1967.

66. **Newhouse, M. T., Sanchis, J., and Bienenstock, J.,** Lung defense mechanisms, *N. Engl. J. Med.*, 295, 990, 1976.

67. **Niewoehner, D. E., Kleinerman, J., and Rice, D. B.,** Pathologic changes in the peripheral airways of young cigarette smokers, *N. Engl. J. Med.*, 291, 755, 1974.

67a. **Patterson, R., Talbot, C. H., and Booth, B. H.,** IgE mediated respiratory responses of subhuman primates, reproducibility and effect of certain pharmacologic agents, *Am. Rev. Respir. Dis.*, 102, 412, 1970.

67b. **Patterson, R. and Kelly, J. F.,** Animal models of the asthmatic state, *Annu. Rev. Med.*, 25, 53, 1974.

68. **Pavia, D., Thomson, M. L., and Phillipakas, D.,** A preliminary study of the effect of a vibrating pad on bronchial clearance, *Am. Rev. Respir. Dis.*, 113, 92, 1976.

68a. **Pepys, J.,** Immunopathology of allergic lung disease, *Clin. Allergy*, 3, 1, 1973.

69. **Pham, Q. T., Peslin, R., Puchelle, E., Salmon, D., Caraux, G., and Benis, A. M.,** Respiratory function and the rheological status of bronchial secretions collected by spontaneous expectoration and after physiotherapy, *Bull. Physio. Pathol. Respir.*, 9, 293, 1973.

70. **Proctor, D. F.,** The upper airways. I. Nasal physiology and defense of the lungs, *Am. Rev. Respir. Dis.*, 115; 97, 1977; II. The Larynx and trachea, 315.

71. **Puchelle, E., Zahm, J. M., and Have, R.**, Relation des proteins et mucines bronchiques aves les proprietes rheologignes. *Bull. Physio Pathol. Respir.*, 9, 237, 1973.
72. **Reid, L. M.**, Correlation of certain bronchographic abnormalities seen in chronic bronchitis with the pathological changes, *Thorax*, 10, 199, 1955.
73. **Reid, L.**, Measurement of the bronchial mucus gland layer: a diagnostic yardstick in chronic bronchitis, *Thorax*, 15, 132, 1960.
74. **Reid, L. M.**, Secretory cells, *Fed. Proc.*, 36, 2703, 1977.
75. **Rhodin, J. and Dalhamn, T.**, Electron microscopy of the tracheal ciliated mucosa in rat, *Z. Zellforsch. Mikrosk, Anat.*, 44, 345, 1956.
76. **Rhodin, J. A. G.**, Ultrastructure and function of the human tracheal mucosa, *Am. Rev. Respir. Dis.*, 93;(Suppl 3), 1, 1966.
76a. **Roberts, R. C. and Moore, V. L.**, Immunopathogenesis of hypersensitivity pneumonities, *Am. Rev. Respir. Dis.*, 116; 1075, 1977.
76b. **Robertson, D. G., Kerigan, A. T., Hargreave, F. E., Chalmers, R., and Dolovich, J.**, Late asthmatic responses induced by ragweed pollen allergin, *J. Allerg Clin. Immunol.*, 54, 244, 1974.
77. **Ruffin, R. E., Wolff, R. K., Dolovich, M. B., Rossman, C. M., Fitzgerald, J. D., and Newhouse, M. T.**, Aerosol Thearpy with SCH 1000: short term mucociliary clearance in normal and bronchitic subjects and toxocity in normal subjects, *Chest*, 73, 501, 1978.
78. **Sackner, M. A., Chapman, G. A., and Dougherty, R. D.**, Effects of nebulized ipratopium bromide and atropine sulfate on treacheal mucous velocity and lung mechanics in anesthetized dogs, *Respiration*, 34; 181, 1977.
79. **Sadé, J., Eliezer, N., Silberberg, A., and Nevo, A. C.**, The role of mucus in transport by cilia, *Am. Rev. Respir. Dis.*, 102, 48, 1970.
80. **Sadoul, P. and Puchelle, E.**, Transport and rheology of bronchial secretions in chronic bronchitis, *Am. Rev. Respir. Dis.*, (Suppl), 115; 241, 1977.
81. **Sanchis, J., Dolovich, M., Chambers, R., and Newhouse, M. T.**, Regional distribution and lung clearance mechanisms in smokers and non-smokers, in *Inhaled Particles and Vapours III*, Walton, W. H., Ed., Unwin Brothers, Old Woking, Surrey, 1972, 183.
82. **Sanchis, J., Dolovich, M., Rossman, C., and Newhouse, M. T.**, Lung clearance in patients with airways obstruction, *Bull. Physio Pathol. Respir.*, 9, 325, 1973.
83. **Santa Cruz, R., Landa, J., Hirsch, J., and Sackner, M. A.**, Tracheal mucous velocity in normal man and patients with obstructive lung disease: effects of terbutaline, *Am. Rev. Respir. Dis.*, 109, 458, 1974.
84. **Schlesinger, R. B., Lippmann, M., and Albert, R. E.**, Effects of short-term exposures to sulfuric acid and ammonium sulfate aerosols upon bronchial airway function in the donkey, *Amer. Ind. Hyg. Assoc. J.*, 39, 275, 1978.
85. **Serafini, S. M. and Michaelson, E. D.**, Length and distribution of cilia in human and canine airways, *Bull. Eur. Physio pathol. Respir.*, 13, 551, 1977.
85a. **Shih, C. K., Litt, M., Khan, M. A., and Wolf, D. P.**, Effect of nondialyzable solids concentration and viscoelasticity on ciliary transport of tracheal mucus, *Am. Rev. Respir. Dis.*, 115, 989, 1977.
86. **Spicer, S. S., Chakrin, L. W., and Wardell, J. R.**, Effect of chronic sulfur dioxide inhalation on the carbohydrate histochemistry and histology of the canine respiratory tract, *Am. Rev. Respir. Dis.*, 110, 13, 1974.
87. **Sturgess, J. M., Palfrey, A. J., and Reid, L.**, The viscosity of bronchial secretions, *Clin. Sci.*, 38, 145, 1970.
88. **Sturgess, J. M.**, The mucous lining of major bronchi in the rabbit lung, *Am. Rev. Respir. Dis.*, 115; 819, 1977.
89. **Thomson, M. L. and Short, M. D.**, Mucociliary function in health, chronic obstructive airway disease and asbestosis, *J. Appl. Physiol.*, 26, 535, 1969.
90. **Thomson, M. L., Pavia, D., and McNicol, M. W.**, A preliminary study of the effect of guaiphenesin on mucociliary clearance from the human lung, *Thorax*, 28, 742, 1973.
91. **Thomson, M. L., Pavia, D., Gregg, I., and Stark, J. E.**, Bromhexine and mucociliary clearance in chronic bronchitis, *Br. J. Dis. Chest*, 68; 21, 1974.
92. **Thomson, M. L., Pavia, D., Jones, C. J., and McQuiston, T. A.**, No demonstrable effect of S-carboxymethylcysteine on clearance of secretions from the human lung, *Thorax*, 30, 669, 1975.
93. **Toremalm, N. G.**, The daily amount of tracheobronchial secretions in man. A method for continuous tracheal aspiration in laryngectomised and tracheotomised patients, *Acta Oto-Laryngol. Suppl.*, 158, 43, 1960.
94. **Van As, A.**, Pulmonary airway clearance mechanisms: a reappraisal, *Am. Rev. Respir. Dis.*, 115, 721, 1977.
95. **Wanner, A., Hirsch, J. A., Greeneltch, D. E., Swenson, E. W., and Fore, T.**, Tracheal mucous velocity in beagles after chronic exposure to cigarette smoke, *Arch. Environ. Health*, 27; 370, 1973.

95a. **Wanner, A., Zarzecki, S., Hirscha, J., and Epstein, S.,** Tracheal mucous transport in experimental canine asthma, *J. Appl. Physiol.*, 39, 950, 1975.

96. **Wanner, A.,** Clinical aspects of mucociliary transport, *Am. Rev. Respir. Dis.*, 116, 73, 1977.

96a. **West, J. B.,** Obstructive diseases, in *Pulmonary Pathophysiology—the Essentials,* Williams & Wilkins, Baltimore, 1977, 80.

97. **Wolff, R. K., Dolovich, M., Rossman, C. M., and Newhouse, M. T.,** Sulfur dioxide and tracheobronchial clearance in man, *Arch. Environ. Health,* 30, 521, 1975.

98. **Wolff, R. K., Dolovich, M. D., Obminski, G., and Newhouse, M. T.,** Effects of exercise and eucapnic hyperventilation on bronchial clearance in man, *J. Appl. Physiol., Respirat. Environ. Exercise Physiol.*, 43, 46, 1977.

99. **Wolff, R. K., Newhouse, M. T., Dolovich, M., and Obminski, G.,** Effect of TLV levels of SO_2 and H_2SO_4 on bronchial clearance in exercising man, *Arch. Environ. Health,* 33, 24, 1978.

99a. **Yamatake, Y., Sasogawa, S., Yanawa, S., and Kobayaski, N.,** Allergy induced asthma with *ascaris suum* administration to dogs, *Jpn. J. Pharmacol.*, 27, 285, 1977.

100. **Yeates, D. B., Aspin, N., Levison, H., Jones, M. T., and Bryan, A. C.,** Mucociliary tracheal transport rates in man, *J. Appl. Physiol.*, 39, 487, 1975.

101. **Yergin, B., Goodman, R. M., Landa, J. F., Golinvaux, M. H., and Sackner, M. A.,** Effects of cigarette smoking on tracheal mucous velocity in young smokers with and without small airway obstruction, *Am. Rev. Respir., Dis.* (Suppl.), 115, 183, 1977.

Chapter 16

PULMONARY NEOPLASIA

J. A. Pickrell

TABLE OF CONTENTS

I. GENERAL

Although little is known about the mechanisms responsible for producing either neoplasia in general or pulmonary neoplasia, one may review a few general facts concerning pulmonary neoplasia. Neoplastic growths are the product of uncontrolled cell division of the transformed cell of origin. As such, they require (1) mutagenesis, (2) low enough injury so that the mutant cell survives and divides, (3) minor enough alteration of the mutant so that the immune system does not recognize and eliminate the mutant cell, and (4) a vascularizing factor so that rapid growth may be sustained.

Mutagenic events are thought to be specific and of extremely diverse etiologies. The nature of such events has not currently been deduced from the known mechanisms of the etiologic agents. A high level of injury would be injurious to the survival and cell division of the mutated cell. Thus, lower levels of lung injury would be favorable to the production of cancer. A major function of the immune system is to eliminate foreign cells, including neoplastic ones. The highly successful mutant cell would be one changed little enough or in such a way that the immune system did not feel compelled to "search and destroy" the newly transformed cell. Recently, a factor which promotes tumor vascularization as a prerequisite to malignant growth and metastasis has been reviewed.[7]

II. CHANGES FROM SELECTED CARCINOGENS

In this section, an attempt is made to illustrate relation of specific types of primary cancers of the lungs and thoracic cavity to interstitial fibrosis by reporting results from two known carcinogens, asbestos and radiation. No attempt is made to review all causes of primary lung cancer or to discuss the wide variety of metastatic ones. This exceeds the scope of the report. Moreover, the types of cancer discussed relate most prominently to development of interstitial fibrosis. Exposure to asbestos is associated with two types of cancer, bronchogenic carcinoma and mesothelioma.[6,23,26] In bronchogenic carcinoma the asbestos may act as a secondary carcinogen or promoting agent. For instance, fibers less than 10 to 20 micrometers induce tissue reaction and fibroblast proliferation in vitro.[16,17] However, in mesothelioma the evidence strongly indicates that asbestos may act as a direct carcinogen. Asbestos may act as a mediator of carcinogenesis by inhibiting the electron transport system so that the intermediate in 3,4 benzopyrene degradation has a longer residence time, raising the dose to adjacent tissue. Note that a characteristic which leads to fibrosis may also enhance the possibility of cancer, possibly for an entirely different reason. Alternatively, it may increase cell permeability so that carcinogens can enter[6] or act as a direct carcinogen.

Tumors are frequently associated with interstitial fibrosis. Fraire and Greenberg[8] reported the presence of one each of pulmonary adenocarcinoma, undifferentiated small cell carcinoma, and squamous cell carcinoma in 16 cases of interstitial fibrosis. All three tumors occurred in regions of severe fibrosis. Meyer and Leibow[19] have observed similar patterns. Cember et al.[3] reported that radioactive cerium fluoride produced a bronchogenic carcinoma in rats. Metivier et al.[18] reported that two epidermoid carcinomas and two secreting adenocarcinomas (muciginous), two cases of malpigian metaplasia and one of bronchial metaplasia were noted in 17 baboons which had 10-100 nCi of alpha emitting radio-nuclide per gram of lung tissue at sacrifice, 30 to 180 days after exposure.

Jones et al.[11] and Benjamin et al.[1] reviewed pulmonary carcinogenesis from chronic beta irradiation of lung and compared it to chronic alpha irradiation of lung in beagle dogs. The pattern of carcinogenesis seems different for beta-gamma irradiation than

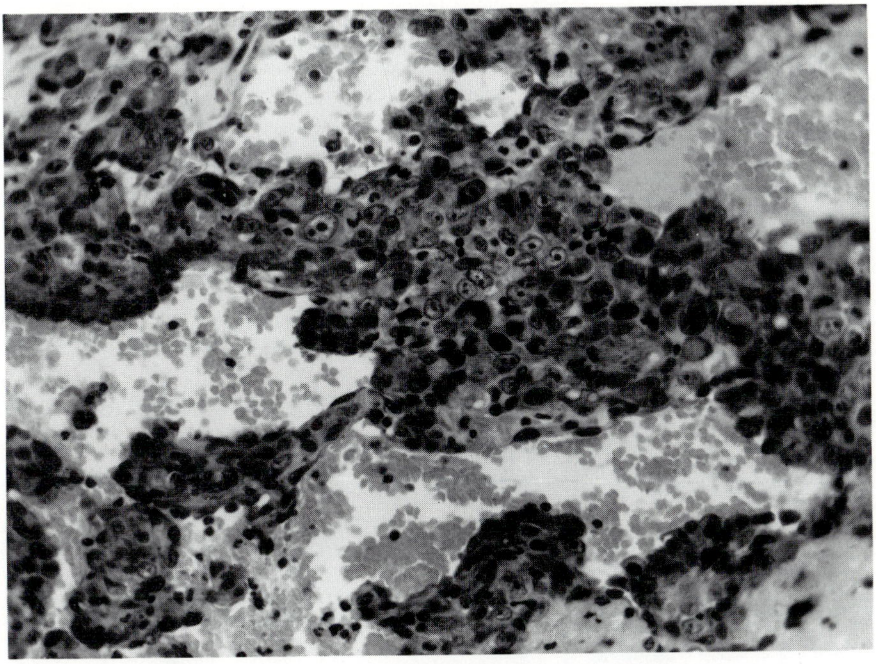

FIGURE 1. Pulmonary hemangiosarcoma induced in dog by inhaled radionuclide. (× 257, H and E stain.)

for alpha irradiation. Beta gamma irradiation produces primarily hemangiosarcomas (21 out of 24) (Figure 1) and only 2 out of 24 bronchoalveolar carcinomas (Figure 2). Alpha irradiation produces mostly bronchoalveolar carcinomas (24 of 36) and only 2 of 36 hemangiosarcomas. The peripheral bronchoalveolar carcinomas are generally associated with significant pulmonary fibrosis, epithelial hyperplasia, and metaplasia. The mechanism is not clear. However, the association may indicate no more than that the level of injury which produced carcinomas was sufficiently high and persistent to produce squamous metaplasia of bronchioles and pulmonary fibrosis (presumably of alveoli). These findings were minimal in dogs with hemangiosarcoma. Perhaps the dogs with hemangiosarcoma did not live long enough to develop carcinomas. If one analyzes our postulated requirements for neoplasia, each of these injury models certainly (1) provides a mutagenic stimulus, (2) provides low enough injury that the tumor can survive and the cells divide, and (3) provides the vascularizing factor necessary for metastasis. Just how much the cells must be altered so that the immune system will recognize it is unclear. For instance, in the case of chronic beta-gamma radiation, Benjamin et al.[1] have shown a lymphopenia and a reduced ability of circulating lymphocytes (on a per cell basis) to respond to phytohemagglutin. He interprets this as one indication of radiation's suppression of immune function. If this is a general phenomenon, then the immune system may be less able to remove foreign cells. Thus, some very different cells may be able to proliferate and form tumors.

Likewise, extremely high level injuries are inconducive to survival and thus multiplication of the existing tumor. This is borne out by many of the experiments reported in this section. For instance in the beta-gamma irradiation and the alpha radiation of Jones et al.,[11] the tumor animals reportedly have higher doses than surviving animals, but lower doses than those which contracted fibrosis. Although the tumors are associated with some fibrosis, indicating previous injury, the level of injury is clearly con-

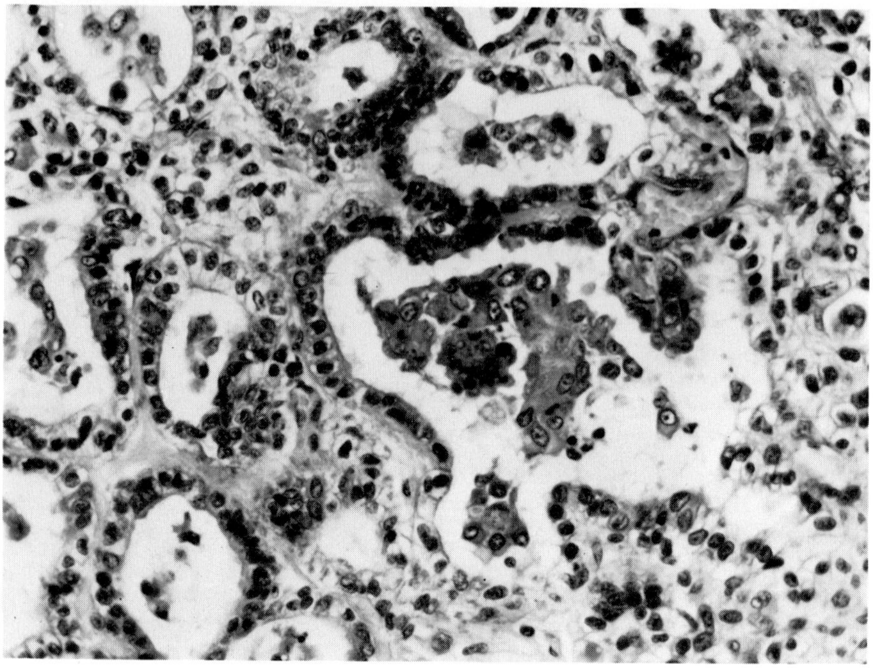

FIGURE 2. Brochioloalveolar carcinoma induced in a dog by inhaled radionuclide. (× 290, H and E stain.)

ducive to mutagenesis since it also has adjacent hyperplastic and metaplastic areas. Although details were not specified, the same reasoning probably applies to the data of Metivier et al.,[18] to Cember et al.,[3] and to Fraire and Greenberg.[8] The relation of asbestos[6] is less clear.

III. BIOCHEMICAL AND CELLULAR CHANGES

Expression of tumor malignancy requires vascularization, which is promoted by tumor angiogenisis factor (TAF).[7] Folkman[7] has reviewed the vascularization of tumors. Each cell division has a possibility for developing malignancy, although only a few develop. They studied the time when a malignant colony of cells was established, but before it had acquired its capacity for rapid proliferation and invasiveness. This is a harmless avascular stage of tumor development where newly generated cells are balanced by dying cells. The micro tumor adheres well to underlying tissue and does not migrate. Only when it induces the host to provide it with its own network of blood vessels does it become invasive. Tumor angiogenesis factor (TAF) induces blood vessels to bud and supply it with vascularity. The vascularized tumor compresses, invades, and destroys neighboring tissue. This budding is accompanied by increased DNA synthesis by 8 to 10 hr after inoculation with TAF, and thus reflects cell division. Moreover, it is unaccompanied by inflammation.

Inhibition of this process has interesting medical applications. Cartilage pieces seem to inhibit this process. Collagenase is associated with rapid fibroblast proliferation. Pinto et al.[21] noted a decrease in collagen in the dermal area painted with 2-aminoanthracene, which may relate to increased collagenase. Kuettner et al.[12] have isolated a low molecular weight collagenase inhibitor from aorta or cartilage (approximately 11,000 daltons) which may modulate the physiological regulation of collagen in vivo.

The possibility that it may be the cartilage factor which prevents neovascularization should be given some consideration in light of its inhibition of tumor collagenases[13] and its ability to inhibit fibrosarcoma and mammary tumor growth in mice.[5] The material injected was a previously isolated inhibitor of collagenase and proteinase[12] which was presumed to be the effector molecule. Normal embryonic tissue vessels attach to those of the host. Graft vessels survive approximately three days while inducing neovascularization from the host. However, tumor vessels disintegrate within 1 day, inducing the same response.[7] This process describes an intriguing mechanism by which the tumors can become invasive. The possibility of connective tissue modulation, via collagenase and its inhibitor, in this process is largely speculative. Especially intriguing in light of Chapter 10 might be the concept of a reduction of collagen but not collagenase production. Thus, collagenase would be free to bind to collagen in the area remote to the rapidly proliferating cell, freeing the way for it to grow still further if any proteolysis were present. Low level proteolysis would be anticipated to be present in developing neoplasia so that this mechanism could provide for rapid growth of the tumor cell. However, Thurlbeck[25] reviewed lung growth mechanisms and indicated that species fibroblasts, not epithelial cells, held the specificity of anatomic configuration in normal budding lung. Likewise the observation that disoriented collagen of bronchial mesoderm is stimulatory to branching of bronchial buds lend support to this importance.[22] Certainly connective tissue strata are important for vascularization and rapid growth in any system.[22]

Boone[2] subcutaneously injected contact-inhibited anchorage dependent Balb/3T3 cells anchored to glass beads into syngenic mice. Hemangiosarcomas associated with the beads developed in 8 weeks. Presumably the higher concentration of serum induced them to divide, overriding the anchorage dependence. The formation of hemangiosarcomas and their morphologic resemblance to endothelial cells suggest that Balb/3T3 cells are endothelial cells. This work provides a potentially correct but simplified concept of an exquisitely specific mutagenic stimulus.

The differences between cell division in normal contact-inhibited 3T3 fibroblasts and transformed ones deserves examination. Normal cells are stimulated to divide. This stimulus triggers a cyclic phosphatidyl inositol response reviewed by Mitchell[20] and Ciechanover and Hershko,[4] which presumably relates to cellular movement or rearrangement of membrane necessary to initiate cellular growth. Secondly, there is an increased cyclic GMP/AMP ratio[24] which may be related to fibroblast growth factor release.[9] Thirdly, inorganic phosphate is increased,[10] which activates glycolysis and, coupled with increased NADP/NADPH, activates the alternate pentose pathway and lipid, nucleic acid, and protein synthesis, leading to cell division.

Some interesting differences are noted between these normal cells and transformed ones. Transformed 3T3 fibroblasts do not have a PI response from serum addition.[4] Likewise, they have no increase in the ratio of cyclic GMP/AMP; however, the ratio which they maintain may be conducive to cell division and presumably to release of fibroblast growth factor.[24] Likewise, there is no increase of inorganic phosphorous prior to cell division, but the amount here is like contact-inhibited 3T3 cells. Presumably an alternate method of activating glycolysis and the pentose pathway to provide the lipids, proteins, and nucleic acids of cell division must be present. Kuhn and deKock[15] reported that alkaline phosphatase is elevated in bronchial aspirates of lung cancer and bronchitis. In bronchitis, it presumably represents death of cells which carry the enzyme. In bronchus carcinoma it may represent cell death or possibly secretion from the tumor. Alkaline phosphatase has the ability to cleave phospholipids and may represent this motility of lipids in membrane of a rapidly dividing cell system.

IV. SUMMARY

The mechanism of pulmonary neoplasia remains unclear. However, low continued stimulus seems to be a common denominator in its development. It is not clear why, with the formidable lung defense mechanisms which exist, such a simple common occurrence should not be dealt with easily. Much future work remains to be done concerning the pathogenesis of pulmonary neoplasia. It is vital that we understand and find a way to manipulate pulmonary neoplasia, because it will become an increasingly severe problem if pulmonary toxicants increase in our atmosphere. One may expect fascinating work concerning pulmonary neoplasia in the future.

REFERENCES

1. **Benjamin, S. A., Hahn, F. F., Chiffelle, T. L., Boecker, B. B., Hobbs, C. H., Jones, R. K., McClellan, R. O., and Snipes, M. B.,** Occurrence of hemangiosarcomas in Beagles with internally deposited radionuclides, *Cancer Res.*, 35, 1745, 1975.
2. **Boone, C. W.,** Malignant hemangioendotheliomas produced by subcutaneous inoculation of BALB/3T3 cells attached to glass beads, *Science,* 188, 68, 1975.
3. **Cember, H., Watson, J. A., and Spritzer, A. A.,** Bronchogenic carcinoma from radioactive cerium fluoride, *Arch. Ind. Health,* 19, 14, 1959.
4. **Ciechanover, A. and Hershko, A.,** Early effects of serum on phospholipid metabolism in untransformed and oncogenic virus-transformed cultured fibroblasts, *Biochem. Biophys. Res. Commun.,* 73, 85, 1976.
5. **Eisenstein, R., Schumacher, B., Meineke, C., Matijevitch, B., and Kuettner, K. E.,** Growth regulators in connective tissue. Systemic administration of an aortic extract inhibits tumor growth in mice, *Am. J. Pathol.,* 91(1), 1, 1978.
6. **Flowers, E. S.,** Relationship between exposure to asbestos, collagen formation, ferruginous bodies, and carcinoma, *Am. Ind. Hyg. Assoc. J.,* 35, 724, 1974.
7. **Folkman, J.,** The vascularization of tumors, *Sci. Am.,* 234(5); 59, 1976.
8. **Fraire, A. E. and Greenberg, S. D.,** Carcinoma and diffuse interstitial fibrosis of lung, *Cancer,* 31, 1078, 1973.
9. **Gospodarowicz, D.,** Purification of a fibroblast growth factor from bovine pituitary, *J. Biol. Chem.,* 250, 2515, 1975.
10. **Gray, P. N., Cullum, M. E., and Griffin, M. J.** Population density and regulation of cell division in 3T3 cells, *J. Cell Physiol.,* 89, 225, 1976.
11. **Jones, R. K., Hahn, F. F., Hobbs, C. H., Benjamin, S. A., Boecker, B. B., McClellan, R. O., and Slauson, D. O.,** Pulmonary carcinogenesis and chronic beta irradiation of lung, in *Experimental Lung Cancer. Carcinogenesis and Bioassays,* Karbe, E., and Park, J. F., Eds., Springer-Verlag, New York, 1974, 454.
12. **Kuettner, K. E., Hiti, J., Eisenstein, R., and Harper, E.,** Collagenase inhibition by cationic proteins derived from cartilage and aorta, *Biochem. Biophys. Res. Commun.,* 72, 40, 1976.
13. **Kuettner, K. E., Soble, L., Croxen, R. L., Marczynska, B., Hiti, J., and Harper, E.,** Tumor cell collagenase and its inhibition by a cartilage-derived protease inhibitor, *Science,* 196, 653, 1977.
14. **Kuettner, K. E., Soble, L., Croxen, R., Hiti, J., Harper, E., and Pauli, B.,** Inhibition of tumor collagenases by a cartilage-derived inhibitor, *Fed. Proc. Abstr.,* 36, 677, 1977.
15. **Kuhn, S. H. and deKock, M. A.,** A preliminary study of elevated alkaline phosphatase and cathepsin in bronchial aspirates of patients with lung cancer and bronchitis, *Chest,* 68, 326, 1975.
16. **Kuschner, M. and Wright, G.,** The effects of intratracheal instillation of glass fiber of varying sizes in guinea pigs, in *Occupational Exposure to Fibrous Glass,* symposium sponsored by National Institute of Occupational Safety and Health, College Park, Md., June, 1974, U.S. Government Printing Office, 1976, 151.
17. **Maroudas, N. G. and O'Neill, C. H.,** Fibroblast anchorage in carcinogenesis by fibres, *Lancet,* 1, 807, 1973.

18. **Metivier, H., Nolibe, D., Masse, R., and LaFuma, J.,** Cancers provoked in the babboon monkey (*Papio papio*) by the inhalation of PuO_2, *C. R. Acad. Sci.*, 275; 3069, 1972.
19. **Meyer, E. C. and Liebow, A. A.,** Relationship of interstitial pneumonia honeycombing, and atypical epithelial proliferation to cancer of the lung, *Cancer*, 18, 322, 1965.
20. **Mitchell, R. H.,** Inositol phospholipids and cell surface receptor function, *Biochim. Biophys. Acta*, 415, 81, 1975.
21. **Pinto, J. S., Dobson, R. L., and Bentley, J. P.,** Dermal collagen changes during 2-aminoanthracene carcinogenesis in the rat, *Cancer Res.*, 30, 1168, 1970.
22. **Reddi, A. H.,** Collagen and cell differentiation, in *Biochemistry of Collagen*, Ramachandran, G. N. and Reddi, A. H., Eds., Plenum Press, New York, 1976, 449.
23. **Reeves, A. L., Puro, H. E., and Smith, R. G.,** Inhalation carcinogenesis from various forms of asbestos, *Environ. Res.*, 8, 178, 1974.
24. **Rudland, P. S., Seeley, M., and Seifert, W.,** Cyclic GMP and cyclic AMP levels in normal and transformed fibroblasts, *Nature (London)*, 251, 417, 1974.
25. **Thurlbeck, W. M.,** Postnatal growth and development of the lung, *Am. Rev. Respir. Dis.*, 111, 803, 1975.
26. **Wagner, J. C., Berry, G., Skidmore, J. W., and Timbrell, V.,** The effects of the inhalation of asbestos in rats, *Br. J. Cancer*, 29, 252, 1974.

Chapter 17

SUMMARY

J. A. Pickrell

TABLE OF CONTENTS

I. LOCATION AND STRUCTURE

Collagen is found in the interstitium and basement membrane of large and small airways, in vessels, and in cartilage plates. Tropocollagen is a triple helix, a rope-like spiral of three linear alpha chains, each of approximately 1050 amino acids. Hydroxyproline and glycosylation of hydroxylysine stabilize the helix, which may contain intra- and intermolecular cross-links. Collagen is heterogeneous, consisting of at least four types.[6,7,9] Type I collagen is composed of two α_1-chains, and one α_2-chain $[\alpha_1(I)]_2\alpha_2$, and located in airways, alveoli, and blood vessels. It is produced by mesenchymal cells (fibroblasts, contractile cells, and pericytes) and by a cell resembling alveolar type II epithelium.[6,7] Type II collagen is composed of three identical α_1-chains $[\alpha_1\ (II)]_3$, does not form prominent fibrils, and requires high salt concentrations for precipitation. It is synthesized primarily by chondrocytes[9] and located in cartilage plates. Type III collagen is also composed of three identical α_1-chains $[\alpha_1\ (III)]_3$, located with and synthesized by the cells which produce type I collagen. Type IV collagen, found in basement membranes, is composed of three identical α_1-chains $[\alpha_1\ (IV)]_3$. These chains contain large amounts of hydroxylysine and carbohydrate and a modest amount of 3-hydroxyproline.

Bundles of elastic tissue fan out over alveolar ducts and margins, sweeping across several alveoli, providing elastic support for the alveolar capillary sinuses, and preventing excess bronchodilation. Demosine and isodesmosine, elastin cross-links, confer unique features to elastin and reflect its content in lung; extensive hydrophobic regions account for its elasticity.[13] The smooth muscle cell, the fibroblast, and possibly the contractile cell synthesize elastin. The proteoglycan glycocalyx covers the entire alveolar surface epithelium. Proteoglycans, composed of glycosaminoglycans and protein, are interspersed between collagen and elastin in bronchial and vessel walls.[6,7] Mucoproteins or glycoproteins are part of a mucus blanket which clears particles up the bronchial tree. Although similar to proteoglycans, mucin glycoproteins have shorter carbohydrate side chains, lack uronic acids, are resistant to hyaluronidase, and are somewhat more neutral than proteoglycans.[6,7]

II. METABOLISM

Collagen metabolism (biosynthesis and breakdown) encompasses events between transcription of the collagen genome and degradation of the collagen fibril. Each type of collagen probably has its unique genome[9] whose rate of transcription is under control. Collagen, a protein destined for cellular export, is most likely translated on a complex of ribosomes and messenger (m) and transfer (t) RNA which are bound to the rough endoplasmic reticulum (RER); nascent chains are vectorally secreted into the cisternae of the RER.[4a,12] Monocistronic mRNA are the most likely codes for a single pro-α chain. The helical portion of procollagen is translated at about 200 amino acid residues per minute, and the entire molecule is produced in $\simeq$ 6 min.[3,4,4a] Proline and lysine in the newly translated chain are hydroxylated and hydroxylysine glycosylated by enzymes bound to the ribosomes of the RER. The three amino terminal extensions of secreted chains combine in registration and disulfide bonds and the triple helix forms probably as a concerted process. Procollagen has a triple helical portion ($\simeq$ 66%), a nonhelical amino terminal extension without disulfide bonds ($\simeq$ 10%), and nonhelical disulfide bonded carboxy terminal extension ($\simeq$ 24%).[3,4,4a] The Golgi apparatus packages procollagen in secretory vesicles. Microtubules provide transcellular movement to the plasma membrane,[1,2,4a] an energy-requiring process. Prior to or immediately following exocytosis of the procollagen, it is converted to P_c-collagen, through the cleavage of the amino terminal extension by one form of procollagen peptidase. Possibly after microfibril formation, polymerized P_c-collagen is converted to polymerized tropocollagen through excision of the carboxy terminal extensions[1,2,4a] in three steps by procollagen peptidase. Lysyl oxidase catalyzes the initial step of collagen cross-linking, leading to the formation of inter- and intramolecular cross-links. Collagen synthesis decreases as a function of increasing age.[6,7,10] However, noncollagenous protein incorporation of proline, collagen breakdown (low molecular hydroxyproline), and collagen content do not. The reduction of collagen synthesis in the face of constant collagen breakdown may reflect a decreasing instantaneous growth rate. Maturity is reflected by a constant synthesis at later times, indicating the minimal pulmonary collagen turnover.

Although native collagen is resistant to digestion by most proteases, it is digested by vertebrate collagenase into two tropocollagen (TC) fragments, TC^a (three fourths) and TC^b (one fourth), by cleavage at a specific gly-ile bond.[8] Pulmonary alveolar macrophages, neutrophils, and platelets contain collagenase, as do rapidly dividing cells in wound healing and in rheumatoid nodules.[8] Collagenase is inhibited by an α_2 globulin ($\simeq$ 500,000 daltons), reversibly by α_1 antitrypsin (AAT), and by a low molecular weight inhibitor ($\simeq$ 11,000 daltons) from cartilage. Following collagenase action, monomeric TC^a and TC^b denature, because their denaturation temperatures (32 and 29°C) are below body temperature. Fragments which have been digested by collagenase but remain cross-linked are endocytized by fibroblasts and degraded by lysosomes. Some forms of collagenase exist as inactive procollagenase which may be activated by a variety of procedures.[8]

Proelastin[5] is apparently synthesized on the ribosomes of the RER, much like collagen. Some proline residues are hydroxylated, but apparently the extent of hydroxylation has little structural effect. Precursor microfibrillar elastin[7] is presumably produced with distinct but similar steps to proelastin. Both are probably packaged in secretory vesicles, utilize microtubules, are secreted, and are cleaved by an uncharacterized enzyme. Tropoelastin is attached by disulfide bonds to the scaffolding, microfibrillar elastin, making it a particulate substrate for lysyl oxidase and aligning it so that cross-linking will produce mature amorphous elastin containing demosine and isodesmosine. Continuous proteolysis of newly synthesized, but incompletely cross-linked elastin is probable;[7] however, turnover of mature elastin is also suggested. Pancreatic proelastase will bind but not cleave elastin until a single tryptic cleavage of proelastase occurs. AAT and an α_1 globulin distinct from AAT will inhibit elastase.[6,7]

Cells producing proteoglycans segregate enzymes of precursor production (soluble cytoplasm) from those of protein synthesis (ribosomes of RER) and of macromolecular assembly (Golgi). The protein backbone is probably synthesized on ribosomes of the RER. This protein is secreted into the cisternae of the RER and attaches to the primer in the smooth endoplasmic reticulum (SER), where polymerization using the UDP-sugar bases and sulfation with 3′-phosphoadenosine 5′-phosphosulfate (PAPS) occur as a concerted process. Modifications of the product occur in the Golgi, after which secretory vesicles form and the product is extruded.[14] Hyaluronidase, which is present in rat lung, degrades the polysaccharide portion.[15] Mucus glycoproteins are probably synthesized like protein. However, incorporation of sialic acid makes them acid rather than neutral glycopeptides. The carbohydrate portion is most likely attached in the SER or Golgi, and the mucoprotein processed and secreted as usual.

III. RESPONSE TO INJURY

Alveolar epithelial type II cells, endothelial cells, smooth muscle cells, fibroblasts, and contractile cells produce connective tissue. Since their proportions in lung determine quality and quantity of connective tissue production, factors influencing proliferation of those cells are of interest. Fetal lung fibroblasts are influenced by their culture substrata; removal by collagenase stimulates cell division. Increasing serum concentrations in media increases the number of diploid lung fibroblasts entering cell division. This increase evokes a cyclic phosphatidylinositol response followed rapidly by an increased cGMP/cAMP ratio, a probable secretion of fibroblast stimulating factor, and a rise in intracellular phosphate which activates glycolysis and precedes cell division. Only when these cells reach saturation density do they make appreciable quantities of collagen. A cell matrix composed of fibronectin, collagen, collagen bound collagenase (in the "pro" form or with bound inhibitors), elastin, elastin bound elastase (inhibited same as collagen), dermatan sulfate, and perhaps other proteoglycans, fibrinogen or fibrin connects with the cell microfibrils directly or indirectly. Fibronectin, the connecting protein, is extremely sensitive to proteases, providing a mechanism for freeing the cell from the matrix (and degrading the matrix) so that it can proliferate rapidly to fill the gap produced by injury and thus influencing the proportion of mesenchymal cells after injury. Alternatively, the intact matrix presumably signals the cell to make connective tissue. After the cell is contact inhibited, secreted procollagen may be attracted to either cell surface heparin or matrix fibronectin proportionate to their relative abundance. The type of procollagen bound may be proportional to synthesis rate. Thus, in excess proteolysis, procollagen will mostly be bound to cell surface heparin. Since type III procollagen is protease sensitive, the procollagen will be mostly type I. Thus, type I collagen will be produced rapidly. Following protease decrease and matrix buildup, there will be a gradual return to a more normal collagen synthesis rate, and type III collagen will increase. These and other data suggest the possibility for transcriptional and translational control of collagen production. The possibility for a parallel mechanism for elastin and proteoglycans must be considered.

Changes in lung connective tissue metabolism may be induced by a variety of inhaled toxicants. Although deposition and clearance of the inhaled material may influence the pattern of response, development of alveolar injuries contains many common features. These include endothelial and type I epithelial damage, fibrin deposition, proliferation of endothelium and type II epithelial cells, interruption of basement membranes, proliferation of fibroblasts, and development of pulmonary fibrosis. Whether fibrosis or emphysema is produced is largely a function of severity of local pulmonary injury. Emphysema is primarily associated with lower injury levels than is fibrosis. The relationship between either condition and pulmonary neoplasia is uncertain. However, the existence of "scar cancer" in both animals and man does suggest some association. Alveolar injury may also include edema, complement activation, coagulation, fibrinolysis, proteolysis, and collagenolysis. Neutrophil and macrophage accumulation and the effect of collagen and cold insoluble globulin on cell mediated immunity has significant impact on the production of these diseases. This may reflect the interaction of the cell with the extracellular matrix under a set of circumstances unique to the disease.

Injury to the bronchus and bronchioles usually involves injury to the ciliated epithelial cells. Hypersecretion of mucus and goblet cell hyperplasia and retrograde mucus flow may lead to granuloma formation. Hyposecretion of viscous mucus may lead to obstruction, bronchoconstriction, hypoxic vasoconstriction, and either alveolar injury or asthma, usually with an immunologic component. Squamous metaplasia or Clara cell hyperplasia may have successful resolution.

Specific alterations in collagen metabolism have been described for a number of conditions or disease states. Idiopathic pulmonary fibrosis is a hypercellular response with an apparently normal whole-lung collagen metabolic pattern.[6,7] Silica alters oxidative phosphorylation of macrophages, discharges proteolytic enzymes, and produces accelerated collagen metabolism, indicated by increased hydroxyproline, and accelerated proteoglycan metabolism. Hyperoxia and hypoxia produce increased lipoperoxidation, lung lactate, and prolyl hydroxylase, leading to pulmonary fibrosis. Additional oxidizing substances or conditions capable of inducing pulmonary fibrosis include assorted mineral dusts, paraquat, bile duct obstruction, histamine and histamine releasers, cigarette smoke, platelet mitogenic factor, and radiation. The amount of dermatan sulfate may closely parallel collagen changes; however, collagen is the most important altered constituent following fibrogenic doses of radioactive aerosols.[10] All changes of collagen metabolism were similar, differing only in time and magnitude. Early increases of noncollagenous protein incorporation of ^{14}C-proline and collagen breakdown preceded any increase in collagen synthesis. Subsequently, increased collagen synthesis predominated over increased collagen breakdown. The positive balance of collagen metabolism led to increased collagen content and pulmonary fibrosis. This was observed earliest in hamsters exposed to ^{90}Y in fused aluminosilicate particles due to a high dose rate and a rapid accumulation of dose. Increased collagen metabolism was observed somewhat later in animals exposed to 100 nCi of $^{238}PuO_2$ and still later in hamsters exposed to 50 nCi of $^{238}PuO_2$. Later reductions of collagen content in hamsters exposed to 50 nCi of $^{238}PuO_2$ were due to a negative collagen balance, reflected by reduced collagen synthesis relative to breakdown. The reduction of collagen content is less in hamsters exposed to 100 nCi of $^{238}PuO_2$. The consistently elevated collagen synthesis observed in these animals at later times appeared to maintain the elevated collagen content. Animals exposed to $^{238}PuO_2$ illustrate a clear-cut radiation dose-effects relationship for pulmonary fibrosis. Steroids block fibrogenesis in vivo and fibroblast proliferation in tissue culture. Thus, the possibility that fibroblast and mesenchymal cell proliferation constitutes an important determinant of pulmonary fibrosis must be considered.[10,11]

Proteolysis is a feature of emphysema, which leads to losses of connective tissue (collagen and elastin) of alveolar septa, to proliferation of type II alveolar epithelial cells to replace the damaged type I cells, and to production of more surfactant to counter the proteolytic changes. Apparently, the collagen is replaced, but the elastin is variably deficient by later times, suggesting that the efficiency of connective tissue production, especially elastin, influences the severity of emphysema. Emphysema is associated with the inhalation of numerous oxidants which reach the deep lung: NO_2, O_3, 100% O_2, Cd^{2+}, other pollutant gases, and numerous other causes, such as smoking.

Mucoproteins are altered by a number of conditions, including bronchitis and asthma. Increased quantities of mucoproteins are associated with hyperplasia of goblet cells and submucosal glands and loss of cilia. This leads to impaired clearance and alterations of the quality and quantity of mucus. Retrogression of mucus to terminal bronchioles and alveoli may cause emphysema or fibrosis secondary to alveolar hypoxia induced by airway blockage. Following SO_2 exposure, the PAS staining is reduced, suggesting an alteration in quantity or composition of mucus.

The review goes beyond defined mechanisms of connective tissue metabolism in health and disease. Speculation concerns the relationship of altered connective tissue metabolism to developing pulmonary injury. Especially important is the interaction of the mesenchymal cells with the extracellular matrix in various conditions of injury to establish relative proportions of mesenchymal (connective tissue producing) cells at the site of injury. Following this establishment it is quite important to understand how the level and type of collagen is controlled, i.e., what turns it on and off or modulates it. This book speculates on such possible controls, considering the available evidence. These important questions should be considered and matched to the known anatomic and biochemical changes in each disease condition. This is somewhat difficult, since measurements often relate to only a small portion of the connective tissue metabolism picture and are frequently rather general. Much progress remains to be made in this exciting field. Such speculation is included in an attempt to define more completely the sequence of biochemical changes in pulmonary injury leading to each of these disease entities. Understanding these sequences of events greatly enhances the possibility of successfully manipulating injury to lung.

REFERENCES

1. **Bornstein, P.,** The biosynthesis of collagen, *Annu. Rev. Biochem.*, 43, 567, 1974.
2. **Bornstein, P.,** The structure and assembly of procollagen — a review, *J. Supramol. Struct.*, 2, 108, 1974.
3. **Fessler, L. I. and Fessler, J. H.,** Protein assembly of procollagen and effects of hydroxylation, *J. Biol. Chem.*, 249, 7637, 1974.
4. **Fessler, L. I., Morris, N. P., and Fessler, J. H.,** Procollagen: biological scission of amino and carboxyl extension peptides, *Proc. Natl. Acad. Sci. U.S.A.*, 72, 4905, 1975.

4a. **Fessler, J. H. and Fessler, L. I.,** Biosynthesis of procollagen, *Annu. Rev. Biochem.*, 47, 129, 1978.

5. **Foster, J. A., Mecham, R. P., and Franzblau, C.,** A high molecular weight species of soluble elastin, *Biochem. Biophys. Res. Commun.*, 72, 1399, 1976.
6. **Hance, A. J., Bradley, K., and Crystal, R. G.,** Lung collagen heterogeneity. Synthesis of type I and type III collagen by rabbit and human lung cells in culture, *J. Clin. Invest.*, 57, 102, 1976.
7. **Hance, A. J. and Crystal, R. G.,** The connective tissue of lung, *Am. Rev. Respir. Dis.*, 112; 657, 1975.
8. **Harris, E. D. and Krane, S. M.,** Collagenases (I, II, III), *N. Engl. J. Med.*, 291, 557, 605, 652, 1974.
9. **Miller, E. J. and Matukas, V. J.,** Biosynthesis of collagen — the biochemist's view, *Fed. Proc.*, 33, 1197, 1974.
10. **Pickrell, J. A., Harris, D. V., Mauderly, J. L., and Hahn, F. F.,** Altered collagen metabolism in radiation-induced interstitial pulmonary fibrosis, *Chest*, 69, 311, 1976.
11. **Pickrell, J. A., Straus, F. C., Halliwell, W. H., and Jones, R. K.,** The relation of pulmonary collagen metabolism, inflammation and therapy to radiation-induced pulmonary fibrosis, *Fed. Proc. Abstr.*, 36, 607, 1977.
12. **Sabatini, D. D., Ojakian, G., Lande, M. A., Lewis, J., Mok, W., Adesnik, M., and Kreibich, G.,** Structural and functional aspects of the protein synthesizing apparatus in the rough endoplasmic reticulum, *Adv. Exp. Med. Biol.*, 62, 151, 1974.
13. **Sandberg, L. B.,** Elastin structure in health and disease, *Int. Rev. Connect. Tissue Res.*, 7; 159, 1976.
14. **Silbert, J. E.,** Biosynthesis of mucopolysaccharides and protein-polysaccharides, in *Molecular Pathology of Connective Tissues*, Vol. 3 of *The Biochemistry of Disease*, Pérez-Tamayo R., and Rojkind, M., Eds., Marcel Dekker, New York, 1973, 323.
15. **Silbert, J. E.,** Catabolism of mucopolysaccharides and protein-polysaccharides, in *Molecular Pathology of Connective Tissues*, Vol. 3 of *The Biochemistry of Disease*, Pêrez-Tamayo, R., and Rojkind, M., Eds., Marcel Dekker, New York, 1973, 355.

INDEX

D

E

F

G

H

I

K

L

M

N

O

P